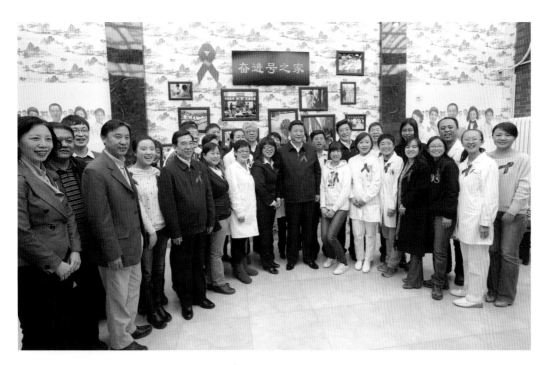

On November 30, 2012, with the 25th World AIDS Day coming, Xi Jinping, General Secretary of the CPC Central Committee and Chairman of the Central Military Commission, attended the activity of World AIDS Day at Puhuangyu Community Health Service Center in Fengtai District of Beijing. The picture shows that Xi Jinping took a group photo with the CDC staff, volunteers and social organization staff at the workroom of volunteer organization—the Home of Endeavour.

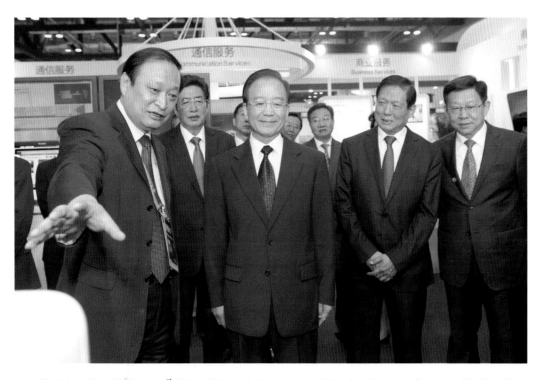

On May 28, 2012, the 1st China (Beijing) International Fair for Trade in Services (Beijing Fair) was inaugurated at China National Convention Center, Beijing. The picture shows that Wen Jiabao, member of the Standing Committee of the Political Bureau of the CPC Central Committee and Premier of the State Council, visited the pavilion of traditional Chinese medicine under the theme of health and social services at the core subject area.

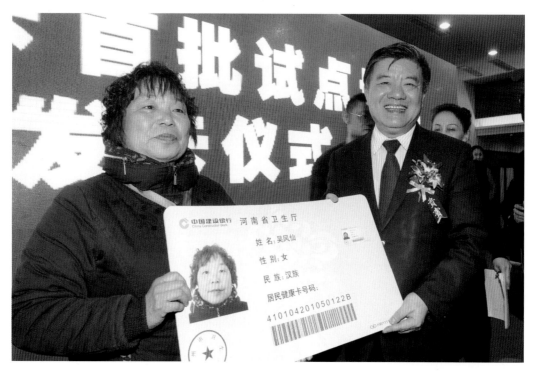

On March 1, 2012, at the issuing ceremony of the first residents health cards held in Zhengzhou, the capital city of Henan Province, Health Minister Chen Zhu issued the first residents health card to the residents' representative.

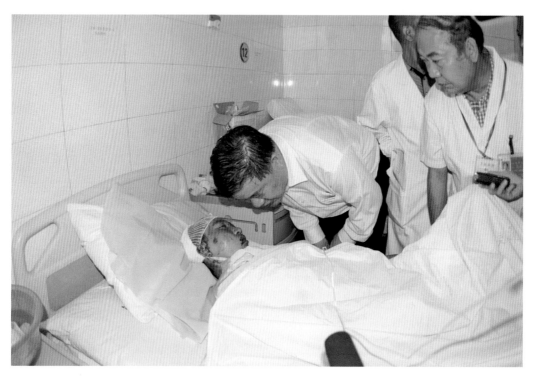

At 11:19 on September 7, 2012, a 7.5-magnitude earthquake occurred at the border of Yiliang County in Zhaotong of Yunnan and Weining Autonomous County of Yi, Hui and Miao nationalities in Bijie Prefecture of Guizhou. The picture shows that Health Minister Chen Zhu visited a victim at the People's Hospital of Yiliang County in the city of Zhaotong in Yunnan Province on September 8.

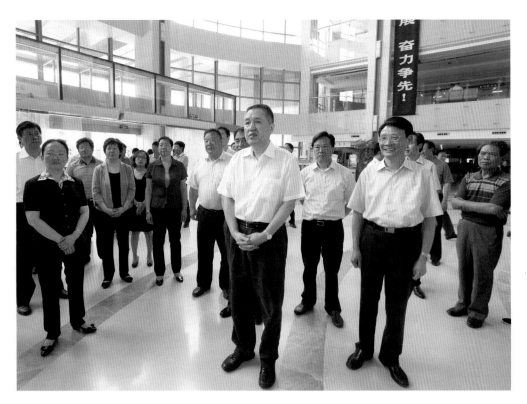

On June 13, 2012, Zhang Mao, deputy head of the Leading Group on Medical Reform under the State Council, Secretary of Party Leadership Group of the Ministry of Health and Vice Health Minister, researched medical reform in Zhenjiang, the riverside city of Jiangsu Province.

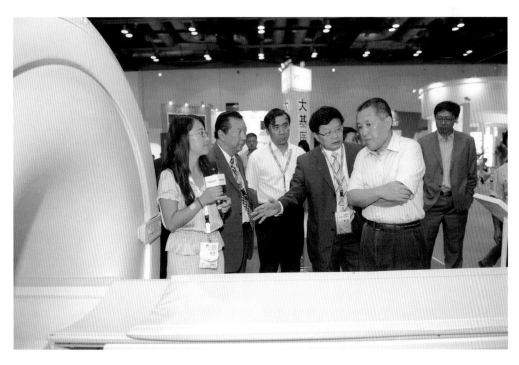

On August 16–18, 2012, China International Medical Equipment Exhibition & Scientific Conference (CHINA-HOSPEQ 2012) was held at China National Convention Center. The picture shows that Secretary of Party Leadership Group of the Ministry of Health and Vice Health Minister Zhang Mao researched the Exhibition and held cordial exchanges with the enterprises.

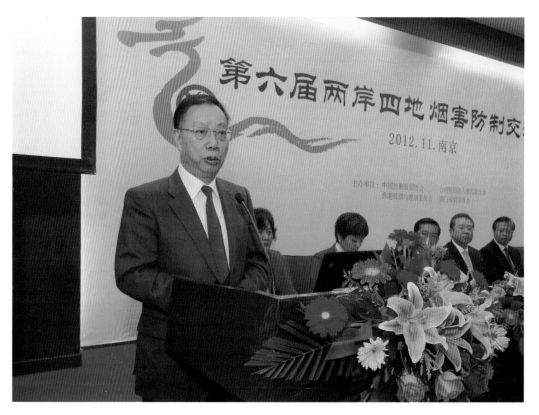

On November 5–6, 2012, the 6th Cross–Strait Conference on Tobacco Control was held in Nanjing, the capital city of Jiangsu Province. Vice Health Minister and President of Chinese Association on Tobacco Control (CATC) Huang Jiefu addressed the opening ceremony.

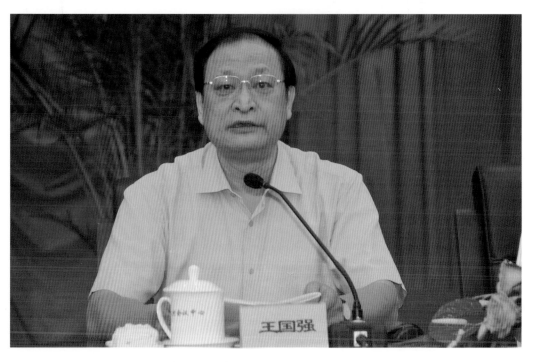

On August 20, 2012, the Summary Commendation Congress for Excelling in Competition in National Medicine and Health Care Circles was held in Beijing. The picture shows that Vice Health Minister Wang Guoqiang addressed the Congress.

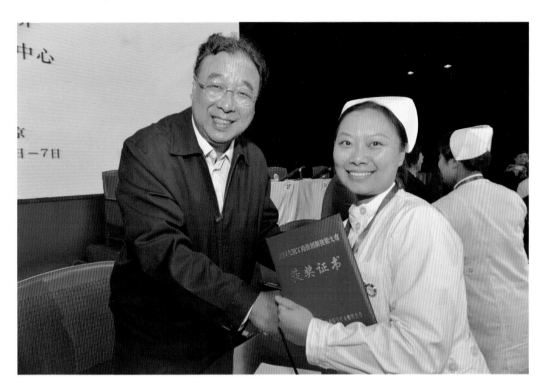

On November 6-7, 2012, the final of innovation skill competition of nursing position of national health care circles, co-sponsored by the Ministry of Health and All-China Federation of Trade Unions (ACFTU), was held in Beijing. The picture shows that Vice Health Minister Ma Xiaowei awarded the prizes to a winner

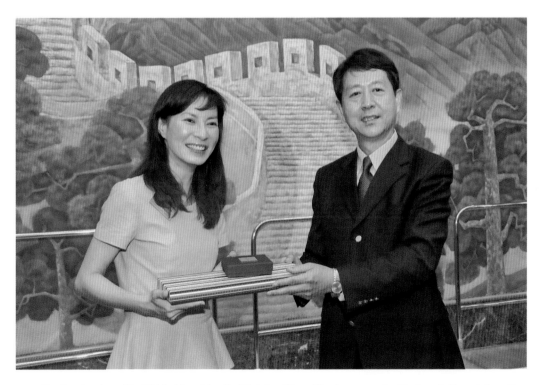

On September 19, 2012, Vice Health Minister Chen Xiaohong met with the visiting delegation headed by Chairwoman of Hong Kong Tung Wah Group of Hospitals CHAN MAN Yee Wai in Beijing.

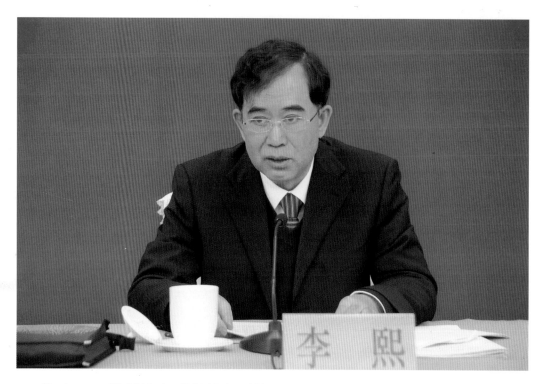

On January 15, 2012, the 2012 National Meeting on Discipline Inspection and Supervision & Check of Unhealthy Tendencies and Malpractices in Health Care Circles was held in Beijing. The picture shows that Li Xi, Team Leader of the Discipline Inspection Commission in the Ministry of Health, was giving the work presentation.

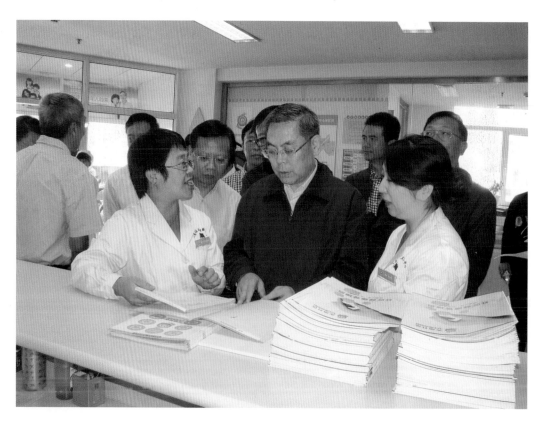

On September 25, 2012, Vice Health Minister Liu Qian paid an inspection visit to Danan Community Health Service Center in Shenyang, the capital city of Liaoning Province.

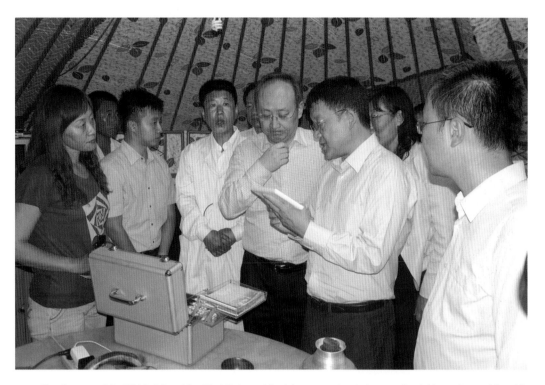

On August 24, 2012, Vice Health Minister Yin Li researched the medical kit project of health security in Hulunbuir, the border city of Inner Mongolia Autonomous Region.

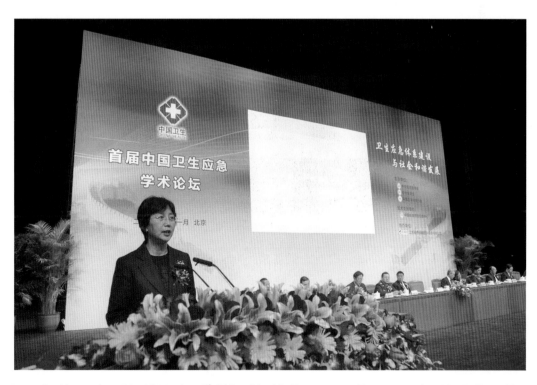

On November 28, 2012, the 1st China Health Emergency Forum was held in Beijing. The picture shows that Vice Health Minister Xu Ke addressed the opening ceremony.

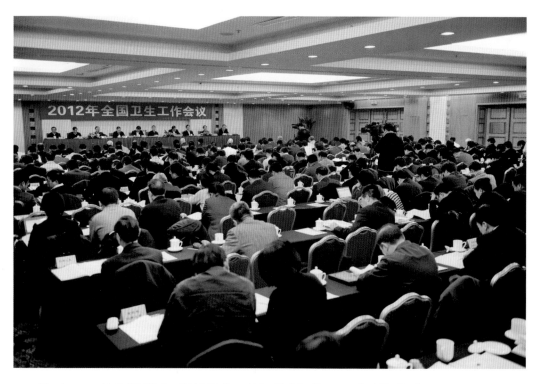

On January 5–6, 2012, the 2012 National Health Meeting was held in Beijing.

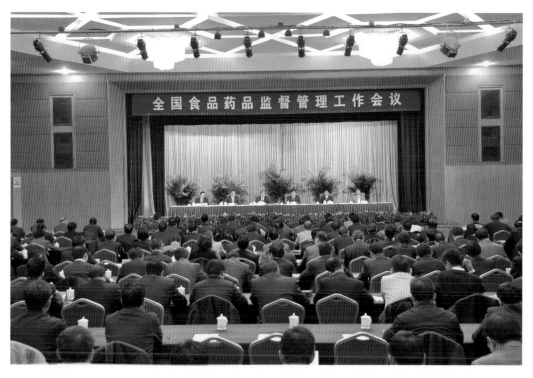

On December 20–21, 2011, the 2012 National Meeting on Food and Drug Regulation was held in Beijing.

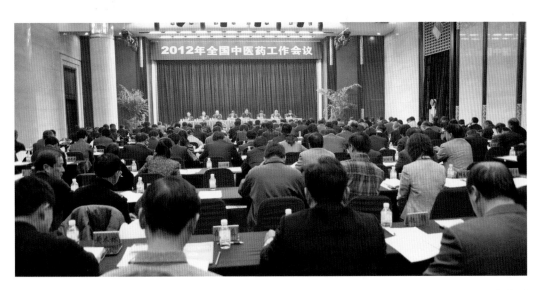

On January 10–11, 2012, the 2012 National Meeting on Traditional Chinese Medicine (TCM) was held in Beijing.

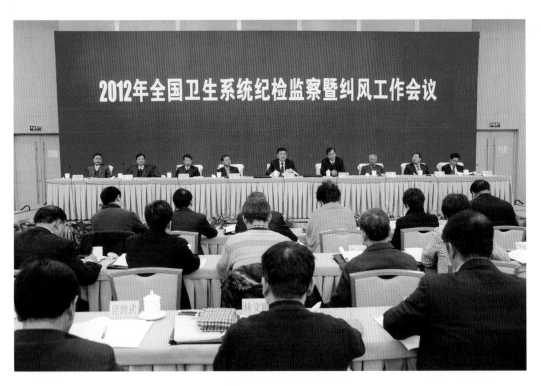

On January 16, 2012, the 2012 National Meeting on Discipline Inspection and Supervision & Check of Unhealthy Tendencies and Malpractices in Health Care Circles was held in Beijing.

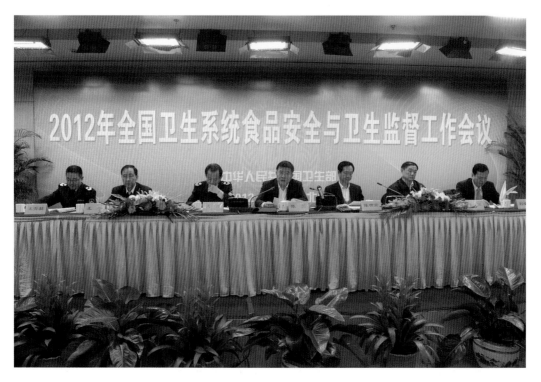

On January 13, 2012, the 2012 National Meeting on Food Safety and Health Supervision in Health Care Circles was held in Beijing.

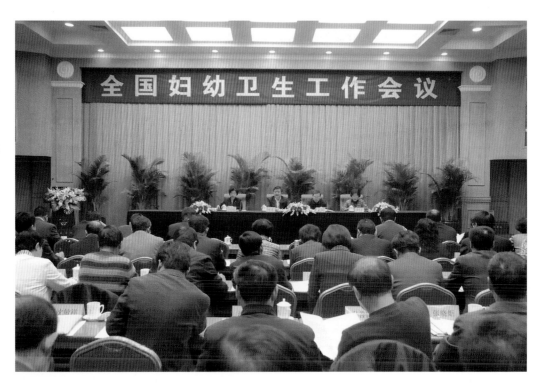

On February 23–24, 2012, the 2012 National Meeting on Maternal and Child Health was held in Beijing.

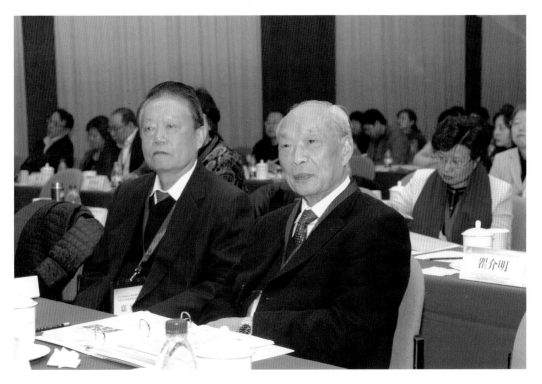

Since February 2012, the Ministry of Health had started great discussions on medical professionalism, and held intensively seven symposiums. The picture shows the meeting site on February 25, 2012.

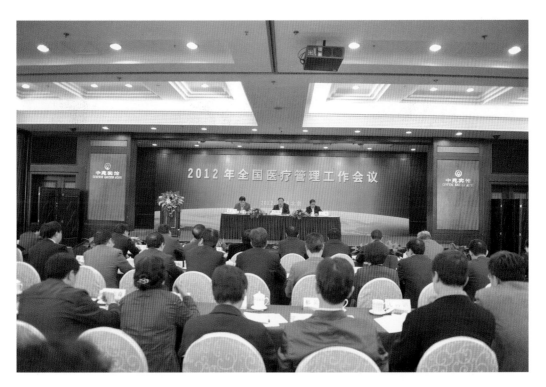

On March 20, 2012, the 2012 National Meeting on Medical Management was held in Beijing.

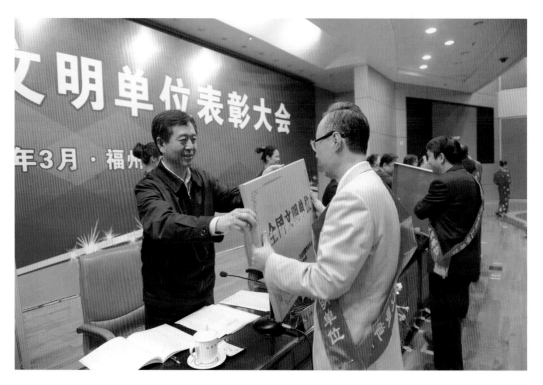

On March 22, 2012, the Office of Spiritual Civilization of the Ministry of Health held the Commendation Congress on National Civilized Unit of Health Care Circles in Fuzhou, the capital city of Fujian Province.

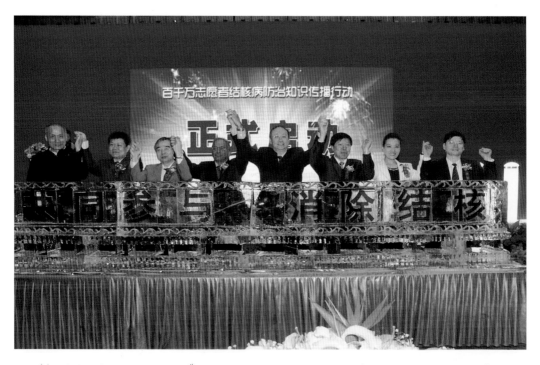

March 24 of 2012 was the 17th World Tuberculosis Day. China's publicity theme was "We are all involved in eliminating TB harm". On March 22, the launching ceremony for the theme activity of the 2012 World Tuberculosis Day and millions of volunteers' TB knowledge dissemination action was held in Beijing.

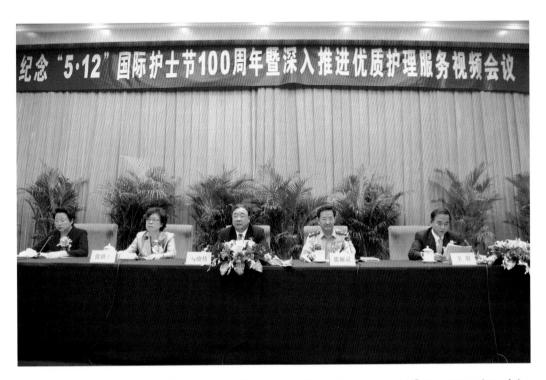

On May 11, 2012, the Ministry of Health held the Video Conference in Commemoration of the 100th Anniversary of 5.12 International Nurses Day and on Deepening the Promotion of High-quality Nursing Service in Beijing.

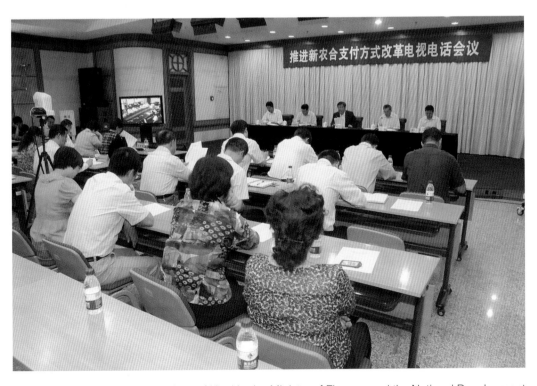

On May 15, 2012, the Ministry of Health, the Ministry of Finance and the National Development and Reform Commission jointly held the Video and Telephone Conference on Promoting the Reform of Payment Mode of the New Rural Cooperative Medical System (NCMS).

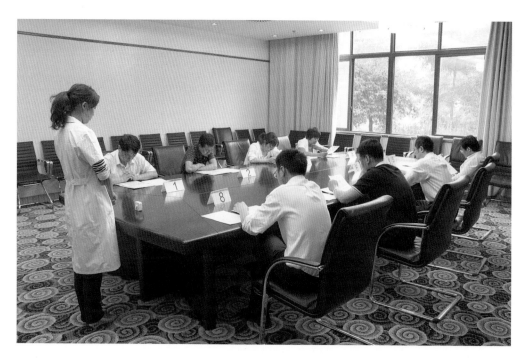

On May 18-20, 2012, the Ministry of Health organized the examination for specialist physicians' access to our country's cardiovascular medicine and interventional diagnosis and treatment of cardiovascular disease. Physicians passing the examination would be the first to become qualified for specialist physicians in our country. The picture shows that the candidates were preparing for the examination at the examination site of Sichuan University-West China Center of Medical Sciences.

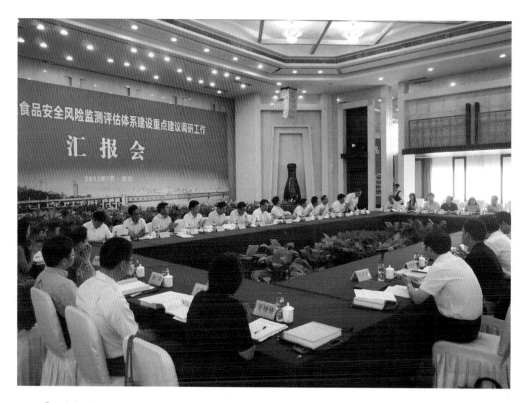

On July 20-22, 2012, the group of key proposals management of the Ministry of Health researched the construction of the monitoring and evaluation system of food safety risk in Hubei Province.

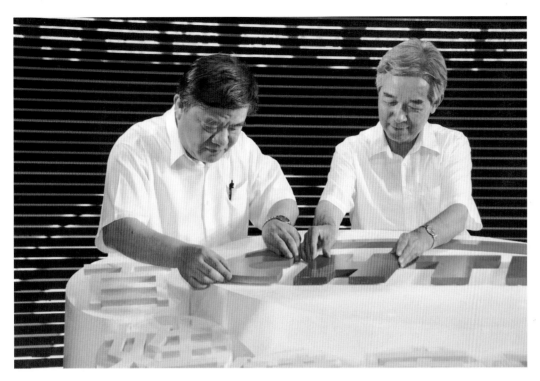

On August 6, 2012, the Citizens' Health Television Channel was inaugurated in Beijing. The picture shows that Health Minister Chen Zhu and former Vice Health Minister Wang Longde started the launching ceremony.

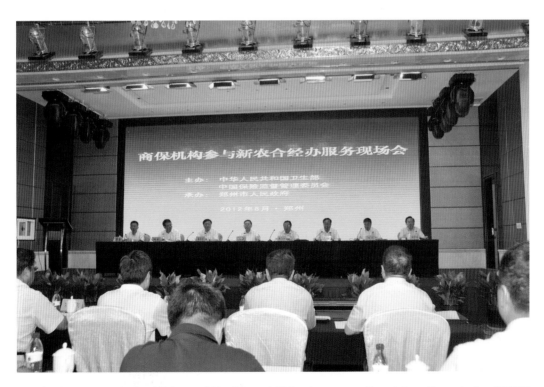

In August 2012, the Ministry of Health and China Insurance Regulatory Commission (CIRC) held the On-the-spot Meeting on the Involvement of Commercial Insurance Institutions in the Handling Service of the New Rural Cooperative Medical System (NCMS) in Zhengzhou, the capital city of Henan Province.

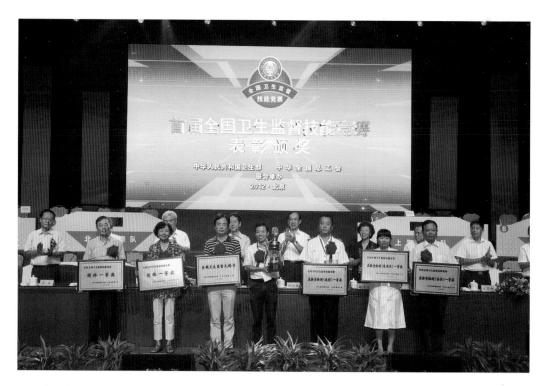

On September 1, 2012, the Ministry of Health and All-China Federation of Trade Unions (ACFTU) held jointly the 1st National Skill Competition of Health Supervision in Beijing. The picture shows the site of prize-awarding ceremony.

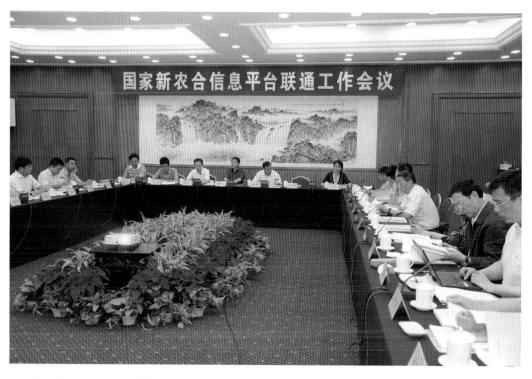

On September 6, 2012, the Ministry of Health held the 2012 National Meeting on the Information Platform Unicom of the New Rural Cooperative Medical System (NCMS).

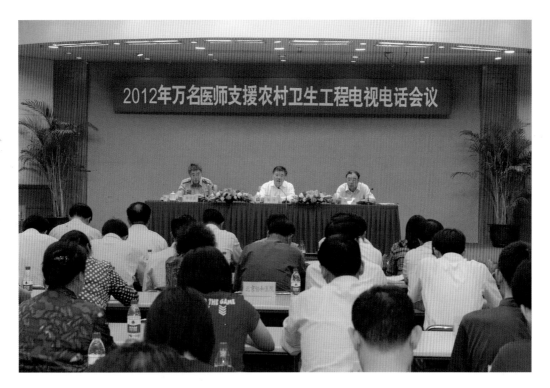

On September 19, 2012, the 2012 Video and Telephone Conference on the Project of Thousands of Doctors' Supporting Rural Health was held in Beijing.

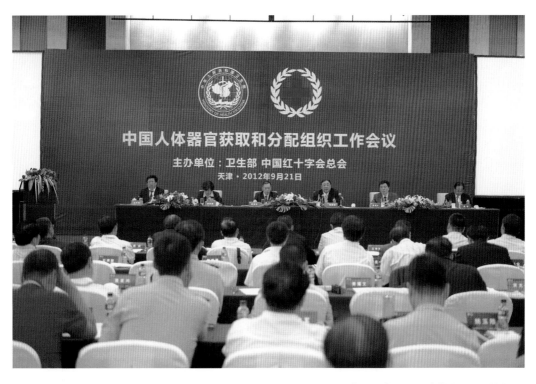

On September 21, 2012, the Ministry of Health and the Red Cross Society of China held jointly the Organizational Meeting on China's Human Organ Acquisition and Allocation in Tianjin.

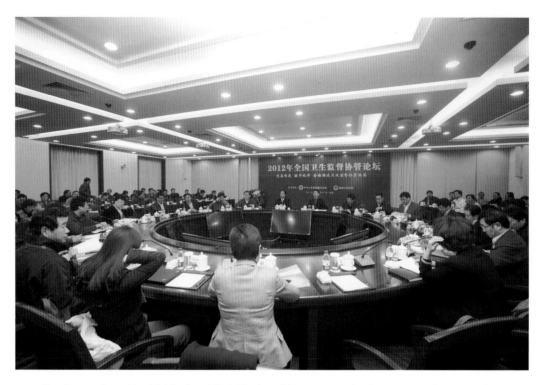

On December 11, 2012, the 2012 National Forum on Assistance in Charge of Health Supervision was held in Beijing.

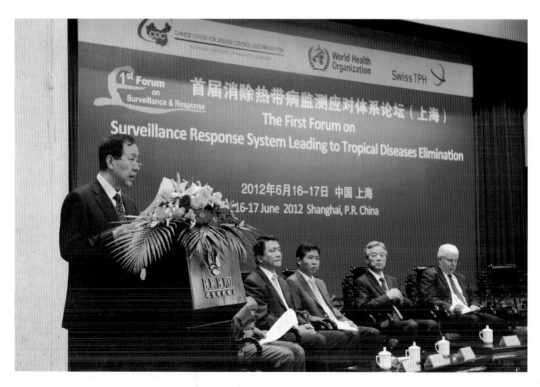

On June 16–17, 2012, the Institute of Parasitic Diseases, the Swiss Tropical and Public Health Institute and the World Health Organization (WHO) held the First Forum on Surveillance Response System Leading to Tropical Diseases Elimination in Shanghai.

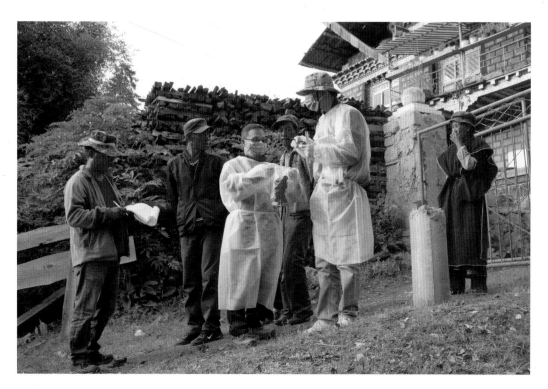

On September 5, 2012, Chinese Center for Disease Control and Prevention (China CDC) conducted epidemiological survey for echinococcosis in Tibet.

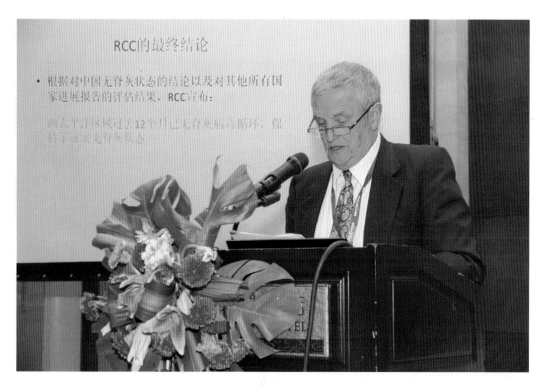

On November 29, 2012, President of WHO Western Pacific Regional Commission for the Certification of Poliomyelitis Eradication Dr. Adams proclaimed China's restoration of polio-free status at the 18th Meeting of WHO Western Pacific Regional Commission for the Certification of Poliomyelitis Eradication (RCC).

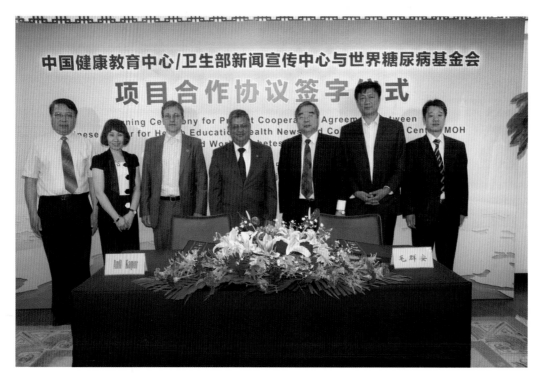

On May 28, 2012, the Health Education Project of Diabetes Prevention jointly carried out by Chinese Center for Health Education (News Center of the Ministry of Health) and World Diabetes Foundation held the Signing Ceremony of Cooperation Agreement in Beijing. The picture shows that Director of Chinese Center for Health Education Mao Qunan, President of World Diabetes Foundation Anil Kapur and Novo Nordisk China Vice President Rao Hong attended the Signing Ceremony.

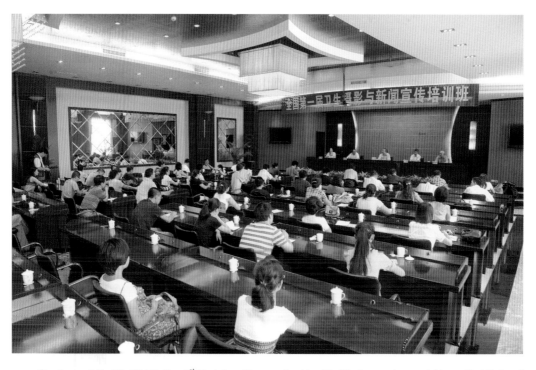

On August 7–10, 2012, the 1st Training Course for Health Photography and News Publicity of National Medical Institutions was held in Taiyuan, the capital city of Shanxi.

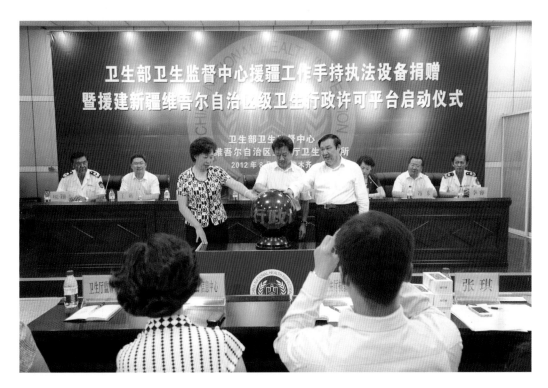

In August 2012, National Center for Health Inspection and Supervision held the launching ceremony for donation of portable law-enforcement facilities of health assistance for Xinjiang and for providing aid in constructing the platform of health administration license at the level of Xinjiang Uygur Autonomous Region in Xinjiang Uygur Autonomous Region.

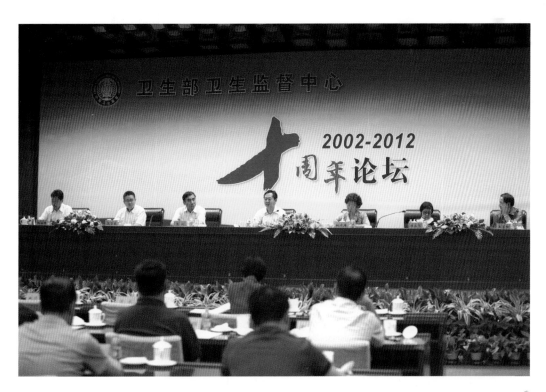

On May 23, 2012, National Center for Health Inspection and Supervision organized the 10th Anniversary of Forum for exchanging the achievements made by all local health supervision and looking to the development prospect of health supervision.

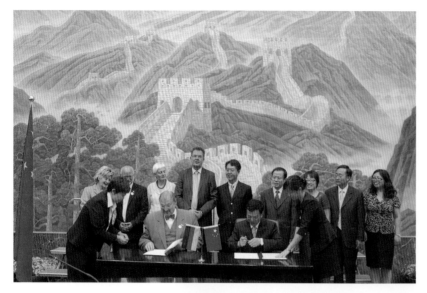

Since its establishment, China National Center for Food Safety Risk Assessment has positively developed its cooperation with the technical agencies of international food safety. The picture shows that, on August 29, 2012, China National Center for Food Safety Risk Assessment and the Federal Institute for Risk Assessment (BfR) in Germany signed the memorandum of understanding on cooperation.

To strengthen the international cooperation in the area of our country's food safety technology, establish a high-level agency of food safety risk assessment, and improve the supporting capacity of food safety technology, National Center for Food Safety Risk Assessment set up an international advisory committee of experts composed of 7 world-renowned experts. The picture shows that Vice Health Minister Chen Xiaohong took a group photo with 8 advisers and experts on September 26, 2012.

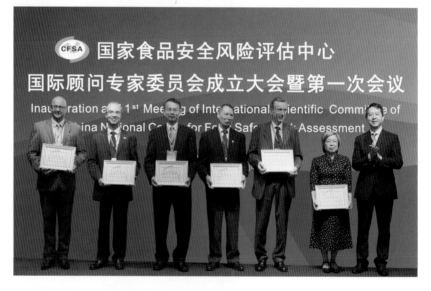

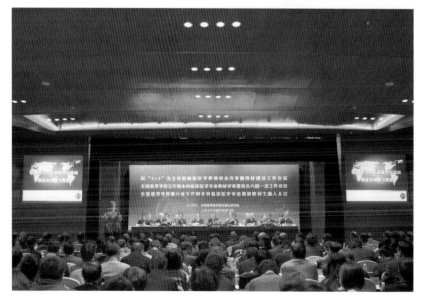

On February 25-26, 2012, the Meeting on the Comprehensive Reform and Textbook Construction of National Clinical Medical Education for Undergraduates was held in Beijing. The Meeting was co-hosted by the People's Medical Publishing House, Co., LTD and the National Research Society of Higher Medical Textbook Construction.

On April 15–18, 2012, the Medical Publishing House, Co., LTD led the delegation to attend London International Book Fair and achieved fruit results. The picture shows that President of the Medical Publishing House, Co., LTD Chen Xianyi and global president of McGraw Hill Professional signed the cooperation agreement.

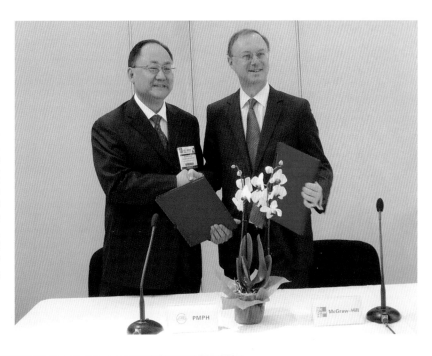

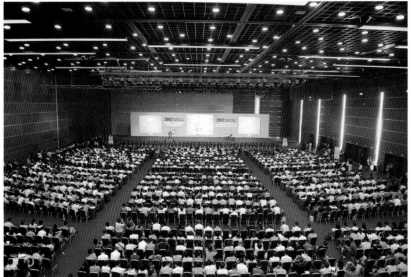

On August 16–18, 2012, the 2012 China Health Forum was held in Beijing. The theme of the Forum was "Deepening Health Reform, Improving Prevention & Control of NCDs (non-communicable diseases) and Pursuing Sustainable Health Development".

On August 30, 2012, Health Express of the Ministry of Health pulled into the old revolutionary area of Baise to perform surgery free of charge for the impoverished cataract patients from all counties of Baise.

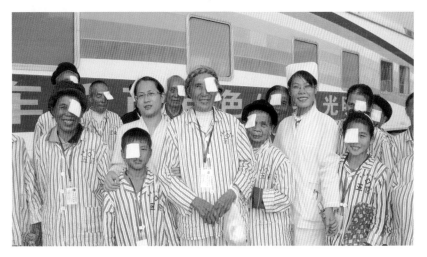

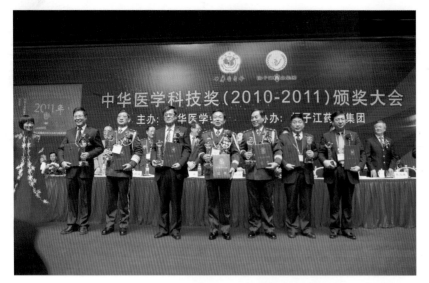

On January 7, 2012, the Award-giving Meeting of the nation's top science and technology award in medical and health field—the Chinese Medical Science and Technology Award—was held in Beijing.

On May 17–18, 2012, Chinese Preventive Medicine Association (CPMA), Chinese Association of Animal Science and Veterinary Medicine (CAAV) and some other organizations held the 2012 Rabies Conference in Beijing, China. The Conference was to strengthen the prevention and control of rabies, promote the trans-department, multidisciplinary cooperation and exchanges, and promote the achievement of the initiative of rabies elimination.

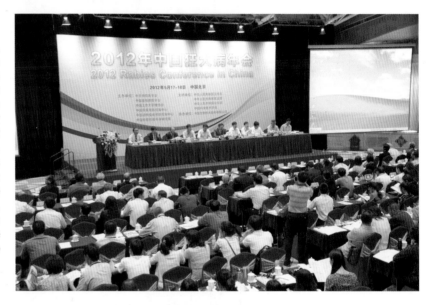

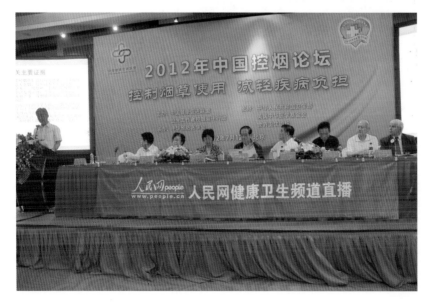

On July 12, 2012, the 2012 China Tobacco Control Forum was held in Beijing. The Forum called on the whole nation to "care for our health, keep away from tobacco".

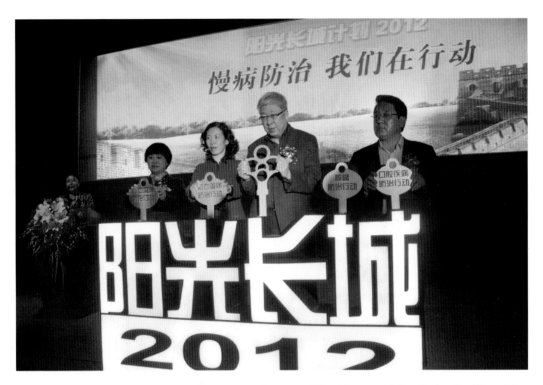

On January 13, 2012, Beijing Municipal Bureau of Health started the Action for "Sunshine Great Wall Plan 2012.The action involved the prevention and control of 4 major chronic diseases including cardiovascular disease, cerebrovascular disease, tumor and oral disorders.

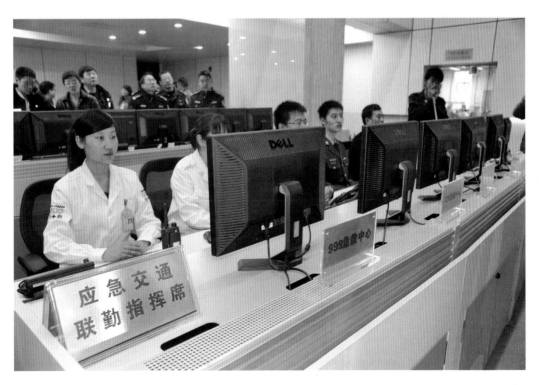

On December 14, Beijing's 110, 119, 122, 120 and 999 started the service mechanism for emergency traffic.

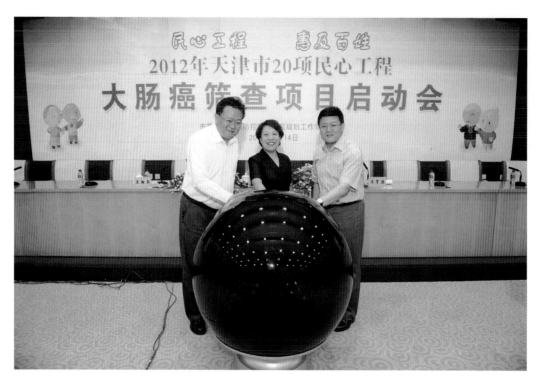

On May 14, 2012, the Launching Meeting of Colorectal Cancer Screening Project—one of 2012 Tianjin's 20 projects in the public interest—was held in Tianjin. The Project conducted colorectal cancer screening free of charge for the city's inhabitants at the age of 60–74.

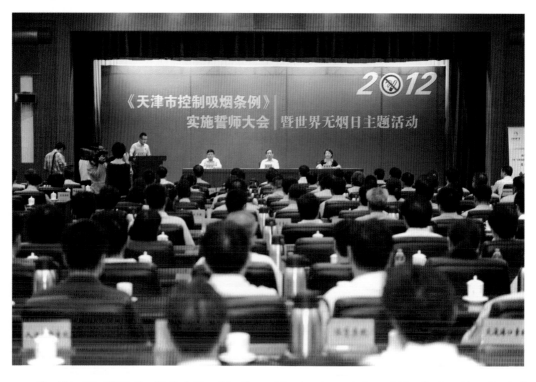

On May 29, 2012, the Oath-taking Meeting of the Implementation of *Tianjin Smoking Control Regulations* and the Theme Meeting of World No-Tobacco Day was held in Tianjin. The campaign was of significance for Tianjin to prevent and control effectively chronic diseases and raise the urban civilization level.

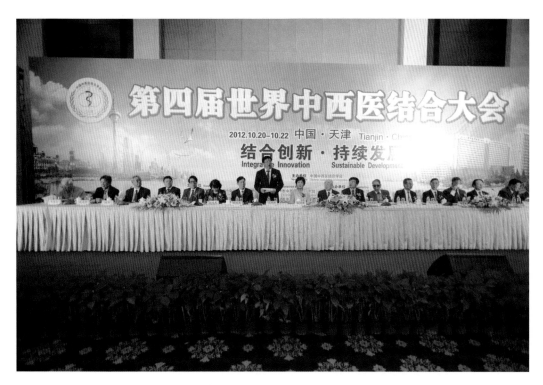

On October 20–22, 2012, the 4th World Integrative Medicine Congress (WIMCO) was held in Tianjin.

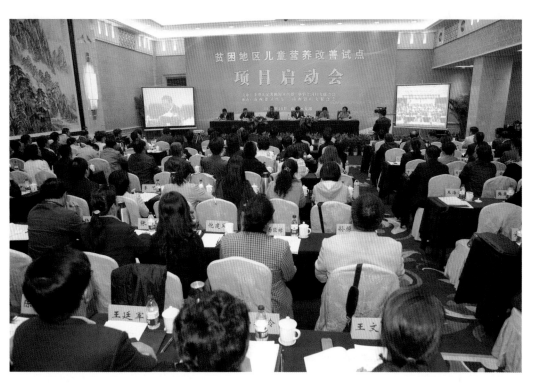

On October 15, 2012, the Pilot Project of Children's Nutrition Improvement in Poverty-stricken Areas co-hosted by the Ministry of Health and the All-China Women's Federation (ACWF) was kicked off in Taiyuan, the capital city of Shanxi Province.

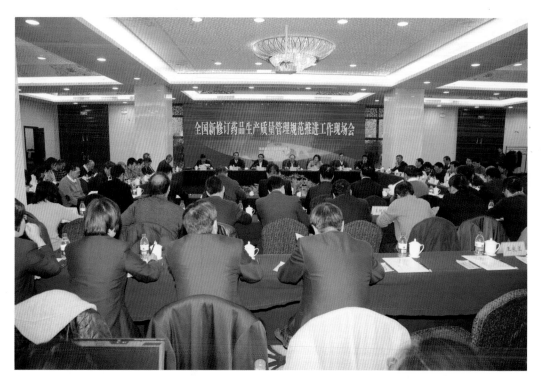

On December 13, 2012, the National On-the-spot Meeting on Promoting the Newly Revised Management Standard of Drug Production Quality was held in Taiyuan, the capital city of Shanxi Province.

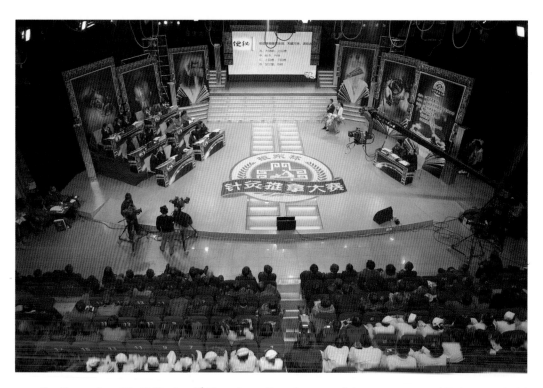

On December 22, 2012, the 1st Zhendong Cup Contest of Acupuncture and Tuina was held in Shanxi Province to further standardize the procedures of acupuncture and tuina in traditional Chinese medicine (TCM), and to improve the theoretical and technical level of acupuncture and tuina in traditional Chinese medicine (TCM).

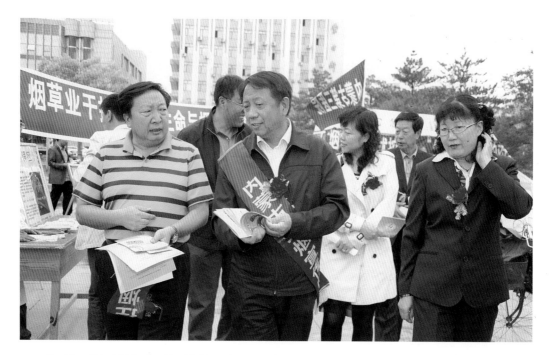

On May 31, 2012, the Health Department of Inner Mongolia held the campaign for the theme of the 25th World No-Tobacco Day in Hohhot, the capital city of Inner Mongolia. The picture shows that Deputy Director-General of the Health Department of Inner Mongolia Yin Chilin attended the on-the-spot campaign.

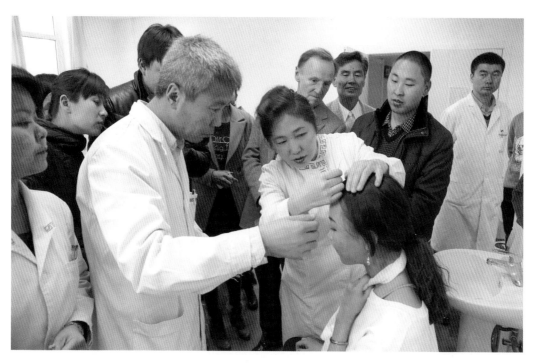

On November 12, 2012, Uland, Deputy Director-General of the Health Department of Inner Mongolia and Director of International Mongolian Medicine Hospital, accompanied Bach, Liaison of the United Nations Human Settlements Program (UN-HABITAT), and Prof. Craig. Lehmann, Dean of School of Health Technology & Management of America's State University of New York at Stony Brook School of Medicine, to visit the Department of Acupuncture and Tuina of International Mongolian Medicine Hospital. Uland introduced the guests to blood-letting therapy.

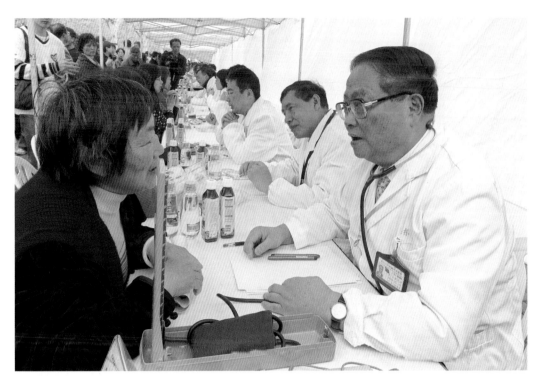

On April 15, 2012, Shanghai Municipal Bureau of Health and Shanghai Medical Trade Unions jointly organized "Guard Life" —a large-scale free medical consultation of Shanghai health care circles.

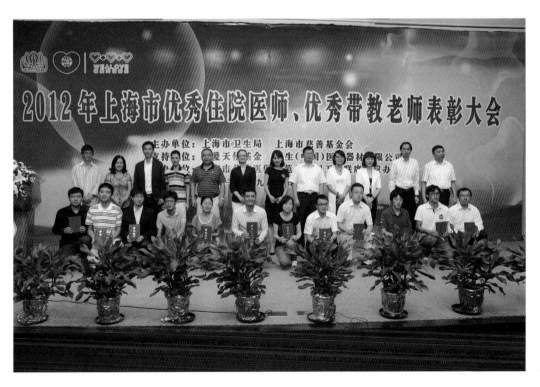

On September 5, 2012, Shanghai Municipal Bureau of Health and Shanghai Charity Foundation jointly held the Commendation Meeting for Shanghai Excellent Resident Doctors and Excellent Clinical Teachers.

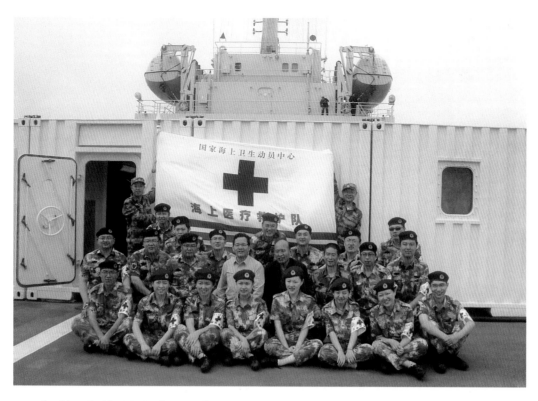

On May 7–16, 2012, Jiangsu Provincial Department of Health organized 10 medical team members to attend the training of transmarine medical rescue of "Oceans Call—2012".

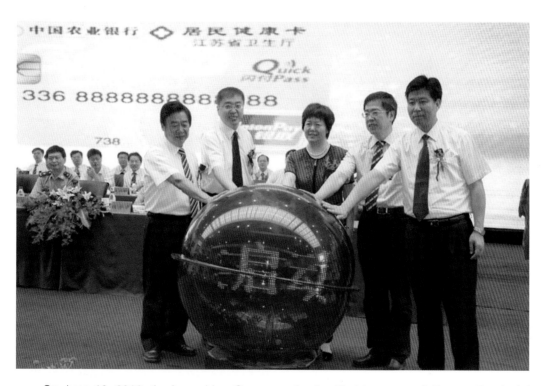

On June 16, 2012, the Launching Ceremony for the First Issuance of Jiangsu Provincial Residents' Health Cards was held in the city of Huaian.

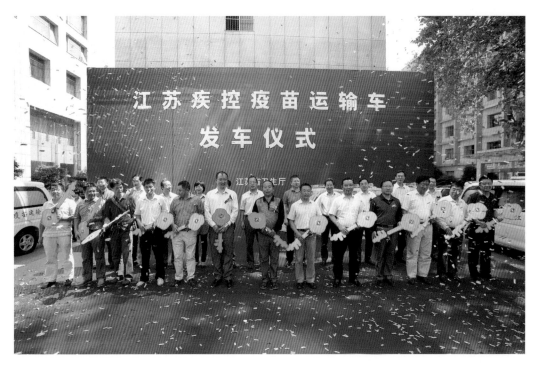

On September 15, 2012, Jiangsu Provincial Department of Health held the Vehicle Distribution Ceremony of Vaccine Trucks in Nanjing, the capital city of Jiangsu Province, to uniformly distribute vaccine trucks to 37 county-level centers for disease control and prevention, including Lishui County of Nanjing.

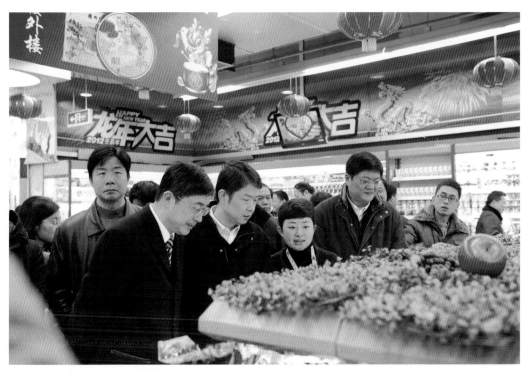

On January 17, 2012, the Office of Zhejiang Triple Food Safety Commission of Province, City and District conducted supervision and inspection for Hangzhou food safety assurance during Spring Festival.

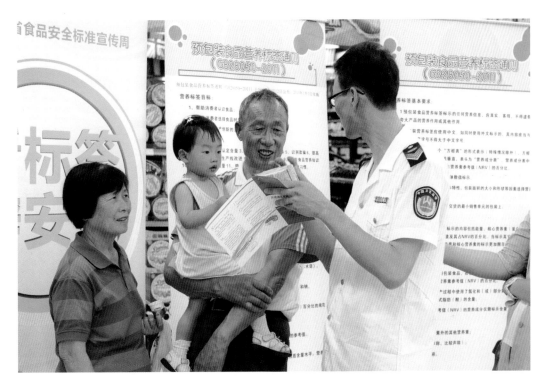

On June 15, 2012, the campaign for food safety standards of "reading labels for safety" was held in Hangzhou, the capital city of Zhejiang Province. The campaign was hosted by Zhejiang Provincial Department of Health and Zhejiang Provincial Administration for Industry and Commerce, and co-organized by Zhejiang Provincial Institute of Health Supervision and Zhejiang Provincial Center for Disease Control and Prevention.

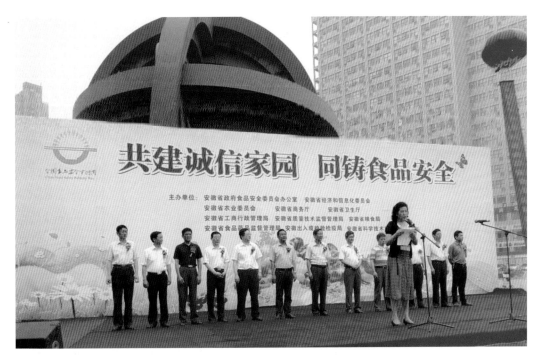

On June 11, 2012, the 2012 Anhui Provincial Publicity Week for Food Safety was kicked off in Hefei, the capital city of Anhui Province.

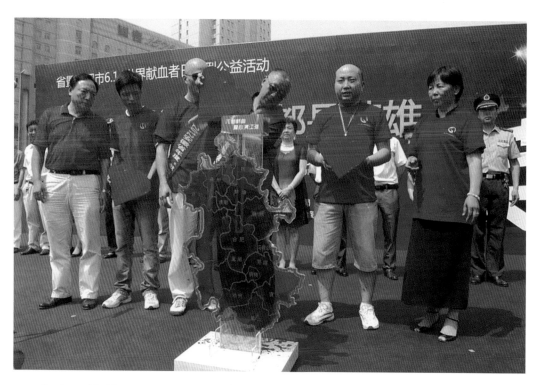

On June 14, 2012, the campaign for "World Blood Donor Day" Was held in Anhui Province.

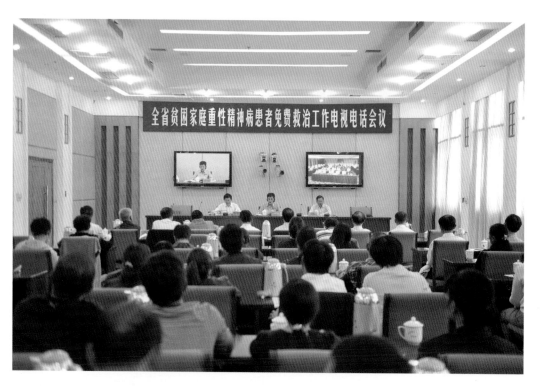

On October 24, 2012, the Video and Telephone Conference on Free Treatment of Severe Psychotic Disorder Patients from Underprivileged Households of Jiangxi Province was held in Nanchang, the capital city of Jiangxi Province, to start comprehensively the Free Treatment of Severe Psychotic Disorder Patients from Underprivileged Households of Jiangxi Province.

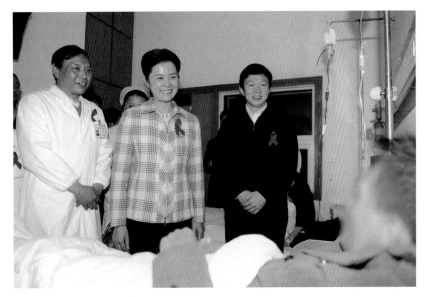

On December 1, 2012, Director of Jiangxi Provincial AIDS Working Committee and Vice Governor of Jiangxi Province Xie Ru visited the HIV/AIDS patients and front-line staff at Wushiqiao Branch of Jiangxi Provincial Chest Hospital and CDC of Xinjian County.

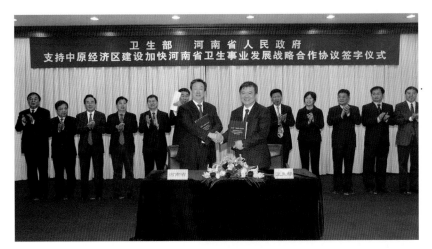

On March 21, 2012, the Ministry of Health and Henan Provincial Government signed the Strategic Cooperation Agreement on Supporting the Construction of Central Plains Economic Zone and Speeding up the Development of Henan Provincial Health Services.

On February 23, 2012, Hubei Provincial Department of Health and Jingzhou Municipal Government signed the Cooperation Agreement on the Implementation of "the Project of Making Jingzhou More Powerful and Stronger".

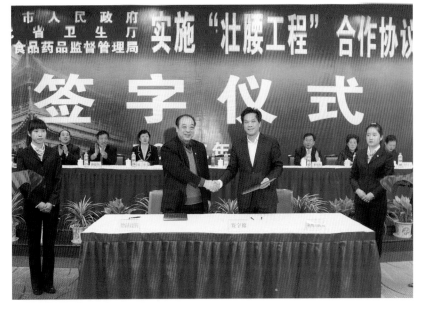

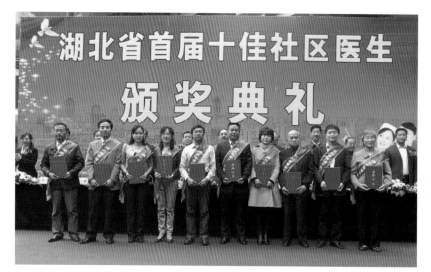

On October 26, 2012, the 1st Award-giving Meeting of Top 10 Community Doctors of Hubei Province was held in Wuhan, the capital city of Hubei Province.

On June 12, 2012, the 2012 Annual Work Meeting on the Collaborative Project of HIV/AIDS Prevention and Control of China's Ministry of Health and the Bill & Melinda Gates Foundation was held in Chongqing, one of the four municipalities directly under the Central Government.

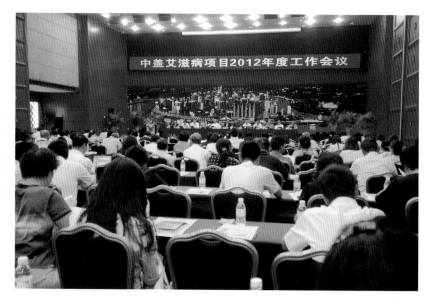

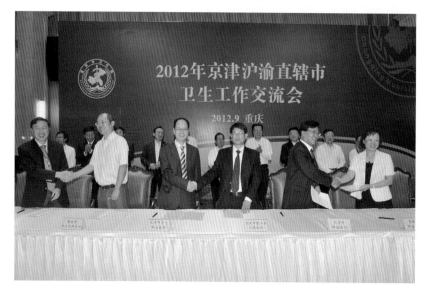

On September 20, 2012, the 2012 Exchange Meeting on Health Work of Beijing, Tianjin, Shanghai and Chongqing was held in Chongqing. The above four cities are municipalities directly under the Central Government.

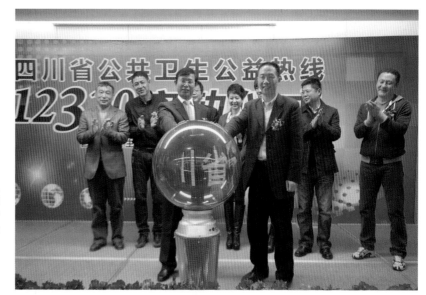

On March 20, 2012, Sichuan Provincial 12320 Hotline of Public Health for Public Benefit was officially launched.

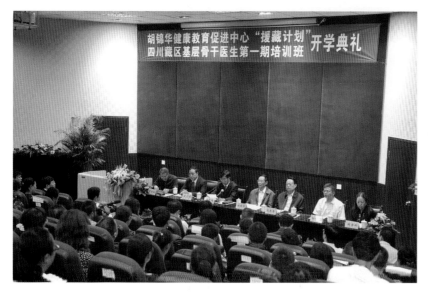

On June 4, 2012, the Workshop for Primary-level Doctors from Tibetan Areas of Sichuan started. The Workshop was funded by Hu Jinhua Health Education Promotion Center and organized by Sichuan University West China School of Public Health. It was also aimed at completing the training for 300 primary-level doctors from the counties and townships of Tibetan areas.

To promote the construction of Sino-Myanmar Ophthalmology Medical Center and improve the technical levels of medical workers, nurses and technicians, China Foundation for Peace and Development invited 10 Myanmar doctors and nurses to Yunnan for a short-term professional training. The picture shows the Closing Ceremony of the Training Workshop for Myanmar Ophthalmologists from the Sino-Myanmar Ophthalmology Medical Center on August 24, 2012.

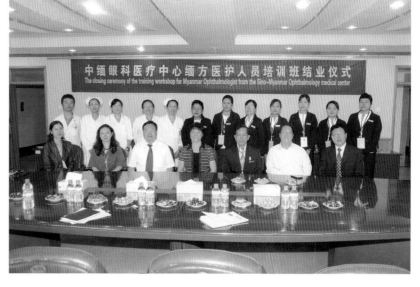

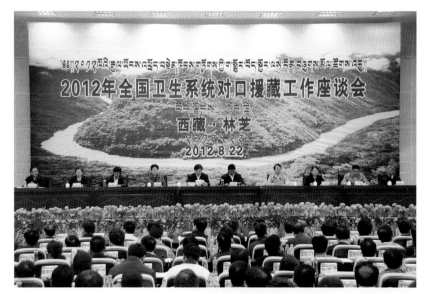

On August 22, 2012, the 2012 National Symposium on the Counterpart Assistance of Health Circles for Tibetan Health was held in Nyingchi, a county in Tibet Autonomous Region.

On September 25, 2012, the Handover Ceremony of Emergency Mobile Hospital of Tibet Autonomous Region was held.

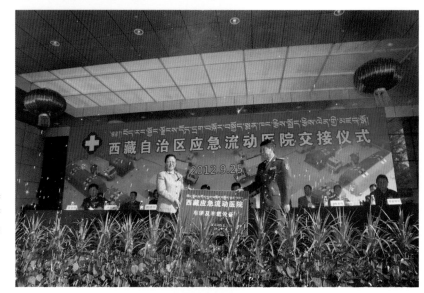

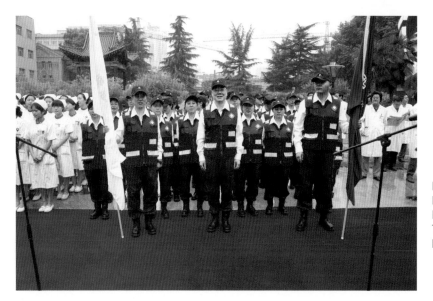

On May 24, 2012, the Handover Ceremony of Mobile Hospital of the National Emergency Medical Rescue Team was held in Shaanxi Provincial People's Hospital.

On July 7, 2012, the Donation Ceremony of Supporting Product of "the Project of Maternal and Infant Nutrition Improvement in Western China" of WHO Children's Health Collaboration Center was held in Xi'an, the capital city of Shaanxi Province.

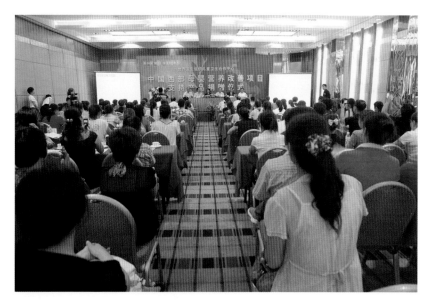

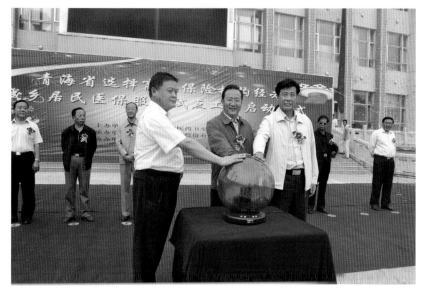

On July 31, 2012, the pilot work for health insurance handled by the insurance company was officially launched in Huzhu County of Qinghai Province.

The Pharmacopoeia of Traditional Tibetan Medicine compiled by Qinghai Provincial Research Institute of Traditional Tibetan Medicine and published by the Ethnic Publishing House was officially published in 2012. So far it is the biggest compilation project of traditional Tibetan medicine literature. The picture shows that the Evaluation Meeting on the Scientific Achievements of the Pharmacopoeia of Traditional Tibetan Medicine was held in Xining, the capital city of Qinghai Province, on December 17.

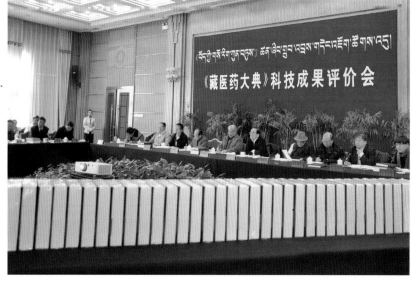

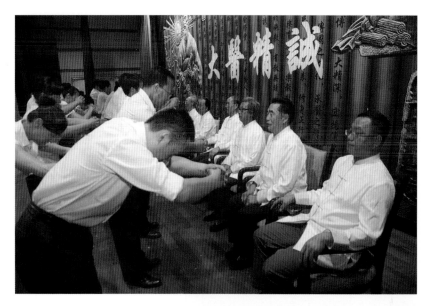

On August 8, 2012, the "36331" talent training, the promotion of scientific achievements and the ceremony of being apprenticed to masters of traditional Chinese medicine and Hui Medicine in Ningxia started in Yinchuan, the capital city of Ningxia Hui Autonomous Region. The picture shows that 54 young doctors of traditional Chinese medicine formally acknowledged 29 prestigious TCM doctors and advisers within and outside the Region in a traditional way of bowing and serving tea.

On July 24, 2012, the 1st Skill Competition for Health Supervision was held in Xinjiang Uygur Autonomous Region to improve the level of health supervision/law-enforcement and the capacity of technical operation.

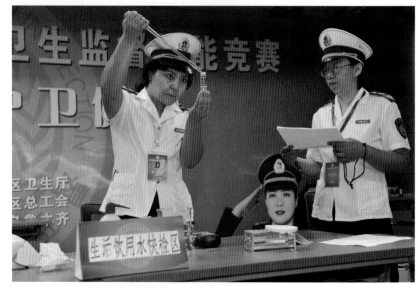

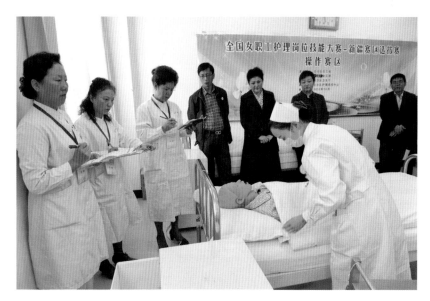

On October 12, 2012, the Department of Health of Xinjiang Uygur Autonomous Region held the national female workers' skill competition of nursing job.

2013
YEAR BOOK OF HEALTH
IN THE PEOPLE'S REPUBLIC OF
CHINA

Editor-in-Chief

Chen Zhu

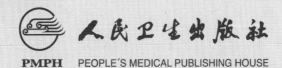

PMPH　PEOPLE'S MEDICAL PUBLISHING HOUSE

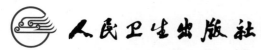

PMPH   PEOPLE'S MEDICAL PUBLISHING HOUSE

http:// www.pmph.com

Book Title: 2013 Year Book of Health in the People's Republic of China
2013 中国卫生年鉴

Contact address: No.19 Pan Jia Yuan Nan Li, Chaoyang District, Beijing 100021, P. R. China
phone/fax: 86 10 5978 7386, E-mail: pmph@pmph.com

First published:
ISBN: 978-7-117-20062-2/R · 20063

Cataloguing in Publication Data:
A catalog record for this book is available from the
CIP-Database China.

Printed in P. R. China

ISBN 978-7-117-20062-2

9 787117 200622 >

Contents

Part II   Policy and Statute   121

Part III   Progress of Work   127

Chapter I   Disease Prevention and Control   133

Section 1   Progress in China Center for Disease Prevention and Control

Chapter XIII Management of Pharmaceutical Industry

Chapter XIV The Basic Medical Security System

Section 2　Important Visits from Other Countries

Section 3   Important International Conferences   *250*

UK Michael Pragnell

Chapter XVII   Construction of Spiritual Civilization

Part IV   Academic and Civil Societies   291

Chapter I   Chinese Medical Association

Chapter II   Chinese Association of Preventive Medicine

Part I
Significant Reports in Conference

1. Focus on Key Areas, Overcome Problems and Fully Implement Medical Reform and Every Task of Health Work
    —A Work Presentation of Health Minister Chen Zhu at 2012 National Meeting on Health Work (January 5, 2012)

Comrades,

This is an important meeting approved by the State Council and convened at the crucial stage of deepening the medical system reform. The theme of this meeting is as follows: Act on the spirit of the 17th CPC National Congress, the spirit of the Third, Fourth, Fifth and Sixth Plenary Sessions of the 17th CPC Central Committee, and the spirit of the Central Economic Work Conference. Under the guidance of Deng Xiaoping Theory and important thought of Three Represents, thoroughly apply the scientific outlook on development; centering round the deepening of medical reform, summarize the health work of the year 2011 and make arrangements for 2012 work and tasks. Strengthen confidence, raise spirits and do solid work to ensure that the people share in the achievements of medical reform and development. Just now, Secretary Zhang Mao conveyed the spirit of Vice Premier Li Keqiang's address when he listened to the report of the Ministry of Health. He fully affirmed the achievements health departments made in medical reform and every work, which indicated the direction for the work this year and the coming period. In seriously studying and having a deep understanding of Vice Premier Li Keqiang's address, we must comprehensively implement it.

Now I will talk about things in three parts for your discussion.

I. The Summary of 2011 Health Work

2011 was a year of hardships for five key tasks of recent medical reform, and it marked the start of health development of the 12th Five-Year Plan. Under the strong leadership of the CPC Central Committee and the State Council, health circles nationwide pooled the wisdom and efforts of everyone, studied the whole situation, and promoted the reform and development. As a result, remarkable achievements were made in medical reform and all the health work.

(1) The tasks for medical reform led by health departments were basically completed.

At the beginning of 2011, the Medical Reform Office of the State Council subdivided the medical reform tasks of the year into 67, 46 of which were in charge of health departments and 18 were finished with the cooperation of health departments. The latest monitoring results have been given out to you as meeting materials. Therefore I will summarize mainly some innovations and work highlights in the fulfillment of medical reform tasks in various localities.

1) The new rural cooperative medical system (NCMS)

The coverage kept on expanding with the level of fund significantly raised. Meanwhile the security level continued to be on the rise, and the management level was constantly improved as well. In Jiangxi, Jiangsu, Liaoning, Hebei, Shandong, Chongqing, Anhui, Hunan, Hubei, Hainan and some other provinces (regions, cities), types of diseases like end-stage renal disease and two cancers of women were added to the scope of major disease security. In Jilin, the range was extended to 20 types of diseases. In Xinjiang, Yunnan, Tibet, Qinghai, Fujian and Hunan, pilot projects for supplemental insurance or commercial insurance purchase of major disease were under way. In Changshu of Jiangsu and Lanshan of Hunan, payment reform was carried out. In Inner Mongolia and Shaanxi, the possibility of raising overall level to city (meng) level was explored. In Guangdong, Henan and Hunan, whether commercial insurance agencies could handle the management of the new rural cooperative system was also explored. In Jiangsu, a mechanism of stable growth for the new rural cooperative medical system was established in the form of legislation.

2) The national system for basic drugs

Universal coverage for basic drug system was attained in government-run medical institutions at the primary level. In all parts of the country, the comprehensive reform for medical institutions at the primary level was promoted in an overall way with the implementation of basic drug system as a breakthrough. In 16 provinces including Anhui, Shandong, Hebei, Sichuan and Hubei, a new round of procurement was completed with the price falling by 30% on average. In Jiangxi, Zhejiang and 9 other provinces, medical institutions of Class II and above were required to prepare and use essential drugs in prescribed proportion. In Ningxia and Henan, centralized bidding and procurement of some of high-value consumables was explored. In Anhui, 30 supplementary policies were issued to consolidate and improve the primary medical reform. In Liaoning, Shaanxi, Qinghai and 13 other provinces as well as Xinjiang Production & Construction Corps, full employment was achieved in all the government-run medical institutions at the primary level. In a great majority of provinces (regions, cities) including Heilongjiang, merit pay in medical institutions at the primary level was attained basically.

3) The medical and health service system at the primary level

With a focus on county hospitals, township hospitals, village clinics and community health services, the renovation project kept carrying forward. Throughout the country, the building of medical teams at the primary level was intensified with a focus on general practitioners. Job-transfer training for general practitioners was carried out while order and directional training programs for medical students were conducted free of charge as well. The project of tens of thousands of doctors aiding rural health was carried out as before. The subsidy policy for village doctors was carried out step by step and the problem of their social pension was solved. In Hebei, college-graduate village doctors were recruited. In Beijing and Shanghai, family doctors services were introduced. And in Inner Mongolia, the implementation of the project of medical kits for health security of herdsman families was explored.

4) The equalization of basic public health services

The project of the equalization of basic public health services was carried out extensively in urban and rural areas at the grass-roots level. Such medical reform task was completed, as the standardized management of residents' health records and patients of hypertension, diabetes and severe mental illness. Some major public health projects were basically completed, such as sight regaining surgery for impoverished cataract patients. In Guizhou, the project for the elimination of the hazard of coal-burning fluorosis was completed one year ahead of schedule. From place to place, new ideas for the management means of public health service were brought forth. In Jiangxi, Qinghai, Tibet and other provinces (regions), the proportions of provincial supporting funds were increased to ease the burden of grass-roots institutions. Cross-departmental projects of social health promotion were launched in Beijing, Hubei and Shandong. And in Jiangxi, the third party assessment mechanism for the equalization of basic public health services was tried out.

5) Pilot reforms of public hospitals

In 17 state-level pilot cities, 37 provincial-level pilot cities and 745 hospitals of 18 provinces, comprehensive trial reform was carried out. Full explorations were started in the areas of planning layout, management system, compensation mechanism, payment system, internal management, service improvement, support for grass-roots level institutions and encouragement for hospital running by non-governmental organizations. Nationwide, some effective and easy-to-operate measures for reform were introduced with a focus on strengthening service. In Class II and Class III hospitals, the services of appointment diagnosis, time-phased doctors visits and high-quality nursing care were under way; besides, the pilot project for clinical pathway and electronic medical records (EMR) was launched. In some of the hospitals in Beijing, the rate of medical appointments reached 40% or so. In Hainan, Shenzhen, Kunming, Chengdu, Luoyang and Beijing, the pilot project for physicians' multi-sited license was launched. Distinctive medical groups were formed in 9 cities including Anshan, Zhenjiang and Wuhu, while the possibility of establishing medical complexes was explored in Shanghai, Beijing and 3 other cities. In Shaanxi, Jiangsu, Zhejiang, Hubei and Shanxi, comprehensive reforms of public hospitals at the county level were started. And in Anhui, payment by type of disease was promoted combined with medical insurance reimbursement policy, and graded diagnosis and treatment was initially achieved.

(2) Remarkable achievements were made in major disease prevention, health emergency and maternal & child health care.

Disease prevention and control was strengthened in an all-round way. Prevention and control measures for such contagious diseases as influenza, hand-foot-mouth disease and brucellosis were carried out effectively. Notifiable diseases of class AB remained stable. The coverage of AIDS surveillance, testing, treatment, intervention and mother-infant block was expanded. The number of HIV testing and the number of antiviral therapy increased by 16% and 37% respectively over the same period. Eight hundred and thirty thousand cases of tuberculosis were found and treated, and the cure rate of infectious tuberculosis was 93%. The incidence of major parasitic diseases including schistosomiasis was in decline. Remarkable achievements were made in the supplementary immunization of measles vaccine (MV), with the morbidity dropped from 25/1,000,000 in 2010 to less than 10/1,000,000, which laid a good foundation for the elimination of measles. We also actively responded to the imported wild-type poliovirus in Xinjiang, and the supplementary immunization for polio was completed through 22,000,000 person-times. In 28 provinces (regions, cities) nationwide, the target of elimination of iodine deficiency was reached. With the prevention and control of chronic diseases continually strengthened, 39 demonstration sites for comprehensive prevention and control of chronic diseases passed examination and acceptance. In 892 counties (cities), campaigns for the lifestyle of universal health were launched, and 200,000 people were screened for early diagnosis and early treatment of major cancers. Key construction projects for professional institutions of mental illness were carried out. A national information management system for major mental illness was set up. In 25 provinces, pilot projects for comprehensive intervention of children's oral diseases were carried out. With patriotic public health campaign launched, there were an increasing number of national hygienic cities (districts) and towns, and staged achievements were made in the problem-addressing action for urban-rural environment. The surveillance of rural drinking water was constantly strengthened with the coverage expanded further.

Health emergency was strengthened in an all-round way. The linkage mechanism for multi-sectored disposal of public health emergencies was improved. A number of contingency plans were made in case of public health emergencies to strengthen the core competence construction for emergency. The establishment of 27 national health emergency teams of 4 main categories was finished. The trainings for management cadres, teachers at the provincial level were intensified. The catalogue adjustment and material preparation for health contingency reserve against terrorism were completed. The early warning and prevention and control of emergent infectious diseases of unknown cause were intensified. Plague control and prevention in key regions was intensified as before. The anthrax emergencies in Liaoning, Jilin and Inner Mongolia were actively dealt with. Fukushima nuclear disaster, the rear-end collision of bullet trains on Yong-Wen Railway and other major emergencies at home and abroad received prompt response and properly dealt with.

Maternal and child health care was strengthened. In the promotion of construction for maternal and child health care system, 4.3 billion yuan were invested to support the basic equipment of county maternal and child health care institutions in central and western regions. The project of reducing maternal mortality and eliminating neonatal tetanus was carried out as usual. The comprehensive prevention and control of birth defects was under way. Free premarital examination was generalized, while antenatal diagnosis was boosted. With the construction for health education system strengthened, professional trainings for health education were organized to push forward the promotion of citizens' health literacy. Banning smoking in public places was carried forward in order to promote the establishment of smoke-free medical system.

(3) The safety of food and drug was further strengthened.

Long-term mechanism and system construction were promoted. *National Drug Safety Program* was worked out and Good Manufacturing Practices for Drugs newly revised in 2010 was enacted. The construction of electronic monitoring system for drugs was promoted. The system of drug quality tracing and safety emergency management was improved. The mechanism of drug examination and approval was reformed. The complaint center was established. The technical support system was strengthened. The action for drug standard improvement was promoted. An information system for drug evaluation sampling was established. The fast drug inspection technique was carried out. The post-marketing drug surveillance and evaluation were strengthened. With the management system of reporting and monitoring of adverse drug reactions (ADRs) improved, decisions were made to handle the drugs with safety risks. Besides, campaigns were launched for drug safety to maintain the public medication safety. The two-year sole rectification for drug safety was completed. Also the sole rectifications were carried out in a deep-going way to crack down on the infringement of intellectual property rights and the manufacturing of counterfeit drugs, medical devices and health care products. And illegal drug ads were seriously governed while food and drug market order was standardized.

The two-year task for food safety rectification was completed. With the special campaign launched against adding non-food substances illegally, a list was released for 64 types of non-food substances and 22 types of easy abuse of additives. Such food safety affairs of public attention as problem milk powder were handled properly in response to social hot issues. With the strengthening of technical regulations and standard construction of food safety, 124 national standards of food safety were reviewed and passed while 21 national standards of food safety were promulgated. Ninety-six product standards for food additives were set. Food additives including benzoyl peroxide were repealed while a notice was issued to forbid the use of bisphenol A in baby bottles. The national center for the risk assessment of food safety was set up, while the monitoring system for food safety risks was established, covering 244 cities nationwide. Through active surveillance, we notified the Food Safety Office of the State Council of food safety problems for 7 times successively. Efforts were pooled to crack down on the unlawful acts including the additives of food, health food and cosmetics. A special campaign was launched against adding non-food substances illegally in the catering service.

(4) Health supervision and law-enforcement was constantly strengthened.

Regular health supervision/law-enforcement was carried out in a deep-going way. Eight hundred thousands medical institutions were inspected with 41,000 medical practices without licenses clamped down. One hundred and forty-six thousand schools were supervised and examined. A national surveillance network for drinking water hygiene in urban-rural areas was established, covering 620 counties (cities) in 110 cities at prefectural level nationwide. Nearly 20,000 surveillance sites were set up. With a general survey for water quality of municipal water supply in urban areas conducted, 28,000 water supply units received supervision and inspection. The quantitative and level-to-level management for over 500,000 public places was conducted. The supervision and inspection for concentrated disinfection of tableware were strengthened with an 86% qualified rate. The special examination for illegal blood collection and supply was carried on. A number of institutions at the municipal and county level for occupational disease prevention and control were newly established. As a result, some occupational hazards including pneumoconiosis and occupational poisoning were properly handled. Jointly with relevant departments, we conducted a national survey of occupational health. In 17 provinces pilot programs were carried out for the surveillance of medical radiation protection. Great progress was made in the construction of health supervision system. The central government invested 5.6 billion yuan for the housing construction and equipment configuration of law-enforcement of over 2,000 health supervision institutions at the county level.

(5) New achievements were made in the work on Traditional Chinese Medicine (TCM).

Several Opinions of the State Council on Supporting and Promoting Traditional Chinese Medicine was actively carried out and implemented around the country to give full play to the role of Traditional Chinese Medicine. The capacity building of 1,814 county TCM hospitals, 58 ethnomedicine hospitals at the prefectural and municipal level and 88 TCM hospitals at the prefectural and municipal level in the west area was started. The work mechanisms of TCM emergency and the prevention and control of emerging infectious diseases were improved. The health project of preventive treatment of disease was pushed forward and menu-style preventive services for 10 chronic diseases were under way. Policies for comprehensively promoting the development of TCM and ethnomedicine were introduced in Guangxi. In Zhejiang, Fujian and Shandong, pilot programs were carried out for chronic disease prevention and control with TCM or integrated management. In Gansu, Hebei, Zhejiang and Ningxia, TCM services were put into the range of basic public health services projects. In Tianjin, Beijing and Shanghai, the TCM Hall construction of medical institutions at the primary level was strengthened to develop the characteristics and advantages of TCM. Pilot programs were launched for the survey of TCM resources. The authentication of staff with special trade skills in TCM was promoted. The research-based results of inheritance from veteran doctors of TCM were abstracted and spread. In addition, the veteran and renowned TCM experts nationwide were advised to established inheritance workshops to promote TCM inheritance. In Gansu, 1,000 veteran TCM doctors were selected for the handing-down teaching supported by the local government to speed up the TCM talent building. The constructions of key disciplines, vocational education and culture of TCM were strengthened. Tu Youyou won the 2011 Lasker Award for clinical research, which showcased the potential value of TCM. TCM standard internationalization was promoted to construct the rights of TCM discourse and domination.

(6) Medical quality/safety and medical services regulation were further strengthened.

The campaign for "good services, good quality, good medical ethics and public satisfaction" and "quality promotion" was launched in a deep-going way. A special rectification for clinical application of antibacterial drugs was carried out. The regulation of such clinical services as organ transplantations and assisted reproductive technology was strengthened. The constructions of 110 regional medical centers in the Midwest got started, while 316 construction projects for national key clinical specialties came into being after appraisal. Pre-hospital first aid and the construction of pediatrics at the municipal level were strengthened. Clinical pathways for 109 kinds of diseases were newly mapped out and issued. Standardized diagnoses and treatment for such major diseases as children's congenital heart disease and children's leukemia were implemented. In medical institutions at the primary level, standardized diagnoses and treatment for 20 kinds of common diseases got started. In January-September of last year, the number of blood donors and the amount of blood collection/supply increased by 5.1% and 5.8% respectively over the same period, which basically met the need of clinical use of blood.

Results were achieved in the control of medical expenses. In January-November of last year, the average cost of outpatient and hospital discharge rose 3.4% and 2.6 respectively, and the amount of increase was significantly lower than the previous two years, which basically achieved the cost control goal set at the beginning of last year and made contributions for the maintenance of general price level. In Fujian, Guangdong, Gansu, Ningxia, Zhejiang and Shanghai, great efforts were made for cost control and valuable experience was accumulated.

(7) The progression of health informatization construction was significantly accelerated.

Both central and local treasuries appropriated special funds for health informatization to strengthen the platform construction of the NCMS information system, residents' electronic health records (EHR) and electronic medical records (EMR), tele-consultation system and regional health information. From place to place, with electronic medical records as the basis, business processes were optimized while some convenience-for-people measures were carried out, like integrated services of appointment outpatient, diagnosis and payment, which made it convenient for people to seek medical advice. Tele-consultation system in Xinjiang had been connected to 88 counties and cities with over 20,000 cases of consultation. In Shanghai, Jiangsu, Zhejiang, Henan, Hubei and Jiangxi, the constructions of regional health information platform were quickened. As a result, the following functions had been achieved: real-time updates on residents' electronic health records, patients' appointment registrations and queries of health records, work performance appraisal of medical staff and the regulation of medical services.

(8) New Progress was made in other health work.

Activity carriers were innovated and the focal points of serving the people were highlighted. The campaign for "good services, good quality, good medical ethics and public satisfaction" was carried out in a deep-going way, which promoted the implementation of every task. The publicity for health policies, medical reform results and role models of industry was strengthened. Hot public opinions of concern were actively guided in order to create a good atmosphere of public opinions for health work and medical reform. The punishment of health system and the construction of anti-corruption system were strengthened. In the departments of health administration and health law enforcement, the monitoring mechanism construction of power operation was carried out in a deep-going way as usual. Centralized drug procurement was greatly standardized. The special assignment of the control over commercial bribery in the area of drug procurement and sales and the rectification of the evil trends in medical services was consolidated and deepened as always. The accountability of work style rectification and the system of medical ethics assessment for medical workers were carried out. A risk evaluation mechanism of health system for maintaining social stability was established. And so were the mediation mechanism for medical disputes and the long-term working mechanism for letters and calls concerning health. As a result, conflicts had been resolved and stability was maintained. Health care for cadres was actively improved to enhance constantly health care level. We cared for the veteran leaders' lives and health, and support them in playing a role of reference and consultation.

The funds for medical reform and financial management were strengthened effectively. The way of fund appropriation was innovated to promote a full coverage for the regulation of medical reform funds. New regulations for finance and accounting were carried out. An Outline of Health Program in the period of the 12th Five-Year Plan was formulated. Regional health planning, the configuration of large-scale medical equipments and the management of basic construction were strengthened as usual. The centralized procurement of large-scale medical equipments and high-value hospital consumables was promoted. Health assistance to Xinjiang, Tibet and Qinghai as well as poverty relief by health was strengthened effectively. The post-disaster reconstruction in Wenchuan was completed and the post-disaster reconstructions in Yushu and Zhouqu were promoted smoothly.

A Mid-long Term Plan for Talent Development in Medical and Health Services (2011-2020) was mapped out and carried out. Some talent projects were launched, such as health talents at the primary level, outstanding medical talents, professionals with special skills, TCM talents and doctors' standardized training. The inter-departmental coordination for medical education was strengthened. *The Twelfth Five-Year Plan for the Development of Medical Science* was mapped out and carried out. The two major special projects of science and technology, namely the prevention and control of major infectious diseases such as AIDS and viral hepatitis and the development of major/new drugs were carried out effectively. Therefore the supporting role of science and technology in research and development was further enhanced.

Interstate and interregional exchanges and co-operations were widely conducted. Through the diplomatic platforms including international organizations, international conferences and multilateral/bilateral activities, the ideas and progress of medical reform in our country were publicized. Moreover, international technology and funds were introduced to support health development. Actively involved in global major health actions, we played a positive role in the promotion of the prevention and control of chronic disease, improvement of social determinants of health and improvement of international food safety. International organizations were invited to conduct independent evaluations for our country's medical reform. The regulation system of vaccines of our country received the pre-accreditation of WHO. The high-level dialogues and technical collaborations in health with developing countries, neighboring countries and countries with emerging economy were strengthened. The construction and innovation of medical teams for foreign aid were strengthened as well. Deep-level co-operations in health with Hong Kong and Macao regions were pushed forward as usual, and so were the cross-Straights exchanges on health.

Comrades, over the past year, medical reform and all health work had been smoothly promoted, which had played an important role in maintaining the people's health benefits and promoting the coordinated economic and social development. Hereby, on behalf of the Ministry of Health, I would like to express our heartfelt thanks and highest respects to Party committees and governments at all levels and departments concerned which attach great importance and support health service development. Also, our thanks and respects go to various circles of the society, the news media and the people who support health work. Finally, the country's health workers deserve the heartfelt thanks and respects.

II. Be Clear about the Situations and Tasks for the Priorities of Medical Reform in the Period of the Twelfth Five-Year Plan

With great progress made in three years' medical work, medical reform in next four years will soon start. We should seriously sum up the results, analyze the new situation and new challenge, clarify our thinking and try hard to make new breakthroughs in key fields and key links.

(1) Great progress was made in three years' medical reform.

Under the correct leadership of the Party Central Committee and the State

Council, Party committees and governments at all levels and departments concerned were well-organized and conducted close co-operations. Medical workers gave full play to the role of main force. As a result, outstanding achievements were made in medical reform.

1) People have benefited more from medical reform.

Over the past three years, the issue of difficult access to medical services has been eased to some extent. The situation, in which medical services facilities in rural and remote areas were poor and the service ability was weak, was changed significantly. The issue that, in large urban hospitals, it takes a long time for patients to register, pay fee and pick up medicine while it takes a short time for doctors to give medical advice has been eased step by step. As a result, the people's experience of seeking medical advice has improved a lot. The proportion of residents' reaching medical institutions within 15 minutes was raised from 80.3% in 2008 to 83.3% in 2011, while in rural area the proportion was raised from 75.6% to 80.8%.

Over the past three years, the issue of high cost of obtaining medical service has been alleviated, because urban-rural residents have begun gaining access to basic medical insurance with low level and universal coverage. The proportion of medical cost at their own expense of rural residents participating in NCMS dropped from 73.4% in 2008 to 49.5% in 2011. So the financial burden of seeking medical advice has been greatly reduced. Based on the special study of the Ministry of Health on 2011 medical reform, the rural residents' proportion of seeking medical advice on Saturdays and Sundays dropped from 12.4% in 2008 to 6.1% in 2011, while the urban residents' proportion dropped from 6.4% to 4.0%. Calculated at comparable prices, the growth rates of outpatient and hospitalization costs in public hospitals were controlled within 7%, thus slowing down the momentum of rapid growth of medical costs since the mid-1990s of the last century.

Over the past three years, urban-rural residents have gained access to equitable basic public health service. More and more residents have got into the healthy lifestyle; more and more patients with chronic diseases have gained access to systematized, standardized health management; and more and more focus groups have gained access to major public health service projects. As a result, remarkable improvement has been made in the equity of basic public health service. Based on the assessment on ten provinces (regions), the people's satisfaction with the basic public health service was above 90%.

Over the past three years, the national health indicators have been improved as usual. During 2008-2011, the maternal mortality dropped from 34.2/10 to 26.1/10, while the infant mortality dropped from 14.9‰ to 12.1‰. With all tasks of medical reform carried out, the national health indicators of our country have entered the period of faster improvement, which is the greatest benefit for the people.

2) The framework of basic health care system with Chinese characteristics has been initially established.

The coverage of basic health care system has reached more than 95%. Such achievements have been made in a large developing country with a population of 1.3 billion, which was hailed as a wonder of the world by international community.

Stage progress has been made in basic drug system. WHO experts believe that no such large-scale reform of drug system has been carried out in such a short time in any other country.

Medical reform has been restructured in a certain sense, which adjusted the health care service system of our country. A service pattern has initially taken shape, in which there are functional complementation and upper/lower linkage between primary health care institutions and top/middle grade hospitals and professional public health agencies, traditional Chinese medicine institutions and western medicine institutions are paid equal attention to, and the collaboration between public medical institutions and non-public medical institutions coexists. It is a component with Chinese characteristics in basic health care system.

There has been institutional arrangement in the country's long-held policy of "prevention first" due to the equitable public health service, which is a prominent highlight of medical reform.

After a few years' endeavor, our country's basic health care system has been initially established, and has become an important component of socialist system with Chinese characteristics. It will not only benefit the nation's health but explore the Chinese solution for the worldwide problem of medical reform.

3) Structural changes are taking place in health service.

With all tasks of medical reform carried out, an improving trend has appeared in some structural problems plaguing the scientific development of health service for a long time. Changes are taking place in some problems, while major structural improvement have been made in some other problems, which is the reform result we have hoped to witness over many years.

Firstly, more marked changes have taken place in the structure of health resources allocation. The problem is being reversed that more attention was paid to cities than to the countryside, more attention was paid to medical treatment than to prevention, more attention was paid to the high-end than to the primary end, and more attention was paid to western medicine than to traditional Chinese medicine. The guiding role of public finance tilting toward the primary level, the countryside and public health has been constantly enhanced. In 2009 and 2010, the net capital of urban community health service agencies reached 55%, while in county hospitals it increased by 39%, both of which were higher than that of urban hospitals. Meanwhile, there was a good trend of the number, educational background and knowledge structure of the talent team of primary-level health. In 2011, the staff of township health centers reached 1.20 million, increasing by 18.7% over 2005, among whom the proportion of staff with college degree or above increased from 23% to 40%. Over the past five years, the proportion of TCM doctors has increased from 10.3% to 12.2%.

Secondly, changes have taken place in the structure of health service utilized by the people. People still further recognize and trust the primary-level health services, so there has been an increasing trend in the utilization of service. In recent years, people have increasingly taken advantage of the primary-level health services. The number of outpatients in 2011 increased by 1.19 billion over 2005, an increase of 45.7%; the number of discharged patients increased by 20.22 million, a 1.2 fold increase.

Thirdly, the gap of health development between urban area and rural area has been narrowed step by step. The survey shows that in 2003 the proportion of medical insurance of urban-rural residents were 55% and 21% respectively, markedly higher in urban area than in rural area. In 2011, the proportions increased by 89% and 97% respectively, showing that the latter overtook the former. The surveillance shows that the gap of health indicators between urban area and rural area has also been narrowed. The maternal mortality rate between urban area and rural area was narrowed from 1:2.15 in 2005 to 1:1.01 in 2010. The urban-rural gap of infant mortality dropped from 7.2‰ to 5.9‰. The rural hospital parturition rate between the western region and eastern region dropped from 34% in 2003 to 2% in 2010. The above progress shows that the pace of urban-rural overall development of health has been quickened, and profound changes are taking place in the long-standing urban-rural dual structure and regional health disparities.

Fourthly, major structural changes have taken place in total health expenditure. In 2011, the proportion of individual health expenditure of our country amounted to 60%, while the proportions of health expenditure of governmental budget and social health expenditure accounted for 16% and 24%. The 2010 proportion of individual health expenditure dropped to 35.5%, while the proportions of governmental budget and social health expenditure rose from 28.6% to 35.9% respectively. This major structural change shows that our country's health financing structure tends to be reasonable, the residents' burden is relatively eased, and the equity is markedly improved.

We must also see that, in recent years, the business volume of health and medical workers was close to saturation. Therefore we should explore the internal potential and carry out a series of measures for the convenience of people, which is not only the medical workers' dedication to medical reform, but pulls them closer to patients, thus improving the satisfaction of service targets. According to the survey, comparing 2011 with 2008, the dissatisfaction of urban inpatients dropped to 7%, while that of rural counterparts dropped to 13%.

Seeing medical reform from a more macroscopic perspective, we find that medical reform plays an important role in macroscopic economy. Medical reform has built up a safe net for people to seek medical advice, relieved their worries, and expanded the immediate consumption, thus boosting domestic demand. Medical reform has promoted relevant industry development of national economy, spurred the growth of manufacturing industry and service industry, and promoted technical progress and product innovation. All those have made important contributions to the building of harmonious socialist society and the boost of national soft power. In the meantime, the health financing and service system with Chinese characteristics, the evaluation system of health economics and the decision-making mechanism of evidence-based health have become increasingly mature in the endeavor to make explorations. It has embodied the major innovation from theory to practice of public services and social management in the area of people's livelihood.

All in all, the practice and results of three years' reform show that the goal, the orientation and the principle of our country's medical reform set by the CPC Central Committee and the State Council are feasible, and accord with the law of health development, China's national situation and the people's will. I believe that these major changes will surely rouse the confidence of medical reform workers and inspire us to push medical reform into a deeper stage with even higher morale.

(2) Fully understand the situation facing medical reform in the period of the Twelfth Five-year Plan.

In the period of the Twelfth Five-year Plan, both internal and external environments of deepening medical reform present new features.

Seeing from the internal and external environments of health development, firstly the economy develops rapidly and lifestyle changes quickly. As a result, the rapidly aging population and the transformation of disease pattern have brought the country's residents a heavy dual burden of infectious and non-infectious diseases. Secondly the residents' living standards continue to rise, the social security system improves gradually, urban-rural residents' consumption concept and consumption structure transform and upgrade rapidly, the demand for health care services is growing, and the expectations of fitness and medical and health services are higher.

Thirdly our country's medical and health services as a whole lag behind the socioeconomic development. As important social services, their internal structure is not very reasonable. Moreover, the scale, function, structure and service pattern of health services are yet to be ready to meet the above challenges.

Seeing from medical reform itself, the institutional contradictions of the system have become prominent. Firstly, there remains imbalance of health resources allocation, and excellent resources in particular are in short supply, which still cannot meet the people's demand for basic medical and health services. Secondly, the deep-level system-mechanism reform advances slowly, and the transformation of health development pattern requires continuous exploration in the area of recognition and practice. Thirdly, there is imbalance of reform progress among various regions, some key links has not yet to make a breakthrough, and there exist a gap between medical reform results and social expectations.

But we should be aware that the period of the Twelfth Five-year Plan is still a period of strategic opportunity. There remain a sound political climate, material conditions, social atmosphere and mass base for pushing forward sound development of medical reform and health services. It shows the strong leadership of Party committees and governments at all levels, the positive teamwork of all departments, the ever-growing economic power, the people's understanding and support, and the successful experiences accumulated by three years' medical reform. All cadres and workers of health circles must understand the situation clearly, seize the opportunity, advance despite difficulties, meet new challenges, and struggle for the new victory of medical reform.

(3) Make a key breakthrough to complete fully the medical reform task for the Twelfth Five-year Plan.

As for the key tasks and requirements of medical reform in the period of the Twelfth Five-year Plan, Zhang Mao will comprehensively expound them in his concluding remarks. Here I will put forward some views on a number of focus issues concerning further breakthroughs for deepening medical reform.

1) Cancel comprehensively the system of "subsidizing hospitals by charging more medicine fees" and straighten out the compensation mechanism.

If asked what are the institutional maladies which need most to be abolished in current medical and health area, I think the answers of a majority of you will be: subsidizing hospitals by charging more medicine fees. This mechanism has pushed forward the unreasonable rise of medical costs, caused drug abuse, distorted the medical workers' behavior, and corrupted our team. Therefore it must be eradicated. For quite some time, medical and health institutions have really relied on the system of "subsidizing hospitals by charging more medicine fees" to maintain operation and development. Currently drug income continues to be an important channel of compensation. Reforming the system of "subsidizing hospitals by charging more medicine fees" inevitably touches on the practical interests of medical and health care institutions. We must make a choice whether to continue to maintain this unreasonable mechanism or to be determined to do away with it. We think that this mechanism will be reformed sooner or later for the maintenance of the interests of the general public, for the sound development of medical and health services and for the long-term construction of health team. It is much more active and beneficial to reform thoroughly the system now than to do it sloppily in the future. All local health administrative departments in various local regions should, according to the arrangements and requirements of medical reform planning for the Twelfth Five-year Plan, strive for the governmental leadership actively, work hard to create conditions, carry out relevant policies of abolishing subsidizing hospitals by charging more medicine fees, ensure that the subsidizing policy for public hospitals is in place, give full play to the role of Medicare reimbursement, steadily promote price reform, and strive for the orderly abolishment of disadvantages of subsidizing hospitals by charging more medicine fees in the whole system during the period of the Twelfth Five-year Plan. This year the practice will be tried out in 300 pilot counties, universally promoted in county hospitals in 2013, and comprehensively launched throughout all public hospitals in 2015.

2) Comprehensively push forward the system of payment system.

The combination of the system of paying fee according to medicine items and subsidizing hospitals by charging more medicine fees is the main reason for excessive prescriptions and examinations. The current pricing mechanism of paying fee according to medicine items makes it hard to reflect the technical value of medical work. This payment system not only wastes health resources but also goes against arousing the enthusiasm of medical workers. We should take the reform of payment system as the key link of institutional mechanism reform and push it forward vigorously. In accordance with the experiences at home and abroad, payment system is an important means for fee control of medical insurance agencies. With the total coverage of our country's basic medical insurance system completed, the conditions of payment system reform have become ripe. Health administrative departments should give full play to the advantages of managing both the new rural cooperative medical system (NCMS) and service delivery, and take the lead in promoting the payment system reform of the new rural cooperative medical system (NCMS). In the meantime, they should coordinate with other relevant departments of medical insurance and price, summarize the pilot experiences in recent years of various regions, map out implementation plans, determine the payment mode suitable for medical institutions at all levels and services of different types, and replace paying fee according to medicine items with global budget, disease entities, the fee for service and capitation. They should also combine clinical pathway with the payment system reform, do well the fundament work such as cost measurement, and ensure that the payment system reform and the elimination of subsidizing hospitals by charging more medicine fees are carried out simultaneously.

3) Reinforce the risk protection mechanism for the new rural cooperative medical system (NCMS) and set up reasonably the management system.

As a basic healthcare system, the new rural cooperative medical system (NCMS) has achieved broad coverage. In the period of the Twelfth Five-year Plan, with the financing level rising constantly, we should take the reinforcement of risk protection of rural residents' health as the special focus of consolidating and perfecting the system. On the basis of universally raising the benefit degree of the rural residents participating in the new rural cooperative medical system (NCMS), we should also make effective institutional arrangements, and establish a stable safeguard mechanism for major serious diseases. This year the government's subsidy for the new rural cooperative medical system (NCMS) will be raised to 240 Yuan. All regions should divide certain proportions from the newly increased funds to establish pooling funds at the provincial level used as the safeguard for major serious diseases, linking up effectively with medical assistance so that the compensation level of major serious diseases can reach 90% or so. By the end of the year, the safeguard for major diseases including children's leukemia will be carried out comprehensively. In 1/3 or so of the regions as a whole, 12 diseases will be brought into the safeguard range, including lung cancer, esophagus cancer, stomach cancer, colon cancer, rectal cancer, chronic granulocytic leukemia (CGL), acute myocardial infarction, cerebral infarction, hemophilia, Type 1 diabetes, hyperthyroidism, and cleft lip and palate. Meanwhile the cost control should be under way through the implementation of standardized treatment. They should also explore how to form a multiple supplementary mechanism with commercial insurance to share the high medical cost for major serious diseases. All local authorities should positively coordinate with the departments of finance and civil affairs to carry out the above tasks. In addition, they should minimize catastrophic medical expenditures of those involved in the insurance in order to prevent illness-related poverty.

Currently, in some regions, explorations are being made into the integration of urban-rural residents' basic medical insurance system. It surely involves the issue of management system of medical insurance. We think that it benefits the principle of simplification, unity and efficiency as well as cost control to plan as a whole the insurance system and the management of service delivery under the system of major health system. But considering the current status quo of management, the form of "unified management, co-located offices" of relevant administrative departments can be carried out after the system integration. The integration of urban-rural basic medical insurance system and the adjustment of management system matter so much that they must be proven scientifically at the level of provincial government, undergo prudent decision-making, and seek the approval of competent authorities of the State Council. From the basic national conditions, most of the regions should keep the existing management system unchanged in accordance with the departmental division of responsibilities determined by the State Council in order to maintain the steady operation of the system.

4) Consolidate and perfect the new operative mechanism of primary-level medical and health institutions.

We should continue to adhere to the fundamental principle of "safeguarding the basic medical and health system, reinforcing the primary-level health care and building the mechanism". We should also continuously consolidate the comprehensive reform results of urban-rural primary-level medical and health institutions. This year, all local authorities should launch a "looking back" for the primary-level comprehensive reform. They should also conduct a comprehensive inspection for the implementation of the policy, measures, tasks and job targets of every link to find out the weak links, and make clear the focus tasks and policies/measures for further perfecting the new operative mechanism of primary-level medical institutions. Moreover, they should earnestly consolidate the implementation results of basic drug system, carry out the input policy, standardize procurement and supply, make strict the key links including zero-profit sales, and promote the realization of normalized sound effective operation of basic drug system in urban-rural primary health care institutions. According to the requirements of relevant documents of the State Council, they should continue to promote the standardized construction of village clinics and carry out every policy for village doctors. Village doctors have always been an important part of our country's primary-level medical teams. In the period of the Twelfth Five-year Plan, they should further study their identities and safeguard benefits, continuously strengthen their cultivation and training, raise their service capacity, and ensure the primary-level base.

5) Comprehensively establish an information closure system and promote a healthy competition among medical institutions.

The most prominent feature of medical and health services is the information asymmetry of supply and requisitioning parties. The most effective measure to solve the problem is to let the people increase their right to be informed and choices through convenient smooth channel and sufficient information, which can promote the healthy competition among medical and health institutions. In recent years, there has appeared rapid development of hospital information technology, which has played a positive role in improving the internal management and service efficiency of hospitals. But the standardized open information system for medical service not yet established not only goes against being subject to public supervision, but also makes it hard to let the general public obtain effective information, based upon which to make judgment and choice for the service qualities of different medical institutions. As a result, the promoting role of normalization in the healthy competition among medical institutions has yet to be given full play to. In the period of the Twelfth Five-year Plan, health administrative departments at all levels should establish release system for information disclosure of medical services, sort the safety, quality and cost of the service of medical institutions within the jurisdictions, so as to notify to the public and be associated with the assessment system of hospitals. We should transform the management concept, understand the importance of the work from a height of maintaining patients' interests, take the reform of supervision pattern as an important measure for deepening the reform, promote medical institutions to improve their services, and form healthy competition.

The diversified patterns of running hospitals are to the advantage of satisfying people's demands at different levels, promote the competition, improve the efficiency, and control the cost. We should carry out every policy of encouraging social funds to run hospitals. In the newly added medical service resources, priority will be given to social funds and paid equal attention to in terms of policy and management. Social capital is encouraged to run non-profit medical institutions.

6) Bring forth new ideas to work style, and carry out comprehensively the equitable basic public health service.

Health administrative departments at all levels should understand the significance of the equitable basic public health service from the perspective of strategy. The equitable basic public health service is a system carrier of carrying out the policy of prevention first as well as a major institutional innovation of deepening medical reform. It is also the most effective institutional arrangement coping with the aging population and the transformation of disease mode. During the period of the Twelfth Five-year Plan, they should bring forth new ideas to organizational leadership, and use the practices of Beijing and Chongqing. In addition, they should integrate the nation's health into every social policy, with the establishment of healthy cities (towns, communities and villages) as a system platform and work focus. As a result, a work mechanism will take shape of governments taking the lead, departmental collaboration and social involvement. They should also bring forth new ideas to work manners, use the practices of Hubei and Shandong for reference, integrate management, service, technique and financial resources, so order that the group-oriented, community-oriented, family-oriented and highly efficient service teams will be formed. Bring forth new ideas to service contents, increase step by step service items of basic public health service and major public health, and expand the scope of people's benefits. Give full play to the role of Traditional Chinese Medicine (TCM) in prevention and health care, and disseminate appropriate technique of the prevention of Traditional Chinese Medicine (TCM). Stress should be put on inflow areas, and pay special attention to and give priority to the issue of the equity of basic public health service which the shifting populations including rural migrant workers are entitled to. Further perfect standardized refined work standards, technical regulations and service process, intensify performance assessment, and link the assessment results to funds investment and individual rewards & punishment. By solid effective work, lay a solid foundation for "Healthy China 2020".

7) Comprehensively promote drug procurement.

Centralized drug procurement is a key link of the chains of production, circulation, price and use, which concerns the people's medical burden. Improving unceasingly the centralized drug bidding and procurement counts for much to the realization of every medical reform target. During the period of the Twelfth Five-year Plan, perfect and push forward the system on the basis of summarizing the past experiences of centralized drug bidding and procurement. Unify the platform of drug procurement, procurement method, and give priority to the quality, the combination of bidding and procurement. Bring consumables and equipment procurement into the scope of centralized bidding and procurement. For some of the patent drugs, high-value consumables and large equipments, make explorations into domestic and foreign manufacturers for centralized procurement. And for imported products, conduct centralized procurement based on international procurement prices.

8) Bring forth new ideas to talent training and the distribution-incentive system.

Over the past three years of medical reform, there has been much searching for the innovation of talent training pattern and encouragement for medical workers. Therefore positive results have been achieved and valuable experiences have been accumulated. But the issue of talent training remains to be a bottleneck of health reform and development. During the period of the Twelfth Five-year Plan, We should continue to make explorations and seek for greater breakthroughs. Further improve the medical education system. Intensify the training of general practitioners and increase the number of general practitioners, so that there will be at least one practitioner in every community health service center and township hospitals. Establish and carry out the system of resident doctors' training. Bring forth new ideas to the utilizing system of primary-level talent training, establish the system of specially contracted doctors, and expand the scale of order training and directed training. Meet the requirement of health reform and development, and devote major efforts to training various talents of nursing, public health, Traditional Chinese Medicine (TCM), pharmaceutics and health management as well as high-level talents of medical teaching and research.

During the period of the Twelfth Five-year Plan, bring forth new ideas to the distribution-incentive system of medical workers. In combination with the reform of public institutions, establish a salary system fitting in with the features of medical and health industries, perfect the income distribution system embodying medical labor value, and improve the overall income level. Expand the implementation scope of post merit pay. Conduct the post management and equal pay for equal work. Raise the percentage of hospital staff's appropriation expenditure in business expenses. Hospital balance of payments should be mainly used for improving the benefits of medical workers.

(4) Carry out the spirit of medial and health profession and provide medical reform with strong spiritual motive.

The Sixth Plenary Session of the 17th CPC Central Committee requires that the construction of socialist core value system should be taken as a fundamental task running through every field of reform and opening-up and socialist modernization. In the Party and the society, form unified guiding thought, common ideals and beliefs, strong spiritual power and fundamental code of ethics, so that they will become the whole people's conscientious pursuit and spiritual motive.

Deepening medical reform is both a very important livelihood project and a worldwide problem. To solve the problem, we need not only the improvement of hardware but also spiritual guide, value support and ethical persistence. Medical reform at a crucial stage particularly needs to carry forward the professional spirit of health care, which embodies the socialist core values. It can be taken as a bright flag of enhancing the morale and unifying wills, and a strong driving force of promoting the scientific development of medical and health service.

There are profound cultural origins in our socialist health service. They inherit the fine traditions of traditional Chinese medicine and western medicine's virtue of great physician and those of respect for life. Also they carry forward the revolutionary humanitarianism of healing the wounded and rescuing the dying as well as the innovative spirit of medicine in the new period. In addition, they unceasingly breed the professionalism of modern health care. Currently we need to centralize the wisdom of the whole industry to solidify the professionalism of health care. In the 1st half of the year, health circles of various regions should carry out a discussion on the health care professionalism embodying the socialist core value, in close combination with studying the spirit of the Sixth Plenary Session of the 17th CPC Central Committee and the cultural construction of health care industry. It is both a process of widely gathering consensus and an educational process of improving ideological and moral consciousness, which is very necessary. During the discussion, be sure to grasp and guide a few problems.

Firstly, fully understand the important role of carrying forward professionalism in achieving the medical goal in close combination with the reality of medical and health care reform. Everybody's access to basic medical and health service is the goal of medical reform. It is the embodiment of common will of the CPC and the nation, the people, and medical workers, and medical workers' responsibility and mission as well. To achieve the goal, we must not only rely on the construction of system and mechanism, but also have strong cultural support and strong spiritual power. We must also rely on a team with belief, pursuit and public trust to fight for it. Through the discussion, medical workers should have a deeper understanding of the close relationship between their own job and carrying out medical reform task and achieving the goal of medical reform from the perspective of the interests of the country and the people. Arouse their senses of social responsibility, and lead them to be more motivated to get involved in and promote medical reform, so that they will realize their value of life at a higher level.

Secondly, fully understand the important role of carrying forward professionalism in arousing medical workers' enthusiasm in close combination with the reality of health team construction. It is a new issue posed for health team construction under the condition of socialist market economy to how to protect, give full play to and arouse the enthusiasm of medical workers. Although some problems have been effectively solved through many years' exploration, yet some other problems have not been fully settled, and there has been even no solution to some problems. For example, how to establish the effective incentive mechanism meeting the requirements of the new situation, how to establish the wages and welfare system embodying the features of medical labor, so that medical workers can have decent income and dignified source of income, how to resist the erosion of money worship and hedonism to the team. Those questions or problems are all needed to be answered or solved in the real world. In the discussion on professionalism, we should carry out the distribution system reform with post responsibility and performance assessment as the core, and intensify financial incentive to improve the income level, in accordance with the requirements of medical reform documents. In addition, we should always remain sober-minded, and stick to both money-material incentive and professionalism incentive. Currently what needs to be specially emphasized is that money incentive is not unique, not even omnipotent. The social value of healing the wounded and rescuing the dead and professional dignity of poverty alleviation cannot be measured by money. It eventually depends on great moral and spiritual power to arouse and mobilize medical workers' enthusiasm. We must adhere to carrying forward noble professionalism accompanied by reasonable material incentive, really arouse the enthusiasm of medical workers, and throw themselves into medical reform with more upward spirits.

Thirdly, fully understand the important role of carrying forward professionalism in establishing a harmonious doctor-patient relationship in close combination with the need to improve the practicing environment. With the boost of medical reform, there has been a positive trend for the medical practicing environment and doctor-patient relationship. However, some recent serious doctor-patient disputes remind us that improving the doctor-patient relationship continues to be an important task facing us, and needs the concerted efforts of both doctors and patients and different sectors of the society. Medical workers in particular should take the initiative to play their role. They should also carry forward professionalism, improve morality, technical level and ability to communicate. Moreover, they should strive for patients' understanding, coordination and support, and give patients more care and comfort with superb technique and excellent service. Meanwhile, news media and health dissemination & health education agencies should not only disseminate the painstaking efforts of medical workers in healing the sick, but also publicize the characteristic feature, law and limitation of medicine. Therefore the people will be aware of the natural law of development that the current medical technique can neither guarantee to cure all diseases nor change life cycle. In addition, they should reasonably guide the people in seeking medical advice expectedly and rationally and improve the mutual understanding of doctors and patients. Currently, health administrative departments and health care institutions should establish and perfect specialized agencies for receiving and dealing with patients' complaints, based on the new features of doctor-patient relationship. They should also give full play to the role of organizations in maintaining the doctor-patient harmony, and create conditions to universally establish a new mechanism of dealing doctor-patient relationship, including the third-party mediation and hospital liability insurance. Through the concerted efforts of parties concerned, the doctor-patient relationship is expected to change for the better during the period of the Twelfth Five-year Plan.

III. Prepare Well for 2012 Health Work

In 2012 firmly grasp the central work, and drive the implementation of every task of health work.

(1) Carry out the annual reform task to have a good start for medical reform in the period of the Twelfth Five-year Plan.

Continue to improve the security level of the new rural cooperative medical system (NCMS). Consolidate the coverage rate, and raise the fund-raising standard to

300 yuan or so per capita. The reimbursement proportion of hospitalization expenses within the policy range will reach 75% or so, and the maximum payment limit will not be lower than eight times of annual per capita income of rural residents and not less than 60,000 yuan. Conduct universally outpatient service as a whole. Establish insurance funds for major diseases and expand the range of diseases. Push forward the reform of payment mode. Make explorations concerning improving the overall level of the new rural cooperative medical system (NCMS), and the commercial insurance agencies' being involved in the service. Perfect the management operation mechanism of the new rural cooperative medical system (NCMS), improve the service, and guarantee the fund safety.

Consolidate and perfect the primary-level comprehensive reform. Organize the "looking back" of the comprehensive reform of primary-level medical and health institutions. Perfect the multi-channel compensation mechanism, put into effect the governmental investment, carry out the ordinary medical fee system, and give play to the compensation role of medical security system. Push forward the reform of personnel distribution system, and put into effect the system of merit pay. Carry out *The Outline of Rural Basic Medical and Health Development (2011-2020).* Push forward the development of community health care service of small-medium cities, and popularize the team service mode of general practitioners.

Continue to perfect the national system for basic drugs. Further expand the range of system implementation. Map out the basic drug catalogue of 2012 edition, and standardize the non-catalogue drugs of local supplement. Standardize the procurement of basic drugs, perfect the comprehensive evaluation index system of pharmaceutical manufacturers and drug quality, and do well the delivery work in rural and remote areas. Try out the state regulated price and designated production for exclusive varieties, varieties in shortage and children's drug dosage form. Formulate the administrative measures for the use of basic drugs, and standardize step by step their dosage form, specifications and packaging. Put forward the policy of encouraging the priority use of basic drugs. Perfect unceasingly the monitoring and evaluation system of basic drugs.

Positively push forward the reform of public hospitals. Strengthen the summary evaluation of the reform pilot cities strive to form experiences spread across the country. Determine about 300 counties (cities) for promoting the comprehensive form of county hospitals. Reinforce the capacity construction of county hospitals, and continue to put into effect the counterpart assistance project. Strengthen the management of establishment and planning of medical institutions. Speed up the construction of job-division and cooperation mechanism between public hospitals and primary-level institutions. Perfect the personnel distribution system of public hospitals, and continue to push forward the doctors' multi-sited license. Continue to carry out the measures benefiting the people, including high quality nursing, appointment diagnosis and treatment and clinics for the convenience of the people. Promote the management of clinical pathways, conduct strict management of cost accounting, and control any unreasonable rise of medical expenses. Perform hospital review and assessment.

Push forward gradually the equal access to basic public health services. Prepare well for the state basic and major public health service projects. Perfect the management system of basic public health service project, and intensify the central government assessment for local authorities. Perfect the job-division and collaboration mechanism of primary-level health institutions and professional public health institutions, and improve the quality of basic public health services. Comprehensively evaluate the implementation of major public health service projects, promote the newly added items including the assistance service for health supervision, and study the formulation of project implementation plans in the new cycle.

In accordance with the unified deployment of the State Council, do well the other health work.

(2) Do well the work of major disease control, health emergency and maternal and child health.

Push forward the standard construction and scientific management of disease control agencies, intensify talent training and talent team construction, and improve the capacity of prevention and control. Give play to the role of disease control agencies in business management and technical guidance, and carry out the basic public health service project. Perfect the monitoring system and direct network report system of infectious diseases. In accordance with relevant prevention and control plans and program of AIDS and tuberculosis, Prepare well for the AIDS prevention and control in the key areas and focus groups, and intensify the management of standardized treatment and prevention & control results of tuberculosis. Prepare well for the prevention and control of key infectious diseases, including cholera, hepatitis B and hand-foot-mouth disease. Carry out the target tasks set by the national action plan for the elimination of measles. Prepare well for the routine immunization and supplementary immunization of poliovirus vaccine, and block the transmission of imported wild poliovirus to restore our country's polio-free state. Steadily improve the national immunization program, and perfect the compensation mechanism of adverse events following immunization. In March of this year, a campaign of supplemental immunization focusing on measles and polio will be launched nationwide. Start comprehensively the campaign for eliminating the hazard of leprosy. Push forward the implementation of control program for key parasitic disease and endemic disease, including schistosomiasis, malaria and echinococcosis. Perfect the prevention and control system and work mechanism of chronic disease, popularize the experiences of demonstration area construction for comprehensive prevention and control of chronic disease, and push forward the action for the healthy lifestyle of the whole nation. Strengthen the early detection, standard management and effective intervention for chronic disease and high-risk population, and conduct early diagnosis and early treatment for cancer and stroke screening among high-risk population in key areas. Strengthen the surveillance, medical care and service management of serious mental disease. Strengthen the system construction of the prevention and treatment of oral diseases, and intensify the prevention and control of children's oral diseases. Continue to conduct the creation and environment renovation of national health towns. Push forward the building of rural innocuous sanitary toilets, and strengthen the hygienic evaluation of rural drinking water safety and the surveillance of environmental health hazard factors.

Strengthen in an all-round manner health emergency. Perfect the standards and collaboration mechanism of health emergency. Carry out the construction of the comprehensive demonstration areas for health emergency, and strengthen the drills for the training of health emergency team. Make overall arrangements for on-site emergency management, and push forward deeply the construction of 27 national health emergency teams. Perfect the command platforms at the provincial level and municipal level, and start the construction of decision-making platform at the county level and on-site mobile command. Prepare well for emergency material reserve, and establish the information integration and fund guarantee mechanism of stockpile resources. Push forward the capacity building of emergency medical rescue. Conduct the risk evaluation for public health emergencies, and improve the risk recognition capability and the risk monitoring capability. Prepare well for the response to health emergencies and health emergency security for major events. Competent leaders of health administrative departments at all levels should be concerned about the epidemic situation and public opinion reports everyday, and fulfill the obligations of public health emergencies. They should also fulfill their duties of dealing with public health emergencies.

Strengthen the work of community health, maternity & child care and health education. Continue to carry out the activity of creating demonstration community health service center. Carry out and put into effect, the "Two Outlines", and promote and protect the health of women and children with the focus on the promotion of the system management rate for children under 6 and the promotion of the system management rate for pregnant women. Continue to prepare well for the major public health projects aimed at women and children. Prepare well for premarital health care, prenatal screening and diagnosis and neonatal screening to improve the comprehensive capacity of prevention and control of birth defects. Strengthen the system construction of maternal and child health, intensify the standard management of maternal and child health care institutions, and conduct the performance assessment for county-level maternal and child health care institutions. Strengthen comprehensively health promotion and health education. Strengthen the tobacco control publicity, consolidate the results of smoke-free medical and health institutions establishment, and carry out comprehensively the smoke-free policy in public places.

(3) Conduct strict management to ensure medical safety and quality.

Prepare well for the planning of medical institutions, focus on strengthening the constructions of prehospital emergency system and pediatrics, and continue to carry out the construction of key clinical specialty development. Strengthen critical care medicine and pathology of county-level hospitals and the construction of weak departments closely related to the supply of basic medical services. Develop rehabilitation therapy and long-term nursing care. Standardize the institutional setup, approval and calibration management. Relax the requirements of running clinics according to law for qualified persons, and encourage social capital to run sizeable medical institutions. In all medical and health institutions, launch a campaign of "fine service, fine quality, fine medical ethics and people's satisfaction" and "quality promotion", and strengthen the connotation construction of nursing with "the demonstration project of high-quality nursing service" as the platform. Strengthen the management of medical quality and control, give guidance to the establishment of the centers for medical quality control at the levels of the state, province and city, and continue to carry out the project of the standardized diagnosis and treatment of major diseases, and clinical pathway management. Continue to carry out special rectification for anti-bacterial agents. Prepare well for the admittance management of clinical application for medical techniques, and promote the mutual recognition of test results. Carry out the management system of specialist physicians, and conduct the admittance management of specialist physicians. Continue to strengthen the pharmacy administration of medical institutions, conduct reasonable medication monitoring, and establish an access system of clinical pharmacists. Start the revision of *Blood Donation Law*, establish a long-term mechanism of unpaid blood donation, promote steadily nucleic acid testing, ensure blood safety, and promote clinically reasonable use of blood. Continue to prepare well for blindness prevention and treatment as well as the medical treatment of drug rehabilitation management.

Continue to take the unreasonable increase of drug expenses as the focus of medical service regulation. All local authorities should set targets of expenses control from a practical standpoint. They should also take comprehensive measures and means, including the promotion of clinical pathway, restriction of medical behaviors, standardization of medical instrument procurement, strict regulation of expenses, open information of expenses and payment system reform. Try to bring medical expenses under reasonable level. The medical administrations and medical institutions should take the initiative to cooperate with the administrations of health insurance, and work together for expenses control.

(4) Accelerate the construction of health talent team to improve the science and education of health.

With the health talent projects as the focus, including the primary-level health talent, outstanding health talent, professionals in short supply, talent of traditional Chinese medicine and standardized training of doctors, carry out and put into effect *A Medium- and Long-Term Talent Development Plan for Medicine and Health (2011-2020) and An Implementation Plan for Health Talent Guarantee Project of National Health*. Make arrangements for standardized training of no few than 10,000 5+3 general practitioners, and no fewer than 5,000 resident doctors. Continue to carry out the project of ordered and directed training for medical students in Midwest area. Improve continuing medical education. Promote the implementation of *Educational Planning for National Village Doctors (2011-2020)*, continue to conduct the in-service training of rural health staff, and strengthen the training of primary-level pharmacy staff. Start the ad hoc job project for general practitioners of primary-level health institutions. Implement and improve the merit pay system for public health and primary-level health institutions.

Give full play to the supporting role of health science and technology in the reform and development of health services. Organize the implementation of *A Development Plan of Medical Science and Technology in the Period of the Twelfth Five-year Plan*. Strengthen applied research, and researches of translational medicine and preclinical medicine. Intensify the promotion of research and development of appropriate health technique, and promote the new-type innovation system construction of national medical technology. Start the construction of scientific research base for key laboratories, and intensify the bio-safety management of laboratories. Establish and improve the management system of clinical research for new medical technology.

(5) Speed up the promotion of health informatization with platform construction as the focus.

Strengthen the overall planning and management of health informatization, and speed up the platform construction. Complete and check the construction projects of 13 comprehensive pilot provinces of the 1st and 2nd batches, and start the 3rd batch. Form gradually the basic framework of health informatization throughout the country, province, city, county, township and village, and covering the main business areas, strive to achieve inter-agency and cross-regional interconnection and interworking and information sharing, and strive to make a breakthrough in pilot areas. Accelerate the promotion of the construction of residents' electronic health records and electronic medical records, and promote the mutual recognition of test results, remote consultation and real-time regulation of diagnosis and treatment among medical agencies. Step up the promotion and application of residents' health cards, achieve the recognition, individual basic health information records, inter-agency and inter-area data exchanges and expense settlement in health service activities, and bring convenience to residents' seeking medical advice and conducting health management.

(6) Strengthen food and drug safety.

Improve the regulatory system of drugs. Strengthen the construction of drug testing system, the quality regulatory system of production and operation, and testing system of adverse reaction. Improve drug standard and technical specification. Promote comprehensively the system construction of quality regulation of basic drugs. Strengthen information sharing and linkage mechanism construction of regulation. Establish and improve the traceability system of drug quality, promote the electronic regulatory system of drugs, intensify the spot check of supervision, and expand the coverage of spot check. Give guidance to enterprises to improve the capability of drug research and development, strengthen the relevant technical reserves related to inspection evaluation of new drugs and preventive bio-products. Launch the crackdown on the special operation on posting fake ads via the internet, and selling fake drugs by post. Strengthen the regulation of cosmetics safety.

Intensify food safety. Improve the regulatory system of catering foods and health foods. Work out plans for national standards of food safety, improve the standard system, focus on the formulation and revision of the production and operation standards of basic standards for food additives and food-relate products, and the standards of food testing methods. Strengthen the follow-up assessments of standard implementation. All local authorities should prepare well for local standard construction and enterprise standard filing. Work out and organize the implementation of the monitoring plan of national food safety risks. Conduct the risk evaluation and communication of food safety. Strengthen the system of food safety risk surveillance and evaluation, speed up the construction of national center for food safety risk evaluation, and promote the construction of local agencies of food safety risk evaluation. Standardize epidemiology survey and on-the-spot hygienic processing of food safety accidents. Continue to cooperate with the crackdown on the special campaign of illegal food additives, and publicize any "blacklist" of non-food material possibly added.

(7) Intensify health supervision/law-enforcement.

Strengthen the construction of primary-level health supervision agencies and talent teams. Intensify the law-enforcement, and investigate lawfully any illegal behavior harming people's health and life safety. Positively publicize and carry out *Law on Prevention and Control of Occupational Disease*, prepare well for the survey of occupational health status, and promote the capacity building of occupational disease prevention and control. Strengthen the radioactive pollution monitoring of food and drinking water around nuclear power plants, and expand the pilot areas of surveillance of radiation protection. Improve the health monitoring network, and strengthen the health surveillance and supervision and check of public places, drinking water and disinfection products. Deepen the reform of health administrative license for health-related products. Strengthen school health supervision and surveillance, and guarantee students' health. Strengthen the supervision for infectious diseases and medical supervision and law-enforcement, and continue to work together with police departments to keep cracking down on illegal medical practice and illegal blood collection and donation. Strengthen law-enforcement inspection and carry out the responsibility of law-enforcement.

(8) Do well the work of traditional Chinese medicine (TCM).

Implement and carry out the policies and measures supporting and promoting the development of traditional Chinese medicine (TCM), and promote the completion of all medical reform tasks. Improve the service system of public traditional Chinese medicine hospitals, step up the promotion of renovation and construction of county hospitals of traditional Chinese medicine (TCM), and intensify the service function of traditional Chinese medicine (TCM) of primary-level medical institutions. Promote the health project of preventive treatment of disease. Launch the pilot project of traditional Chinese medicine (TCM) service of basic public health service. Promote the comprehensive reform of county hospitals. Strengthen the emergency rescue of medical institutions of traditional Chinese medicine (TCM) and the capacity building of prevention and cure of major diseases. Do well the work of heritage research of traditional Chinese medicine, innovation of scientific system and ethnic medicine. Strengthen the training of traditional Chinese medicine (TCM) talents and technical backbones, carry out the inheritance project of clinical research of senior TCM doctors, and strengthen the inheritance workroom construction of national renowned senior TCM experts. Explore the establishment of standardized training system of TCM resident doctors, and strengthen the constructions of TCM key disciplines and TCM standardization and informatization. Conduct TCM external exchanges, publicize TCM culture with the help of the platform of Confucius institutes abroad, and enhance international influence of our country's traditional culture.

(9) Launch the activity of excelling in competitions in a deep-going way.

Continue to launch the activity of excelling in competitions in a deep-going way around the central work. Give full play to the main force role of CPC members and medical workers in the promotion of scientific development of health services and deepening of medical system reform. With the activity of "fine service, fine quality, fine medical ethics and people's satisfaction" as the important carrier and grasp of "excelling in competitions for the people", enhance the subject of serving the people. Do practical things for the convenience of people, and promote the comprehensive improvement of service style and quality. According to the deployment of the CPC Central Committee, select in due time exemplary primary-level Party organizations and outstanding Party members emerging in the activity of excelling in competitions. Strengthen comprehensively political and ideological education of health industry, cultural construction of industry, launch an activity of spiritual civilization establishment, and provide a strong driving force and guarantee for the achievement of development targets of health services in the period of the Twelfth Five-year plan.

(10) Make overall arrangements for other health work.

Strengthen the construction of health legal system and health policy research, promote the legislation of basic health care and mental health, and the formulation of the standards of health law and regulations, and strengthen legal popularization and administrative review. Centering on the issue of major theories and practice, conduct health policy research. Pay high attention to health statistical information, strengthen the constructions of institutions and teams, improve the work means and conditions, and give play to the role of policy-making, work guidance, medical reform and management improvement. Health statistical information should meet the requirements of new situation, so that there can be informational integrity, accurate data, timely reporting and reliable of analysis.

Continue to strengthen the system construction of punishing and prevent the corruption in health circles, and deepen the precaution of integrity risks. Further implement the responsibility system of checking unhealthy tendencies and malpractices in health, and the system of medical ethics appraisal. Stick to "zero tolerance" for corruption, intensify the governance of commercial bribery in medicine purchases and sales, and seriously investigate and handle any violations of laws and the rules of discipline. Improve centralized drug procurement, and promote positively the procurement of large-sized medical equipments and high-value consumables.

Do well the work of planning and finance. Organize the implementation of health plan in the period of the Twelfth Five-year Plan, and intensify fund supervision and specific inspection. Reinforce the management of departmental budget and internal audit, and continue to prepare well for specific governance of the prevention and control of "private coffer" and protruding problems in the area of engineering construction. Push forward the formulation and management of construction and equipment standards. Prepare well for health assistance to Tibet, Xinjiang and Qinghai, and reconstruction of disaster areas. Carry out earnestly the essence of the Central work meeting on poverty alleviation and mobilize all forces to put poverty alleviation into effect.

Intensify health publicity through the press, improve the ability of guidance for public opinions, focus on the publicity of medical reform, strengthen typical publicity and risk communication, and establish a favorable environment for public opinions. Make greater efforts to keep the public informed of the government affairs, and establish the government in sunshine, legal system government and service-oriented government. Strengthen and improve the work of complaints about health, promote the innovation of work mechanism, and resolve long-pending cases. Implement the system of leaders' reception of people's visits, push forward the risk evaluation system for major events, and prevent and eliminate labile factors. Make overall arrangements for safety management, maintain the safety and stability in health field, and take effective precautions against work safety accidents and vicious events.

Take care of the lives and fitness of retired veteran cadres and workers, send to them warmth, consideration and loving care, and warmly support them in offering advice and suggestions for health development and deepening medical reform. Do well the work of health care for cadres.

Positively develop international exchanges and collaborations, give play to health advantages, and serve the national diplomacy. Deepen international co-operations and exchanges of health in various areas, and publicize the ideas and results of medical reform via international conferences, and bilateral multilateral co-operation platform, to strive for international technical financial aid. Conduct multilateral diplomacy in health, and create a new situation for foreign health aid. Promote pragmatic exchanges and co-operations in health on both sides of the Taiwan Straits, between the mainland and Hong Kong, and between the mainland and Macau.

Comrades, under the strong leadership of the CPC Central Committee with Hu Jintao as the General Secretary, let us mobilize and rely on all medical workers to make persistent efforts, be united, strive to complete all health tasks for 2012, and greet the successful opening of the 18th National Congress of the CPC Central Committee with excellent achievements.

(Shan Yongxiang)

2. Lift Our Spirits and Have the Courage to Bring Forth New Ideas for Creating a New Situation of Food Safety and Health Supervision
—An Address by Health Minister Chen Zhu to the 2012 Meeting of National Health Circle on Food Safety and Health Supervision (January 13, 2012)

Just now, Comrade Xiaohong's report reviewed 2011 food safety and health supervision, and made arrangements for 2012 priorities, with which I agree. All local authorities should make arrangements for all the work this year as required by Comrade Xiaohong's address.

Now I would like to express my opinions in three aspects.

I. Fully Affirm the Achievements Made in Food Safety and Health Supervision

In 2011, in the face of a very complicated tough situation, hard-won achievements were made in economic/social development and the reform of medical and health care system of our country under the leadership of the CPC Central Committee and the State Council. Over the past year, according to the overall arrangements of guaranteeing basic medical care, strengthening primary care, and establishing medical mechanism by the central government, under the leadership of Party committees and governments at all levels, centering on ensuring and improving the people's livelihood, all local authorities earnestly implemented tasks of medical reform, performed their regulatory duties, and did their jobs solidly. In investigating and punishing the law cases, responding to emergencies, perfecting the monitoring network, and the ability to strengthen primary care, they made remarkable achievements, which played an important role in maintaining the people's health benefits and promoting the economic development, and gained the recognitions of governments at all levels and people.

Firstly, some major law cases were investigated and punished, which greatly safeguarded the people's health benefits. In 2011, centering on the prominent issues that were the biggest concern of and most reflected by the people, including food safety, occupational hazard, drinking water safety and illegal practice of medicine, all local authorities intensified the supervision and law-enforcement, and worked with related departments to crack down on illegal and criminal acts, thus having punished some law-breaking offenders. They also launched a special campaign against illegally added non-food substances, and keep a high profile in the crackdown on law-breaking in food. In addition, they investigated and punished such cases as the problem milk powder, clenbuterol and swill-cooked dirty oil, which eliminated hidden hazards of food safety. Jointly conducting special rectification for occupational hazards and occupational health survey, the local authorities properly handled some occupational hazards, including those in Gulang of Gansu, Chaoyang of Liaoning and Xiushui of Jiangxi, which practically protect the physical fitness of workers. A special campaign of supervision and inspection was launched fully for drinking water, public places, centralized disinfection of tableware, school hygiene, crackdown on unlicensed medical practice and health-related products, which effectively maintained the health, safety and vital interests of the people, and set up a good social image for health supervision.

Secondly, emergencies were actively dealt with to effectively maintain social stability. After the nuclear accident in Fukushima Nuclear Plant in Japan, 22 provinces (regions, cities) nationwide took emergency actions to assemble elites for conducting emergency monitoring of radioactive pollution over the possibly polluted key food and drinking water. They gave accurate reports concerning the monitoring information, and released monitoring results scientifically. With regards to plasticizer pollution in Taiwan, according to the unified deployment of the State Council, the Ministry of Health, Food Safety Office and relevant departments actively and steadily did their jobs of disposal. They adopt such measures as emergency risk monitoring and evaluation, import and export control, screening for production and operation processes, and unified information release, thus minimizing the harm and influence as well as maintaining the normal market order and social stability in our country.

Thirdly, the monitoring network was improved to raise steadily the scientific level of scientific regulation. The monitoring capacity of disease prevention and control agencies at all levels for food and drinking water was improved, and the risk monitoring was enhanced. Currently a risk monitoring system of food safety and drinking water covering the country has been established, with increased monitoring spots, increasingly diverse types and ample indexes. With millions of data obtained in 2011, the hidden hazards of food and drinking water safety were notified to all the relevant departments. Therefore control measures were adopted to effectively enhance the pertinence and timeliness of supervision and law-enforcement. National Center for Risk Evaluation of Food Safety was established, which is in charge of technical support including food safety risk evaluation, monitoring, early warning and communication, thus improving the risk evaluation capacity of food safety. The monitoring of disease prevention and control agencies and radiation monitoring agencies of 32 provinces (regions, cities) was completed for illegal additives in food and radioactive substances, and so were the active monitoring and traceability construction of food-borne disease. Pilot projects for basic occupational health services were launched for rural migrant workers' occupational health care and monitoring of key occupational diseases. The coverage rates of prevention/control and diagnosis agencies and physical examination agencies for occupational disease were constantly expanded. The prevention and control capacity of occupational disease was further strengthened.

Fourthly, the capacity building was reinforced to lay a solid foundation for health supervision. In 2011, the financial fund support for primary health supervision was enhanced by both the central government and local governments, which promoted the infrastructure construction of primary health supervision agencies, and consolidated the basis of urban-rural health supervision system. With the construction of county health supervision agencies nationwide fully started up, the law-enforcement equipments of county health supervision agencies in the central and western regions have been put into use, thus greatly improving the rapid detecting ability to conduct on-site supervision. With the start-up of coordinating service of health supervision, food safety, occupational disease prevention and control, drinking water safety, school hygiene, crackdown on illegal practice of medicine and illegal collection and supply of blood were brought into national basic public health service projects as public health products provided by the government free of charge. The sentinel role of three-level public health network and primary health care institutions was given full play to. It was a fundamental task of deepening medical reform to solve the weaknesses of primary health supervision, especially rural health supervision. The training program for health supervision talents was carried out to strengthen health supervision talent training for food safety and occupational disease prevention and control, which provided powerful guarantee for supervision work.

With the joined efforts of health administrative departments, health supervision agencies and disease prevention and control agencies at all levels, no major accidents ever occurred nationwide in 2011, including food safety, occupational hazards and drinking water contamination. With food safety and health supervision promoted greatly, steadily and in good order, new achievements were made in every task, which maintained the people's health benefits, and promoted social harmony and stability. Hereby, on behalf of the Ministry of Health, I would like to give our cordial greetings to and show high respect for all the supervisors of health supervision and those engaged in food safety and relevant public health. Also, our heartfelt thanks go to the leaders and comrades from various departments, who have long cared for and supported the development of health supervision services.

II. Enhance the Sense of Responsibility and the Sense of Urgency in Food Safety and Health Supervision

Food safety and health supervision concern both the people's health and family well-being of thousands of households. They are also the main contents of basic public health services and major issue of livelihood. Having thought highly of them, the CPC Central Committee and the State Council adopted a series of policy measures, issued *Food Safety Law*, and revised *Law on Prevention and Control of Occupational Disease*, which improved the regulation system and work mechanism. The Fifth and Sixth Plenary Sessions of the 17th CPC Central Committee laid special emphasis on food safety, and brought it into the important contents of strengthening and bringing forth new ideas of social management. General Secretary Hu Jintao, Premier Wen Jiabao, Vice-Premier Li Keqiang and the other leading comrades of the CPC Central Committee have made important instructions repeatedly for food safety, occupational disease prevention and control, and drinking water safety. Attaching great importance to food safety and health supervision, the Ministry of Health strengthens further food safety, occupational disease prevention and control, drinking water safety and crackdown on illegal practice of medicine, based on the decisions and arrangements of the CPC Central Committee and the State Council. The Ministry also held more than once the meetings of leading Party group and ministerial meetings to analyze and study the situations of food safety and health supervision. With arrangements made, the Ministry brought food safety and health supervision into the key items of medical reform for the people as the benefit-for-all system of the equalization of public health services.

Although great progress has been made in 2011 food safety and health supervision, which should be given enough affirmation, yet we should see that there remains a certain gap between our work and the requirements of the CPC Central Committee and the State Council as well as the people's expectations. Just now, Comrade Xiaohong pointed out the existing problems and shortcomings, to which I will add a little. In the first place, our country is still in the primary stage of socialism in the macro environment. The basic conditions for food safety, occupational disease prevention and control and drinking water safety are weak. There is poor management of some production and operation enterprises. There exist objectively hidden trouble and risks for major public health security events. In particular, some lawbreakers have loss of credibility and forsake good for the sake of gold, thus leading to food safety accidents and other criminal offenses, which poses great harm to the society and is hated extremely by the people. In addition, the tendency of overall environmental status to get worse remains uncontained. So the issues of food safety and drinking water safety caused by environmental factors in some places appear from time to time, which has been a matter of great concern in the community. The tasks of health supervision and public health are arduous, and with heavy responsibility. In the second place, there have long been instability and outstanding accounts in health services. And it is an objective reality that the system construction of food safety and health supervision lags behind. There is a great insufficiency in the staffing and law-enforcement input of health supervision, and there is not a high coverage rate for supervision and law-enforcement. The relevant capacity of technical support of public health remains poor, and food safety risk monitoring and evaluation as systemic task has just started out. Therefore there are no capacities of conducting comprehensive detection by the sanitary standard of drinking water in some places. There is also a scarcity of resources for occupational disease diagnosis and occupational health examination in cities and counties, which is an important factor restricting the level and work results of food safety and health supervision. In the third place, from the perspective of our own work, there exist problems of lack of understanding and limited attention to varying degrees. In recent years, there have been frequent responsibility adjustments in the area of health supervision. As a result, some local authorities have failed to meet the requirements of fulfillment of new responsibilities. In addition, there has been lack of sensitivity, and the work has not been strengthened, which will possibly bring hidden trouble to our duty fulfillment. For example, it has been two and a half years since Food Safety Law was put into implementation. But we have learned that the functions of the primary health administrative departments in some regions have not been completely transformed, and the new statutory duties have not been fulfilled. Currently the CPC Central Commission for Discipline Inspection and the Ministry of Supervision are taking the lead in formulating The Provisions of the State Council on Accountability for Food Safety. The accountability system for food safety will be further perfected and strengthened. So please be sure to attach great importance to that.

The situation and challenge facing us are serious, so we must be sure to have a clear understanding of that. Face up to the difficulties, strengthen the consciousness of potential dangers, earnestly seek gaps and shortcomings, and earnestly perform the duties. What's more, see the greater responsibilities that we are shouldering, enhance the sense of mission, and further keep up our spirits. Promote constantly health supervision and related public health work, and strive for improving the capacity and level for serving the people, with the attitude of being highly responsible for the people.

III. In Implementing the Tasks for Medical Reform, Promote Food Safety and Health Supervision to a New Height

The purpose of medical reform is to ensure the people's access to public health and basic medical services and sharing in the fruits of reform and development. Now and for a fairly long time to come, it is and will be the central task to deepen medical reform. Food safety and health supervision are the main content of medical reform concerning the people's health benefits. All local authorities should regard food safety and health supervision as an important task of deepening medical reform and improving the people's livelihood. They should also strengthen the organizational leadership, stick to scientific management, pay special attention to talent team building with the focus on capacity building, and strive for creating a new situation for food safety and health supervision. Hereon, I will make a few demands:

(1) In strengthening the leadership, further reinforce health supervision.

Facing the current arduous task and the responsibilities we shoulder, we must further raise our awareness, and strengthen the organizational leadership over food safety and health supervision. In 2011, after the study of the Ministry's leading Party group, the Ministry of Health decided to establish respectively the Ministry's leading group for food safety and the leading group for the prevention and control of occupational disease. The purpose is to study in time important events, perfect the coordinating mechanism within the Ministry, and further strengthen the leadership over food safety and the prevention and control of occupational disease. Based on the decision of State Commission Office of Public Sectors Reform in the second half of last year, the responsibilities assumed by the Ministry of Health of comprehensive coordination for food safety, taking the lead in organizing investigations for major accidents of food safety, and unified release of major information about food safety, have been included into the Food Safety Office of the State Council, and will be transferred in the near future. We think that it is an important measure for strengthening the regulation of food safety under the new situation. Also it is a major decision of the CPC Central Committee and the State Council for further attaching importance to food safety and paying attention to the people's livelihood improvement. After the adjustment of responsibilities, we will further strengthen the following job functions: standard setting and tracking assessment of food safety, risk monitoring and early warning, epidemiological survey and hygienic disposal for food safety accidents, and inspection specification for food safety. All local health administrative departments should do well and in detail the related work of food safety, find out weak links, eliminate hidden dangers, and mustn't get carried away with the work, under the unified leadership of local governments and according the division of responsibilities. At the end of 2011, the Standing Committee of the National People's Congress approved the amendment to the *Law on Prevention and Control of Occupational Disease*, which defined the responsibilities of health department and related departments. Proceeding from the whole situation, local health administrative departments at all levels should actively perform statutory duties, continue to strengthen the regulation, reinforce the protection of occupational health of workers, and strive to form the work force of the prevention and control of occupational disease, jointly with relevant departments. Health administrative departments at all levels should further strengthen the leadership, and give full play to the roles of agencies for the prevention and control of occupational disease, agencies for disease prevention and control, and comprehensive medical agencies. In addition, they should do well in the monitoring, diagnosis, appraisal and treatment of occupational disease, and occupational health examination. Health supervision agencies at all levels should focus on strengthening the supervision and inspection for occupational disease diagnosis, occupational health examination, and safety of radiological diagnosis and radiotherapy. Meanwhile, we should better the thoughts of those at the grass-roots level as required by the functional adjustment. Seriously study the amendment to the Law on Prevention and Control of Occupational Disease, and make in-depth study of and solve the problems and difficulties at work. Sort out responsibilities, define the tasks, and raise the sense of responsibility. Pinpoint the work focus to reinforce the supervision and law-enforcement in combination with the prominent issues reflected by people. Set up and perfect the performance assessment system, and bring the fulfillment of job responsibilities for food safety and health supervision into the performance assessment index to arouse the enthusiasm of the whole cadres and workers. Be sure to have a keen ear for the voice of people, strengthen the publicity in public, solve problems and doubts in time, and do a good job in public opinion guidance. Food safety and health supervision are of a strong policy-oriented nature, and are also the important content of strengthening and bringing forth new ideas in social management by the government. Therefore I hope that you will keep learning to deepen the understanding of the conditions of the country, society and people. Strive for improving the ability to handle various complex situations and emergencies, and enhance the level of serving the people.

(2) Conduct actively the coordination for health supervision, and promote greatly the implementation of basic public health projects.

For a considerable period of time in the future, we will face such challenges as rapidly ageing population, disease pattern conversion and ecological environment deterioration. Those increased health risk factors have caused rapid climbing of contagious disease and chronic non-infectious disease, which poses a direct threat to the people's health. To resolve the issue of people's medical treatment, we must adhere to the policy of prevention first. By achieving step by step the equalization of basic public health services, we will achieve the strategic goal of people's being disease-free, getting sick less often and getting sick late, which is also a very important system arrangement of medical reform. Playing an important role in the deepening of medical reform, health supervision is the important means of disease prevention and control as well as an important part of the system of basic public health services. Doing well the work of health supervision not only helps achieving better results of every public health measure, but also improves the equity of basic public health services, and let the people have access to the results of reform and development. Currently we have taken the coordination of health supervision as the newly added service item of the equalization of basic public health services, which is an important measure of extending effectively the health supervision system to the grassroots level. It should be seen that, as this work is just at the initial stage, all local authorities should make active explorations and have the courage to bring forth new ideas. They should also further establish and perfect the work mechanism of health supervision coordination, strengthen the guidance over primary health care agencies, and strive for improving their capacities for work. In addition, they should promote the transformation of service pattern, fulfill the task of health supervision coordination, urge the implementation of public health measures, and maintain effectively the health benefits of the people.

(3) Pay special attention to the construction of health supervision system to improve the capacity for regulation.

The period of the Twelfth Five-Year Plan is a crucial stage for the constructions of health supervision system and capacity. We should take full advantage of the opportunity of deepening medical reform, positively enlist the governmental increased input jointly with related departments, and strengthen the capacity building. In the period of the Twelfth Five-Year Plan, the Ministry of Health will work with related departments to continue to enlist support in increasing the input for the constructions of health supervision system and capacity. Based on the construction of the national center for food safety risk evaluation, promote simultaneously the construction of local technical support agencies for food safety risk monitoring and evaluation. The national system for food safety risk monitoring and evaluation will take shape with the national center as the leader and local agencies as the support. The purpose is to give full play to the scientific support role of risk evaluation in the formulation of food safety standards and regulation improvement. All local authorities should earnestly carry out the key programs of health supervision and related plans from the central finance as transfer payment to ensure fund security and substantial fruits of the projects. Standardize further the construction of health supervision agency, in order that the three-level health supervision agencies of provinces, cities and counties as well as the resident agencies will meet the standards of construction in the period of the Twelfth Five-Year Plan. As required by 2011-2020 health talent development plans and the training planning for health supervisors, strengthen the manning and talent training for law-enforcement. Try to meet the target that by 2015 there will be 0.9 supervisors per million people on average as a whole, and by 2020, 1 supervisor and above, to meet basically the demands of health supervision/law-enforcement. As required by the statutory duty of health departments, make overall arrangements to bring the construction of technical support capacity of disease prevention and control agencies and occupational disease prevention and control agencies into local plan for the Twelfth Five-Year Plan, so that inspection agencies at the state level will reach international advanced level, and possess stronger capacity for scientific research and development as well as arbitration inspection. Inspection agencies at the provincial level will meet the needs of test and monitoring of health supervision within the jurisdiction, and possess certain capacity for research and development. Inspection agencies at the municipal-prefectural level will possess the capacity for conducting inspection by inspection methods and standards. Inspection agencies at the county level will possess the capacity for testing common indexes. All local authorities should bear in mind that capacity building must be promoted by project implementation to improve constantly regulation.

(4) Strengthen cultural development to improve the ideological quality.

The Sixth Plenary Session of the 17th CPC Central Committee requires that we must take the construction of socialist core value system as the fundamental task running through all areas of reform and opening-up as well as socialist modernization to form unified guiding ideology, common ideals and beliefs, strong mental strength and basic code of ethics within the whole Party and whole society, so that the construction of socialist core value system will become the conscious pursuit and dynamism of the whole people. All local authorities should seriously carry out the spirit of the Sixth Plenary Session of the 17th CPC Central Committee, conduct in-depth education of anti-corruption and clean government building, deepen the construction of team work style and professional ethics education, and strengthen the risk prevention and control for incorrupt government. As the law-enforcement team with uniforms and conducting health supervision/law-enforcement on behalf of the government, health supervision is the "health police" and "health guardian" of the people. I hope that those working on the front of health supervision will take the lead in the cultural construction of the whole system, and keep a firm grasp on good services, good quality, good medical ethics and public satisfaction. In combination with the industrial characteristics of health supervision, always adhere to the purpose of serving the maintenance of the people's health benefits, dig into and compact the idea of core value, and carry out the construction of industry culture. Regard the maintenance of the people's health benefits as your mission, show your hospitality, intensify the supervision and law-enforcement, dare to face tough things or persons, and enforce the law strictly and punishing all offenders.

In the new year, hopefully all of us will make persistent efforts, be united as one, brave difficulties, further perform every task of food safety and health supervision, and meet the successful convocation of the 18th CPC National Congress with splendid work.

(Shan Yongxiang)

3. Fully Implement Development Outline for Women and Children, and Make Efforts to Create a New Situation of Women and Children's Health Work
—A Speech Made by Chen Zhu, Minister of Ministry of Health at 2012 National Conference on Women and Children's Health Work (February 23, 2012)

The main tasks of this national conference on women and children's health work are: to further carry out Outline for Development of China Women and Children in 2011-2020 and *Opinions of Deepening Medical and Health System Reform* by State Council, implement earnestly the spirits of the 5th National Working Conference on China Women and Children and 2012 National Health Working Conference, summarize experiences, deepen the understanding, grasp the situations, deploy comprehensively work of women and children in the period and speed up the undertaking development of women and children based on Outlook of Scientific Development.

Next, I'll speak out three points of opinions.

I. Affirmation of Significant Achievements in Women and Children's Health Work

Since the new century, the Party and government focused on the promotion of coordinated development of economy and society, and attached more importance to ensuring and improving people's livelihood, the development of health undertaking, and the health of women and children. In the process of deepening the reform of medical health system, the work of women and children has been further strengthened, health rights and interests of women and children further guaranteed and health conditions constantly improved.

(1) Significant Improvement in the Health of Women and Children

In 2011, mortality rate of pregnant and puerperal women nationwide was 26.1/100,000, which was 51% lower than that in 2000. Mortality rates of babies and children under 5 were 12.2‰ and 15.6‰, 62% and 61% lower that those in 2000. Women's common diseases and frequently-occurring diseases were effectively prevented and treated. Significant results were obtained in the prevention of mother-to-child AIDS transmission. The indicators for morbidity of moderately severe anemia among pregnant and puerperal women, the incidence of low birth weight and morbidity of children's malnutrition were constantly improved and the targets of the two Outlines in 2001-2010 were smoothly realized. Mortality of children under 5 covered in UN Millennium Development Goals was realized ahead of schedule. Mortality of pregnant and puerperal women continuously decreased. The average life expectancy of women was 75.2. The gap between the main indicators for women and children and those in developed countries is gradually narrowing, which attracted broad attention and high evaluation by international society.

(2) Gradual Improvement in Laws and Regulations for the Health of Women and Children

Law for Health Care of Women and Babies is the first special law for the protection of the rights and interests of women and children, which jointly provides legal protection for the health of women and children with *Protection of Women's Rights, Law of Juveniles Protection,* and *Regulations for Labor Protection of Female Workers.* In 2001, the State Council issued *Implementation of the Law on Mother and Infant Health Care,* brought Outline for Development of China Women and Children in 2011-2020 into force, and clarified aims, demands and policy measures for development of women and children's health undertaking. Ministry of Health, taking "One Law and Two Outlines" as the core, formulated successively a series of rules and regulations, and documents, like *Special Technology License of Mother and Infant Health Care and Management Methods for Personnel Qualification, Management Methods for Institutions of Women and Children, Management Methods for Neonatal Disease Screening and Management Methods for Prenatal Diagnosis Technology.* Thus the management of women and children's health in accordance with the law was gradually realized in administrative management, supervision and examination and standardized management.

(3) Gradual Establishment of Health Guarantee System for Women and Children

With the establishment of steady mechanism for ensuring funding, the equalization of the basic public health service was constantly promoted. And grassroots medical health institutions provided urban and rural residents services of health care for pregnant and puerperal women, children, and preventive vaccination as public products, which improved the accessibility and fairness of health service for women and children. The expanded program for immunization was implemented based on the original 6 vaccines for the prevention of 7 diseases and was further expanded to 14 vaccines for 15 diseases. Free routine immunization for children was carried out. Medical security system for women and children was constantly improved, the participating rate of the new rural cooperative medical care system has been 97%, fund-raising standard was about 230 and medical security for rural women and children was gradually improved. Medical insurance for urban and rural residents has fully covered primary and secondary school students and young children. By the end of 2011, the improvement in medical security of serious diseases of rural children, like congenital heart disease and acute leukemia was promoted nationwide. The pilot security work of cervical cancer and breast cancer was comprehensively developed in 13 provinces of Hebei, Anhui, Hubei and so on. Accumulatively 7,629 children with leukemia and 26,536 children with congenital heart disease across the country were rescued and treated, and the actual compensation rates were 65% and 78% respectively, which effectively avoided the families of children patients becoming or returning poor due to illnesses. Some provinces, such as Jiangxi Province basically realized the full coverage and all free of children's leukemia and congenital heart disease.

(4) Continuous Solution to Women and Children's Major Health Problems

A series of major public health service projects of "Decrease and Elimination", subsidies for rural pregnant and puerperal women of hospitalized delivery, examinations for rural women with the two cancers, HIV mother-to-child block and others were implemented. By the end of 2011, 11,690,000 rural women of the right age had been given check for cervical cancer and 1,460,000 rural women offered check for breast cancer so that the women patients got the early diagnosis and treatment. 22,630,000 pregnant and puerperal women were provided AIDS consultation and testing, which decreased the rate of HIV mother-to-child transmission from 34.8% before the project implementation to 7.4%. The rate of hospitalized delivery of rural pregnant and puerperal women was 96.7%, which forcefully guaranteed the safety of mothers and babies, and the urban-rural mortality gap of pregnant and puerperal women was basically eliminated, regional gap was gradually narrowing and the good social benefits were obtained. Simultaneously, comprehensive prevention and treatment of birth defects was steadily promoted. All places innovated working mechanism and explored free mode of premarital check-up. The rate of premarital check-up nationwide increased from 2.9% in 2005 to 31% in 2011 and the premarital check-up rate in Fujian Province, Guangxi Province and others reached over 90%. Supplement of folic acid for the prevention and treatment of neural tube defects was practiced. 23,560,000 rural reproductive women got folic acid supplementation, which improved the decrease of incidence rate of neural tube defects. The network for prenatal screening and prenatal diagnosis was constantly improved. The services of prenatal screening and prenatal diagnosis were launched in 511 medical institutions nationwide and the service ability was constantly enhanced. The screening for neonatal diseases was rapidly promoted; the screening rate of inherited metabolic diseases increased from 15% in 2002 to 63% in 2010; and hearing screening was increasingly popularized, which promoted the timely intervention and treatment for the children patients, avoided physical and mental damage and reduced the occurrence of the disabled children. The screening rate for neonatal diseases was over 95% in Heilongjiang, Zhejiang, Shandong and other provinces. Beijing, Tianjin, Shanghai and other places actively launched free screening for neonatal diseases and relief for children patients. Gansu Province covered "Program for the Rescue and Treatment of Children with Hearing Impairment" in the provincial government's 10 people-benefit projects and provided free rescue and treatment for poor children with hearing impairment. Ningxia formulated policies of "Six Frees and One Rescue", free hospitalized delivery, free screening and treatment for neonatal diseases and so on.

(5) Constant Perfection of Women and Children's Health Service System

For years of constructions and developments, China has had women and children's health service system with Chinese characteristics, with women and children's health care institutions as the core, grassroots medical health institutions as the base, large and medium-sized medical institutions, and the relevant teaching institutions of science and technology as technical support so as to provide women and children comprehensive, continuous and humanized health care service. All-level women and children's health care institutions, as the organizers, managers and providers in the administrative areas, acted as the important backbone in women and children's health work. Grassroots medical institutions, as the net bottom of women and children's health service system, undertook women and children's health service and the collection of the basic information. Hospitals of obstetrics and gynecology, children's hospitals and comprehensive hospitals carried out extensive medical care service for the diagnosis and treatment of women and children's diseases. At the moment, there are 3,025 women and children's health care institutions at the levels of province, city and county, 398 hospitals of obstetrics and gynecology and 72 children's hospitals across China. The grassroots health service network was constantly perfected, of which there are nearly 33,000 community health service institutions, 39,000 township health centers and 65,000 village clinics. Nationally, there are 245,000 workers in women and children's health care institutions, 360,000 practitioners and assistant practicing doctors of department of obstetrics and gynecology and department of pediatrics.

(6) Continuous Enhancement of Women and Children's Health Management

All-level women and children's health institutions launched service and management related with reproductive health in accordance with law, strengthened vertical and horizontal professional guidance, personnel training, and technical support. Especially, they not only undertook the organization and implementation of major women and children's health service projects but also technical guidance, examination and management for the basic public health service projects, which intensified the functions of public health. All places feasibly strengthened technical service, and daily supervision and administration of women and babies' health care, standardized the management in baby-friendly hospitals, launched county-level health performance assessment of women and babies, and promoted grade appraisal of women and babies' health care institutions. The connotation construction in women and babies' health care institutions was continuously strengthened. Women and babies' information system was gradually improved, and the monitoring of birth defects, deaths of pregnant and puerperal women and children under 5 was constantly enhanced. The number of the monitored districts and counties is 336, covering 140,000,000 persons, which is the biggest monitoring network for women and babies' health. The monitoring of the annual reports on women and babies health and women and babies' health care institutions were steadily promoted. And the more comprehensive, accurate, and timely relevant information has been adopted by National Bureau of Statistics, Working Committee of Women and Children under the State Council and international organizations, which provided scientific base for the formulation and improvement in health policies, especially health policies for women and children. Heilongjiang, Hunan and other provinces began the appraisal and examination of women and children's health care institutions. Jiangsu Province established the training system to make sure that health workers for women and babies take appointment with certificates and the training system for all the staff members, which promoted the standardized management of women and children's health service.

The great achievements of women and children's health undertaking are the results of high value and scientific policy-making of the Party Central Committee and the State Council, substantial support and close cooperation of all-level Party committees, governments, and all departments, wide public concern and concerted efforts from all walks of life in the society, hard work, plain living and selfless contributions of national health system, especially all the health workers for women and children. Taking the opportunity, I, on behalf of Ministry of Health, express my heartfelt thanks and great respect to all of you, and express our heartfelt thanks for the great help and support given to us by international organizations, such as World Health Organization, and the United Nations Children's Fund!

II. Further Enhancement of Sense of Responsibility for Women and Children's Health Work

(1) Fully Understanding the Significance of Doing a Good Job in Women and

Children's Health Work

Women and children's health is precondition and foundation for human development and it relates to the development of our country and nationality in the future. Doing a good job in women and children's health is of great significance in improving the population quality and promoting the harmonious development in economic society.

Women and children's health is important target of health reform and development. Medical reform should stick to the core concept of providing all people the basic medical health system as the public products. In China, there are 870,000,000 women and children, accounting for two thirds of the whole population, and they are the key target groups of medical health service. Ministry of Health organized the experts to carry out *Research of 2020 Strategies for China's Health*, which shows that during 1990-2005, China's average life expectancy is 4.4 years older and it attributes to 48% decrease mortality of children under 5. Doing a good job in women and children's health and improving indicators for women and children's health play a globally significant role in improving health performance and reflecting the results of health reform and development.

Women and children's health is the important foundation of a harmonious society. Healthy growth of children is the ardent expectations of parents. Nowadays, most families have only one child. Whether the children can grow up healthily relates to the happiness of the families. Women are not only the direct nurturers of the children in the families but play an important role in taking care of the other family members. If women and children are not healthy, there will not possibly be harmony or happiness in families, and the society will be lack of important basis for harmony. Doing a good job in women and children's health and reducing women and children's diseases is of great importance in reducing economic burden of family and mental stress, promoting family happiness and the construction of harmonious society.

Women and children's health is the important guarantee for sustainable development of economy. Women and children are the vital force and reserve forces for building a well-off society. China is one of those with the highest employment rate of women, who hold up half the sky. They play an indispensable role in developing the economy, improving people's livelihood, and promoting civilization progress. The health of children affects both the state of their own survival, mental development, and their future productivity and creativity. Doing a good job in women and children's health can reduce and avoid a lot of deaths of women and children, birth defects, and childhood disability, improve health quality of the nationality, increase health inventory of human resources, and provide important human resources guarantee for the fast and sustainable development of national economy.

Women and children's health is the important embodiment of social civilization and progress. Women and children are relatively vulnerable groups and the groups with the most fragile survival and health in a society. If a country or a region can't meet women and children's needs for basic survival and development or improve the conditions for their survival and health, the development of the country or the region will not be successful. International has put the average life expectancy, mortalities of the pregnant and puerperal women and the children under 5 as the most basic health development and population health indicators, which act as the comprehensive indicators of social development and human development. Women and children have increasingly become important issues and prior field of particular concern by international community. Doing a good job in women and children's health and improving women and children's health is important strategic measures for China to fulfill international commitments, improve international image and international status.

(2) Objective Analysis of the Situation Facing Women and Children's Health Work

Currently, China's economy and society are developing rapidly, and the deepening of medical health reform system is progressing steadily, which provides unprecedented opportunities for women and children's health.

The first one is that the implementation of the two Outlines provides a more favorable political security for women and children's health. Last July, the State Council promulgated formally Development Outline for Chinese Women and Children in 2011-2020, and put health in the primary fields of the development of women and children, which gives full expression to the idea of all-round development based on health, and depicts the grand blueprint for the development of women and children's health. Premier Wen Jiabao pointed out at the 5th national conference on women and children that women and children's undertaking relates to the future of the state and nationality and the inclusion of the development of women and children's undertaking into the system of the overall economic and social development planning and public policy should be taken as the important indicators of government work. All-level Party committees and governments should attach great importance to the implementation of the two Outlines and provide a good political and social environment for women and children's health work.

The second one is that the deepening of medical reform provides a more powerful policy support for women and children's health work. Medical reform intensifies the leading position of the government in providing public health and basic medical services, and clarifies the requirements of "Safeguarding the Basic, Strengthening the Grassroots and Establishing the Mechanism". With the deepening of medical reform, health investment increases gradually, the basic medical security system is further improved, the grassroots health service system is gradually strengthened, medical and health service ability is constantly improved, and the implementation of "Sickness for Treatment and Treatment for Insurance" for women and children will be more guaranteed. The promotion of equal basic public health services, the implementation of national basic public health services such as health care for the pregnant and puerperal women, and children, and other public health service projects such as the subsidy for rural hospitalized delivery and examinations for two cancers have become the important measures in solving the problems of the most direct and most realistic interests for women and children in medical reform of with coverage, which is welcomed by the masses and provides a good mass base and social atmosphere for women and children's health work.

The third one is that the achievement of millennium development goals provides a more powerful motivation for women and children's health work. Many indicators such as child mortality, mortality of pregnant and puerperal women, and reproductive health in UN Millennium Development Goals directly associated with women and children's health work. Therefore, women and children's health work should be increased to the levels of national development and political commitment. In September, 2010, "Global Strategy for Women and Children's Health" was specially launched at the high-level conference of UN Millennium Development Goals in order to ensure the achievement of millennium development goals on schedule. Premier Wen Jiabao, on behalf of China's government, solemnly promised to significantly increase investment in women and children's health, strengthen the ability construction for women and children's health, make women and children enjoy a higher-level health care, make strenuous efforts to protect women's and children's health and fulfill the bounden responsibilities of the government. The goal of 1 year increase in average life expectancy covered in National "Twelfth Five-year Plan" was put forward explicitly, which is the first time for China to list the indicator in national economic and social development planning and embodies the importance of health in the global economic and social development.

In the meantime, we should soberly realize that women and children's health work still lags behind the economic and social development, and faces many difficulties and challenges. The outstanding manifestations are: that the task of reducing mortalities of pregnant and puerperal women and children under the age of five remains arduous, mortalities of pregnant and puerperal women are obviously farther in the distance from the achievement of millennium development goals, and the number of child deaths still ranks the fifth in the world. The development of women and children's health is imbalanced, urban and rural, regional and groups of people's differences are significant, the mortalities of pregnant and puerperal women in the west areas is 2.5 times higher than that in the east, and the mortality of rural children under the age of five is 2.8 times higher than that in the city. Women's and children's health problems are still outstanding and serious diseases such as breast cancer, cervical cancer, leukemia and congenital heart disease seriously threatens women's and children's health. Birth defect, nutritional disease, mental disorder and other diseases have become increasingly prominent public health issues. Women and children's health service ability is obviously deficient so that it is difficult to adapt it to the growing health needs of women and children.

Opportunities and challenges in women and children's health coexist. We must raise awareness, get a clear understanding of the situation, strengthen the sense of mission and sense of responsibility for women and children's health work, change challenges into opportunities, turn pressure into motivation, deepen the reform, face the challenges and move to higher point. There is a brilliant future in women and children's health work and it must be so.

(3) Accurate Grasp of the Development Principles and Direction of Women and Children's Health Work

We have accumulated a lot of valuable experience in the long-term practice of women and children's health work, which is the principles and direction with long-term adherence for women and children's health work.

The first one is to stick to the aim of "Child Priority and Mother Safety". "Child Priority and Mother Safety" has become the global moral concept and rule of action for safeguarding human health and development. Strengthening women and children's health work, and improving women's and children's survival, life and living quality are the priority areas of health development, and the important practice of implementing people-oriented outlook of scientific development. All-level health administrative departments should take the protection of health rights and interests of women and children as a priority while making health policy and planning, and determining the key work. Medical health institutions must set up the consciousness and idea of "Child Priority and Mother Safety" while carrying out business work so as to provide women and children more convenient and more humanized health care services.

The second one is to adhere to the policy of women and children's health work. China's women and children's health undertaking has adapted to the basic national conditions and has distinct Chinese characteristics. In the aspect of law, the working policy of keeping "health care as the center, reproductive health the purpose, health care and clinic combined, geared to grassroots, groups of people, and prevention first" is established. In many areas of health undertaking, work objective, contents and methods for women and children's health were made clear from the height of the working policy. This work policy clarifies the property of women and children's health—public health, i.e. to keep health as the center, and rely on closely clinical service of technology; the key point—to face the groups of women and children and rely closely on the grassroots medical health institutions, root in grassroots and carry out the work deep in communities and families. This work policy is the guideline to ensure the development of women and children's health, which we must accurately understand and firmly grasp.

The third one is to stick to the service model for women and children's health with Chinese characteristics. Facing groups and keeping health care combined with clinics is the effective service model summed up from decades of women and children's health practice. We should take broad masses of women and children for a specific target groups, extend community health care, reduce and prevent the outbreaks of diseases. Meanwhile, guaranteeing ability of reproductive health have been improved by taking the necessary clinical service as the important means of support for women and children's health care. A series of active, continuous, comprehensive, and warm services are provided in the courses of preconception care, antenatal care, institutional delivery, postpartum house visit, postnatal vaccination, disease screening, neonatal visit, children's health management, nutrition guide and common disease prevention and control, which meets the demands of women's and children's health, fully embodies humanistic care in women's and children's health and forms a unique culture of women's and children's health care. This service model effectively bridges the chasm between community health care and clinical services in the field of women and children's health, and realizes the organic combination of prevention and treatment, which is in line with the development law of health undertaking, and we must always adhere to it.

The fourth one is to stick to the working method of the overall planning and coordination, and classified guidance. China's economic and social development has been in the primary stage of socialism for a long time and the differences between urban and rural areas, and regional differences are obvious. Under this national situation, the shortage of the total health resources and unreasonable configuration in women and children's health undertaking coexist and the unbalanced development between urban and rural, regional areas also exists. In advancing women and children's health work, the overall planning and coordination, and classified guidance must be paid attention to and the specific policies and measures must be taken to solve the prominent problems in women and children's health of different areas. The central and western areas and rural areas should be focused on, the intensity of fund investment and policy support be increased, the gaps of women and children's health between urban and rural areas, and between different regions gradually reduced to promote the coordinated development of women's and children's health undertaking and economic society.

The fifth one is to adhere to the working strategy of government leading, department cooperation and social participation. Strengthening women's and children's health work and improving the women's and children's health are the important contents of implementing the two Outlines and the important responsibility of all-level Party committees and governments. In carrying out the two Outlines, government leadership must be upheld, department cooperation of Ministry of Health, National Development and Reform Commission and Ministry of Finance must be close, women's and children's health must be covered in the overall planning of national economic and social development, and women and children's health work must be included in the planning of medical reform and the development of health undertaking, financial investment must be increased, ability construction strengthened and the development of women's and children's health undertaking promoted. Simultaneously, the role of social organizations should be given full play and good atmosphere of care and support by the whole society created for the development of women and children's health. Only by sticking to the working tactics of government leading, department cooperation and social participation and joining forces, can the powerful institutional and organizational guarantee be provided for the development of women and children's health.

Historical experience tells us that as long as we adhere to the people-centered concept, insist on the outlook of scientific development, respect for the development law of women and children's health undertaking, and adhere to the correct development direction, the development road of women and children's health with Chinese characteristics must be wider and wider and the health situation of women and children will be continuously improved.

III. Comprehensive Promotion of the Development of Women and Children's Health Undertaking

The core of promoting women and children's health work is the implementation of the "One Law and Two Outlines". Ministry of Health has printed and distributed *Implementation Scheme for Carrying out Development Outline for Chinese Women and Children in 2011-2020 (hereinafter referred to as Implementation Scheme)*, clarified the guiding ideology, the target principle, primary mission and safeguard measure for women and children's health work in the future period. The "Twelfth Five-year" planning of medical reform passed principally at the routine meeting of the State Council and the "Twelfth Five-year" planning for health undertaking development to be published both put forward clearly the requirements for women and children's health work. Today, mainly responsible comrades of health departments and health bureaus from all provinces (regions and cities) attend the meeting. And I want to single out that the implementation of the two Outlines is an important responsibility of the entire health system and we should organize strength of various aspects, earnestly implement various security measures, sturdily launch actions of mother and child safety, comprehensive prevention and treatment of birth defects, prevention and treatment of women's and children's diseases, system construction of women's and children's health service, and complete the target tasks in the two Outlines on schedule. Here, I'll emphasize the following points.

(1) Clarification of Development Goals of Women and Children's Health

In the next five to ten years, we must make tireless efforts to establish the basic medical health system covering urban and rural women and children, perfect women and children's health service system, guarantee women's and children's equal access to the basic medical health services and constantly improve women's and children's health. By 2015, national mortality of pregnant and puerperal women will be 22/100,000, which is also the requirement of millennium development goals. Mortalities of babies and children under the age of 5 will decrease 12‰ and 14‰ respectively. By 2020, national mortalities of pregnant and puerperal women will reduce 20/100,000, and the mortalities of babies and children under 5 will decrease 10‰ and 13‰. Besides the overall indexes, the *Implementation Scheme* puts forward different goals and objectives for the different development levels in different areas respectively with the purpose of further enhancement of classified guidance, and more targeted promotion of the coordinated development of women and children health. All places must further clarify and refine the targets for women and children health work in accordance with the requirements in the *Implementation Scheme*.

(2) Stressing the Key Points and Carry out the Main Tasks

The first one is to actually ensure the safety of mother and baby and reduce mortalities of pregnant and puerperal women, and babies. In the process of perfecting the new rural cooperative medical care system, women's and children's participations must be paid more attention to, the practical problems of women's and children's participations and the application for reimbursement be solved timely and the newborns covered in the new rural cooperative medical care system. We will continue to implement the subsidies of hospitalized delivery for rural pregnant and puerperal women and the project of reduce and elimination, improve cohesive mechanism for the subsidies of hospitalized delivery, the new rural cooperative medical care and medical assistance system, increase subsidy standards, and promote stability and improvement of hospitalized delivery. The construction of first-aid capabilities of pregnant and puerperal women and the newborns must be strengthened, and the green channels for pregnant and puerperal women, and the newborns in critical stage were established. Effective measures must be taken to focus on the improvement in the abilities of emergency aid and treatment, transfer and management for rural pregnant and puerperal women, and the newborns in critical stage. Meanwhile, the monitoring network construction for mortalities of pregnant and puerperal women, and children must be strengthened.

The second one is to strengthen the comprehensive prevention and treatment of birth defects and the quality of newly-born population. Comprehensive prevention and control measures of the third grade must be actively implemented, propaganda to the society and health education for prevention and treatment of birth defects be extended, free premarital medical examination promoted, the rate of premarital medical examination increased and preconception counseling, early pregnancy, pregnancy health care services standardized. Labor protection of female workers must be strengthened to avoid women in preconception and pregnant women exposed to toxic and harmful substances and radioactive rays. The ability construction of prenatal diagnosis must be intensified, prenatal diagnosis network be perfected, and prenatal screening service coverage and prenatal diagnosis be improved. Neonatal disease screening must be promoted, the construction of provincial neonatal disease screening centers be strengthened, the screening network for genetically metabolic disease and hearing impairments of the newborns improved, the rate of neonatal disease screening gradually increased, and the treatment and intervention of the confirmed cases enhanced. Monitoring network construction of birth defects must be supported,and scientific research of birth defect prevention and the training for professional and technical personnel be intensified.

The third one is to strengthen the prevention and treatment of women's and children's diseases. The project of national basic public health services must be fully implemented, management and examination system be perfected, the services standardized, and the management rate of pregnant and puerperal women's and children's health improved. The prevention and control of major diseases such as tuberculosis and AIDS, and the major public health service projects such as the examinations for the two cancers of rural women must be continuously carried out, and the coverage of free examinations for the two cancers be enlarged. The security work of serious disease rescue and treatment such as childhood leukemia, children's congenital heart disease, breast cancer, cervical cancer and others must be fully implemented and the compensation proportion of hospitalized subsidy be raised. Women and children's health service must be standardized, and the early detection and intervention of common mental health problems of women and children be strengthened. Children's nutrition intervention program in mid-west areas must be implemented to prevent and treat children's nutritional diseases such as malnutrition, anemia and others.

(3) Seizing the Key and Comprehensively Improving the Ability of Women and Children's Health Service

The first one is to improve network for women and children's health service. The construction of institutions for women and children's health care must be strengthened to ensure that there is one standardized institutions for women and children's health care operated by governments in province, city and county. Construction planning and construction standards for all-level institutions for women and children's health care must be studied and established as soon as possible. According to the principle of overall planning and step-by-step implementation, standardized construction of institutions for women and children's health care at city and county levels in the "Twelfth Five-year Plan" must be focused on. The construction of department of pediatrics must be strengthened, the number of children's hospitals be reasonably increased to relieve the difficulty in children's seeking medical care.

The second one is to strengthen the contingent construction of women and children's health. The standards for the size of personnel in all-level institutions for women and children's health care must be studied and implemented. According to the needs of women and children's health work, workers of women and children's health work must be enriched. The contingent construction of women and children's health must be strengthened, full-time personnel of women and children's health care be put in post in community health service centers and township health centers to tamp the net bottom of grassroots women and children's health service, encourage and guide the college graduates and good professional and technical personnel for women and children's health care to work in grassroots and outlying poverty-stricken areas. Key specialty construction of women's and children's health care must be strengthened, and midwife education be intensified to explore an effective way to strengthen the construction of midwife contingent.

The third one is to improve women and children's health service and management. The functions of women's and children's health care institutions in professional guidance, personnel training, technical support and the information management must be reinforced. Professional training for women and children's health care must be vigorously promoted, appropriate technologies be popularized, and the role of national medicine of traditional Chinese medicine in women and children health care be paid attention to. Information construction of women and children's health must be carried forward to promote interconnection and interworking between women and children's health and regional health information platform and improve the management and application of women and children's health information. The establishment of collaboration mechanism for institutions of women and children's health care, and other professional public health agencies, large and medium-sized medical institutions and grassroots medical and health institutions must be explored. The researches of major women's and children's health problems and intervention measures must be reinforced to provide scientific basis for evidence-based decision making.

The fourth one is to intensify supervision and management of women and children's health. Laws and regulations, and professional and technical standards for improvement in women and children's health must be improved, supervision, evaluation system and work specification be perfected according to *Law for Mother and Baby*, and other laws and regulations. The supervision and law enforcement of mother and baby must be included into comprehensive health supervision and law enforcement, supervision and law enforcement of mother and baby health care be feasibly strengthened, strict access of technical service institutions and personnel to mother and baby health care be made, and medical service behaviors related to reproductive health be regulated. Medical practice without license must be investigated and punished, and the "Two Nons" must be cracked down.

(4) To Overcome Difficulties and Promote Balanced Development of Women and Children's Health

The problem of unbalanced development of women and children's health must be placed at the height of the construction of a harmonious society in order to further strengthen the overall coordination and classified guidance.

The first one is the enhancement of women and children's health work in key areas must be intensified, and the key work of women and children's health be placed in the west and vast rural areas. The transfer payment from the Central Finance in the west and especially rural areas must be further increased, and health payment for women and children's health in rural areas, the old revolutionary base areas, ethnic minority autonomous regions, border areas, and less developed areas be gradually increased, and the relevant policies and projects must be slanted to these areas. The lower rate of hospitalized delivery and worse women's and children's physical conditions in some areas must be given special attention to, and policy guide be strengthened. The support of women and children's health from city to countryside and east to west areas must be explored and launched, and the oriented assistance of hardware and software be furnished.

The second one is to ensure the mobile women and children to enjoy the same health care services. The service management must be optimized, settlement procedures in nonlocal places be simplified to ensure the mobile women and children to enjoy reimbursement of the new rural cooperative medical care system and hospitalized delivery subsidy covered in the public policies benefited to people. The new work mechanism must be innovated, the mobile people be made the target groups of people covered in national basic public health services and major public health services, health care, disease prevention and control, planned immunization for the mobile women and children be enhanced, and the health care services enjoyed by the mobile women and children be made the same with that enjoyed by women and children in urban areas.

(5) To Strengthen the Leadership and Organize Careful Implementation

All places must make practical development planning for local women and children's health undertaking, include indicators for women and children's health and working tasks into the overall local planning of the national economic and social development in accordance with the requirements of implementation scheme for the unified deployment and synchronous implementation. Government leadership must be strengthened, close department cooperation be made, and social participation be encouraged. All-level health administrative departments must strengthen communication and coordination, actively strive for the support from relevant departments, intensify propaganda and mobilization, win over the understanding, support and participation from all sectors of society in women and children's health work, give full play to the enthusiasm of all aspects, and form the joint force to promote the development of women and children's health work.

Women and children's health relates to the happiness of millions of families, the coordinated development of the economy and the society, and the rejuvenation of China. Therefore, our responsibility is heavy and our mission is glorious. We should take the outlook of scientific development as the instruction, implement the two Outlines, deepen medical reform, make efforts to create a new situation for women and children's health work, comprehensively improve women's and children's health, make greater contributions for the construction of a harmonious socialist society and take concrete actions to welcome the 18th National Congress of the Communist Party of China.

(Ji Chenglian)

4. Elaborate Organization and Standardized Operation to Promote Sturdily the Payment Reform of the New Rural Cooperative Medical Care System (the NRCMCS)

—A Speech Made by Chen Zhu, Minister of Ministry of Health at the Video and Telephone Conference on the Promotion of the Payment Reform of the New Rural Cooperative Medical Care System (May 15, 2012)

Recently, Ministry of Health, National Development and Reform Commission and Ministry of Finance have jointly issued *Guiding Opinion on the Payment Reform of the New Rural Cooperative Medical Care System (hereinafter referred to as Guiding Opinion)*. The main purpose of today's video and telephone conference is to deploy and accelerate the NRCMCS payment reform to promote deep development of rural health reform in accordance with the requirements covered in 2012 National Health Work Conference and the *Guiding Opinion*. Next, I'll speak out two points of opinions on the NRCMCS payment reform in carrying out the *Guiding Opinion*.

I. Deep Understanding of the Significance of Pushing forward the NRCMCS Payment Reform

Since the implementation of medical reform, all the work has been progressing smoothly, significant results have been obtained and the people get more and more benefits. The new rural cooperative medical care system, as one of the focal points of work in medical reform, makes important contributions to the realization of periodic targets of medical reform. With the overall NRCMCS coverage and the increase in funding, how to promote quickly the payment reform and further improve the utilization efficiency of the funds have been the important and urgent problems of the NRCMCS construction.

(1) The NRCMCS Implementation is the Important Measure for More Efficient Fund Utilization and More Benefits of the Participants

Recently, with the strong support of all-level governments, the NRCMCS funding increases fast from 100 yuan in 2008 to 300 yuan in 2012, about 3 times more in the 3 years. However, the increase of the NRCMCS guarantee is relatively slow and there is room to improve. The reasons are the rapid growing demand of the rural residents for medical service, the price increase in medical service with price growth, and medical service flow direction in seeking medical treatment after the increase of the NRCMCS guarantee, all of which are reasonable increases in medical expenses and the NRCMCS expenditures. However, for a long time there has been unreasonable compensation mechanism in medical health institutions, whose problem of compensation for the insufficient income of technical services by unreasonable drug use and examinations, and excessive medical services hasn't been properly solved. The situations of non-standardized medical service and the unreasonable growth in medical expenses are rather serious in some places. According to the statistics, from 2007 to 2010, the annual growth rate of the average hospitalization cost in hospitals of the second grade nationwide is above 9%, and the annual growth rate of the average hospitalization cost in township hospitals is not lower than 12%, which is obviously higher than synchronous CPI and GDP growths. Unreasonable medical expenses consume the funds and affect utilization efficiency of the NRCMCS fund and the real benefits of the participating farmers. To change the current situation, the operating mechanism of medical health institutions must be changed, the income structure of medical expenses be adjusted, and unreasonable growth of medical expenses be effectively controlled, which is the requirement of comprehensive reform in rural medical health institutions and the NRCMCS requirement for further self improvement.

(2) The Implementation of the NRCMCS Payment Reform Is Effective Measure for the Promotion of Operating Mechanism Transfer in Medical Health Institutions and Reasonable Cost Control.

Payment reform means to transform the traditional individual pay into mixed payment through the promotion of pay by disease, bed and day, and total outpatient pay so as to standardize service and control expenses. Medical service is no longer paid by disease and the total sum is limited, which objectively demands that medical institutions to adjust the structure of medical expenses, control unreasonable examinations, unreasonable drug use on the premise of total amount control, indirectly improve the income for technical labor of medical staff, change the compensation mechanism for the service cost, and the mechanisms for self-discipline in medical expense and self-regulation in cost structure of medical health institutions. The economic lever and guiding functions of the payment reform effectively control the unreasonable growth of medical expense, and reflect the labor value of medical staff and a better implementation of the guiding ideology of "benefits for the masses and encouragement for medical workers" covered in medical reform.

(3) The Implementation of the NRCMCS Payment Reform Is an Important Focus of Reform in Public Hospitals at County Level

In accordance with work deployment of medical reform, the focal point of work in medical reform of this year is the promotion of the reform in public hospitals at county level and the important stage for the pilot reform in public hospitals is going to profundal areas. The bigger interest adjustment range, involvement of more people, and heavier tasks in medical service cost compensation determine that the reform in public hospitals at county level will be more complicated and various policy measures should be given more comprehensive considerations.

With the further increase of the NRCMCS funding in 2012, the payment reform in public hospitals at county level was vigorously promoted by the advantages of the further increase of the NRCMCS paying ability, and the real disposable income of medical institutions, and the NRCMCS utilization rate and guarantee were improved based on the control of the total medical expenses and the structure adjustment, and the reasonable sharing mechanism of medical institution was established by means of medical security, governmental finance and medical income. Only when reasonable compensation problem is solved in the aspect of mechanism, can various reform measures of medical management, personnel allocation and performance assessment be simultaneously promoted and the mechanism of "supplement of medicine by drugs" in public hospitals be broken down.

II. Sturdy Promotion of the Standardized NRCMCS Payment Reform

In recent years, Ministry of Health has guided all places to actively explore the NRCMCS payment reform by means of holding field work meetings, organizing trainings, and researches and guidance by the experts. At the present, the pilot work has been generally carried out in all provinces (regions and cities) nationwide, and the more obvious results have been obtained in many places In Lufeng of Yunnan, Zhen' an of Shaanxi, Lianyungang of Jiangsu and other places, the growths of the average hospitalization cost and outpatient expenditures in medical institutions at county level were effectively controlled through the payment reform of hospitalization by disease and day, and the prepayment of total outpatient expenditures, and the NRCMCS fund utilization and the benefits of the participating farmers were improved. Changshu City of Jiangsu Province, based on the principle of complete coverage of medical institutions and diseases, makes the specified, concrete and detailed implementation plan of payment reform in the whole city, promotes payment reform of hospitalization by disease and day, and the prepayment of total outpatient expenditures of all medical cases in the designated medical institutions of the jurisdictions and formulates a complete set of evaluation methods. Henan Province makes the unified implementation of the payment reform of the total NRCMCS prepayment for hospitalization expenditures in the whole province, covering all designated NRCMCS medical institutions at the levels of city, county and below county , takes second-rate hospitalization cost increase and the proportional drug use outside the directory as the core control indicators to approve the final NRCMCS payments, and establishes the intrinsic motivation and restriction mechanisms of the reward for surplus fund use and the sharing of overspending.

Simultaneously, payment reform is launched in many places but the desired effects is failed to be obtained because of the fewer covered diseases, the non-standardized implementation and the lack of methods for supervision and examination. Therefore, to further standardize and strive for the real results the NRCMCS payment reform, the three ministries like Ministry of Health issued the *Guiding Opinions* to demand all places to do a feasibly good job according to the spirit of the *Guiding Opinions*.

(1) To Define the Fundamental Principles for the Promotion of the NRCMCS Payment Reform

The first one is to adhere to the principle of full coverage. The NRCMCS payment reform should cover all the designated medical institutions, all hospitalized patients and the patients who enjoy outpatient NRCMCS subsidies in the wholly-planned areas. Only when the full coverage is realized, can the selection of patient by medical institutions for the purpose of regulating expenditures and the transfer of the expense cost to the patients who are not covered by payment reform be avoided so as to promote fair competitions among medical institutions and bring the intrinsic motivation and restriction functions of payment reform into effective play.

The second one is to combine with realities and adjust dynamically the NRCMCS payment standards. The direct purpose of payment reform is to control the unreasonable growth of medical expenses. To ensure the maneuverability and sustainability of the payment reform, we should respect for the reasonable reality of medical expenses and the reasonable growth in medical costs in the future. Therefore, the new payment standards should match with the survey of the baseline data and the reasonable estimates of the past medical costs. The definition of the payment standards for medical institutions at different levels should guide the NRCMCS participants with common diseases to seek medical treatment at grassroots. Meanwhile, the payment standards should be given practically routine adjustments in accordance with economic and social development, adjustment of compensation plan, changes in the cost of medical service, high and new medical technology application and the growing demands of residents for health services.

The third one is to give consideration to interests of many parties and ensure the sustainable development.

Whether the payment reform can be promoted smoothly and good effects be obtained relies on the disposition of the interests of the parties involved. The most direct object of the payment reform is medical institutions. Thus, if medical institutions do not actively cooperate, it will be difficult to greet the successful reform. Consequently, the mechanism of negotiation and consultation between the agencies handling the NRCMCS management and the designated medical institutions must be gradually established to negotiate and set the payment standards and other relevant matters. The agencies handling the NRCMCS management should not only consider payment ability of fund and individual burdens of medical expenses, but also give full consideration to the enthusiasm of the medical staff in the reform process so as to guarantee medical institutions to obtain fair compensation and safeguard normal operation and sustainable development in medical institutions.

The fourth one is to strengthen quality supervision and management, and ensure the service level. One of the fundamental targets of the payment reform is to improve the benefits enjoyed by the participants, medical service quality and level at the same time. The agencies handling the management must exploit the advantages of health departments in managing medical service in a wholly planned way and the NRCMCS to the full, jointly with medical management departments set up and improve the payment reform examination and evaluation system combined with handling and service supervision agreements, and make sure that there is no reduce in service contents, service level and guaranteed service quality provided by medical institutions after the implementation of the payment reform.

(2) To Elaborately Design the Implementation Scheme of the NRCMCS Payment Reform

The formulation of the implementation scheme of the NRCMCS payment reform should give the overall, meticulous and comprehensive considerations to the coverage of the people, calculation criteria, incentive and constraint, optimization selection and other factors to ensure the feasibility, maneuverability and effectiveness and give the focal assurance of the following points.

The first one is to maximize the coverage of the payment reform scheme. The payment reform of hospitalization expenses must cover medical institutions at county and township levels. The prefectures with license of handling ability should cover all the designated NRCMCS medical institutions under the premise of unified scheme and unified payment standard. The payment reform of outpatient expense should cover the designated medical institutions with wholly planned outpatient service within the county, and the places with proper conditions may gradually promote the implementation in county-level medical institutions. Simultaneously, the agencies handling urban and rural medical insurance should be invited to participate in the negotiations on some relevant work with the payment reform, and the payment reform of hospitalization expense in county-level hospitals, and the NRCMCS cooperated with urban and rural medical insurance should be launched to cover each hospitalized patient by the new payment for hospitalization expense.

The second one is to select the proper payment reform mode combined with the practical situations of the managing and handling abilities. Because there are greater differences in the NRCMCS managing and handling abilities, the level of informatization, facilities and conditions in medical institutions, the payment reform can't be in a fixed mode. Hospitalization expenses can charged in many kinds of modes such as payment by disease, by bed and day, the total prepayment, and mutual complementation of different modes to ensure each patient covered by rather proper and rather effective payment mode. The places with proper conditions may refer to the payment mode of Diagnosis Related Groups System(DRGs), improve gradually the payment mode by disease and realize the full effective coverage. The outpatient expenditures can give priority to total outpatient prepayment. The payment by capita for service provided by village (general) doctors at village level may be explored for practice. As for the larger outpatient expenses for special diseases, the payment mode of fixed sum of payment for fixed service can be explored for practice. The relatively mature reform pattern can be taken for the NRCMCS payment reform, and the new and effective methods of easy operation can be explored and innovated combined with local practice. No matter which payment mode is taken, we must make sure that the handling agencies are able to implement, supervise and manage, examine and evaluate.

The third one is to do a good job in calculations in a sturdy and meticulous way. Scientific and reasonable calculations is the base for the implementation of the NRCMCS payment reform, the calculation results should guarantee the rational interests of the patients on the one hand and make it acceptable by the two parties of medical institutions and medical insured persons on the other. The calculation on the payment of the total medical expenses should mainly rely on regional service population, outpatient rate, admission rate, the second-rate outpatient expenditure or the second-rate hospitalization expenses in recent 2 to 3 years, and make dynamic adjustment in accordance with economic growth, price fluctuations, and regional population mobility. The calculation on the payment by disease should involve the past average cost and is confirmed rationally combined with clinical pathway of the related diseases, medical resource consumption, and technology service, and the fluctuating space of some expenses should be given according to the changing law of self-development of some related diseases.

The fourth one is to attach great importance to the internal mechanism of incentive and constraint. The internal mechanism of incentive and constraint for medical service behaviors is the core connotation of the payment reform. Whether the payment mode of medical expense has the internal mechanism for automatic constraint of the unreasonable medical service behaviors, or is in favor of improving medical service quality, service efficiency and save medical service cost can determine whether the actual effect of the payment mode reform will be obtained. An effective mechanism will reduce the earnings which are beyond cost standards or from illegal service behaviors in the design. Therefore, only the reasonable and standardized medical service behaviors can maximize economic effectiveness. The payment reform on outpatient cost and hospitalization expenditures should contain this mechanism for the reform scheme for if there is not the internal mechanism of constraint and incentive, the reform must be a mere formality so the only way to go is to promote the changes in medical service behaviors with the help of the mechanism.

(3) To Do a Good Job in the Appraisal of the Supervision and Management of the NRCMCS Payment Reform Mode

A complete set of system of supervision, management and evaluation must be established while the scheme for the NRCMCS payment reform is implemented. The corresponding evaluation index, examining methods, and supervision and management measures should be established according to the characteristics of different payment modes and the key links, and the implementation scheme should be further improved aiming at the problems in the supervision and management.

In total outpatient prepayment, cost control should be supervised and evaluated, and what's more, regular examinations and evaluations should be given to outpatient service quantity, quality, treatment transfer and patients' satisfactory degree. As for the payment for hospitalization expenditures, diagnosis and treatment process should be supervised and managed, the implementation of hospital admission and discharge be examined, the monitoring and the return visit of the discharged patients, and the supervision and control of patients' hospitalization frequency should be done to improve reasonable diagnosis and treatment, and service quality and efficiency. The payment reform can not be obtained at the expense of service quality. Expense shifting to outpatient, upgraded diagnosis, disassembled hospitalization, unreasonable shortening patients' hospital stay and shuffling patients with severe diseases must be avoided. The results of medical service supervision and appraisal should be the fundamental base for the final NRCMCS payment.

The agencies handling the NRCMCS must give the corresponding punishment to the designated medical institutions according to medical service agreement or breach agreement on the appraisal of the payment mode reform implementation for the covert reduce in medical service quality, shuffling patients with severe diseases, purposeful evading payment mode settled by negotiation, and unreasonable cost transfer to patients' own expense in implementation of the payment reform. Medical administration and the departments of medical management must also give the corresponding punishment to the behaviors violating medical service standards and routines on drug abuse and bad check.

(4) To Do a Good Job in Coordination among Departments and Groundwork

Medical departments in each province (region and city) must deeply comprehend the significance of the NRCMCS payment mode reform, and the main leaders of departments and bureaus should be responsible for the implementation of the work. Communication and cooperation with the relevant departments of development and reform, finance must be enhanced to bring the joint force of the departments into full play and ensure the smooth advance of the NRCMCS payment mode reform. At the end of 2012, breakthroughs in coverage and implementing achievements based on the existing NRCMCS payment mode reform will be realized. At the appointed time, Ministry of Health will organize the related departments and experts to make tracking assessment of the standardized mode of payment reform.

Coordination and cooperation among the related departments within Ministry of Health should be done and comprehensive management must be intensified. Rural health (the NRCMCS) departments should take the lead in formulating implementation scheme and methods of supervision and management and the relevant trainings. Departments of medical administration and medical management should provide necessary technical support for payment mode reform from the aspects of clinical pathway selection and standards for diagnosis and treatment service, link payment mode reform and the reform in public hospitals, and enhance the supervision and management of medical service. Departments of finance should coordinate with the relevant departments to improve the measures for the implementation of the financial and accounting system in hospitals and grassroots medical institutions in accordance with the requirements of payment mode reform and provide necessarily basic conditions for the promotion of the new payment mode. Medical institutions and the agencies handling management should further improve information network connection and provide powerful support of information technology for the payment mode reform. Simultaneously, a good job should be done in the necessary propaganda to improve the understanding the significance of payment mode reform of the relevant departments, guide the masses to learn about the work, let the patients participate in, and cooperate with the advance of payment mode reform and bring the promotion of social supervision on the reform into full play.

The implementation of one reform measure progresses relatively smooth in the early pilot stage but it will face greater difficulties and more problems with its gradual promotion. Medical reform follows the pattern so does the implementation of a concrete policy. It is rather easy for the NRCMCS pilot payment mode reform to happen in a small scale with small resistance and advance smoothly. However, we should make greater efforts and do more work to guide the medical institutions from industry level to optimize management, standardize service, control cost, improve efficiency and obtain real effects of reform. The payment mode reform is the key of the NRCMCS work in 2012 and one of the important contents of medical reform. All provinces (regions and cities) must focus on the standardized promotion of the NRCMCS payment mode reform as an important task of medical reform of this year, arrange in a wholly-planned way, make progress in a planned step-by-step way, scheme, standard and examination, do a good job in accordance with the Guiding Opinions and make greater contributions to the further NRCMCS consolidation and development.

(Ji Chenglian)

5. Maintain Confidence, Focus on the Key Issues and Push forward the Comprehensive Pilot Reform of the Public County Hospitals Actively and Steadily
—A Speech of Health Minister Chen Zhu Delivered at the Video and Telephone Conference on the Comprehensive Pilot Reform of the Public County Hospitals (June 19, 2012)

The Central Committee and the State Council have attached great importance to the reform of the public hospitals. After 3 years' piloting, the reform of the public county hospitals is further taken as the key point to guarantee the rural residents' health and push forward the balanced economic and social development of urban and rural areas. On February 22nd, premier Wen Jiabao presided over the committee meeting of the State Council and studied the deployments for deepening the reform of the medical and pharmaceutical systems during the 12th Five-Year Plan. The periodic goals for the reform of the public county hospitals by 2015 were set. At this year's national meeting on the health care reform, vice premier Li Keqiang emphasized that the reform of the public county hospitals should be put at the prominent position in the reform of public hospitals to lessen the problems of poor affordability and accessibility in seeking medical service for the residents in counties. Today, Ministry of Health, the Health Care Reform Office of the State Council, the State Commission Office for Public Sector Reform, Ministry of Finance and Ministry of Human Resources and Human Security jointly held the video and telephone conference to fix the arrangements for the comprehensive piloting reform of the public county hospitals. I would like to speak 3 opinions for reference.

I. The importance of the reform of the public county hospitals should be fully realized

The public county hospitals are the important places to provide medical service for the rural residents and the foremost part of the three-tier rural medical service network. In the deployments for the medical reform of the State Council for the 12th Five-Year Plan, the reform of the public county hospitals will be put at a more prominent place, which shows the determination of the central government to build the grassroots medical service network and to realize the universal coverage of primary health service.

Pushing forward the reform of the public county hospitals is the necessary path to realize the goals of China's health care reform. The county hospitals provide medical service for more than 900,000,000 residents. Only by pushing forward the reform and promoting the overall development of the urban and rural areas can the county residents enjoy the accomplishments of the reform, the public service be accessed fairly and the universal coverage of the basic medical service be realized. Pushing forward the reform of the public county hospitals is the breakthrough point for the reform of public hospitals. The county hospitals are at the dominant position in the public hospital system but they are also the weakest link. Pushing forward the reform of the public county hospitals will elevate the ability of the service system, even the distribution of patients and provide experience and favorable condition for the reform of public hospitals in the cities. Pushing forward the reform of the public county hospitals is the necessary requirement for the health care reform in the counties. With the perfection of the basic medical insurance system, the mass people's needs for medical service are released and higher requirements are raised for the medical service of the public county hospitals. Pushing forward the reform of the public county hospitals is also the important move to strengthen the accomplishments in the comprehensive reform of the county medical institutions. Pushing forward the reform of the public county hospitals is a great impetus to the economic and social development in the counties. At present, the position of the counties in the overall economic and social development is increasingly prominent. The reform and development of the public county hospitals is not only the urgent need for the improvement of the people's livelihood and the construction of the harmonious socialist society but also the guarantee to the economic and social development of the counties.

The 3 years' practice of the health care reform has proofed that "satisfying the basic needs, strengthening the grassroots institutions and establishing mechanisms" is a path that suits China's situation. The establishment of the basic medical service network with the county hospitals as the foremost part and the improvement of the medical service quality in the counties are the basic measures to solve the problem of poor medical accessibility of rural residents. According to the important instructions of the Central Committee and the State Council, Ministry of Health and the Health

Care Reform Office of the State Council have been highly concerned with the exploration in pushing forward the reform of the public county hospitals by the local departments. Since the on-the-spot meeting of Zichang county of Shaanxi province was held in November of 2011, the experience of Shaanxi and other provinces/regions/municipalities has been summed up and popularized. Up till now, over 600 county hospitals in 19 provinces/regions/municipalities have participated in the pilot reform, which has laid foundation for deepening the reform of the county hospitals.

The reform of the county hospitals involves profound readjustments of the benefit structure. Because the economic and social development of the urban and rural areas is not balanced, the service ability of county hospitals varies greatly from place to place and the reform cannot be done overnight. Therefore, 311 counties of 18 provinces/municipalities are selected to carry out the pilot reform and then the policies would be perfected and the reform will be popularized based on the experience of the reform.

II. The overall requirements and policies for the pilot reform of the public county hospitals should be properly comprehended

A few days ago, *The Opinions of the State Council on the Pilot Reform of the Public County Hospitals* (hereinafter referred to as *The Opinions*) was issued by the general office of the State Council, which closely follows the overall deployments of the Central Committee and the State Council for deepening the reform of the medical and pharmaceutical systems and the main spirits for pushing forward the reform of the public sectors. *The Opinions* also clarifies the overall requirements and policies for the pilot reform of the public county hospitals.

We should grasp the basic goals of the comprehensive pilot reform of the public county hospitals. The reform and development of the county hospitals should be in line not only with the overall requirements for the reform of public hospitals but also with the characteristics and functions of the county hospitals. The public nature should be upheld to satisfy the basic medical needs of the county residents. Thus, the problems of poor affordability and accessibility in seeking medical service will be solved and the rate of outpatient within the counties will reach 90%. In addition, the experience will be accumulated and paths will be explored for the public hospital reform in cities.

We should clarify the overall requirements for the comprehensive pilot reform of the public county hospitals. Abolishing the compensation system for the medical cost through drug-selling profits is the key point. The compensation system should be reformed, the administration and supervision should be implemented, the comprehensive reform should be pushed forward according to plans and the mechanisms that boost the public nature, the initiative and the sustainable development of the county hospitals should be established. We should stick to the reform to promote development, strengthen the capacity building and formulate the overall plans for the development of the health system in the counties to make sure that the major diseases can be treated within the counties. We shall deal well with the relations among reform, development and management. For the goals that will benefit the general public, the reform is the foundation and guarantee. The development and the management are the foothold of the reform, for the development will improve the ability and the management will improve service. The mechanism innovation, the capacity building and the enhancement of collaboration are the 3 key links that should be made full use of. While reforming the systems and mechanisms, the capacity building for the weak departments of pediatrics, gynecology, psychiatry and infectious diseases should be intensified to increase the general service ability of the county hospitals. The collaboration of departments at different levels should be promoted to elevate the overall service ability of the health system and to satisfy the people's basic needs for health service within the counties. The public nature of the county hospitals and the initiative of doctors should be maintained. The doctors should take initiative in the health care reform and without their enthusiasm the public nature can't be realized. The harmonious doctor-patient relationship is the basis for all the policies to work well.

We should do well the main task of abolishing the compensation system for the medical cost through drug-selling profits. It is the key link in the comprehensive reform of the county hospitals. The experience of the health care reform at the grassroots level should be used for reference. We should adjust the prices of medical service, reform the insurance payment models and implement the fiscal policies to ensure that the drug-selling profits will be eliminated in the over 600 piloting hospitals. Efforts should be made to implement the basic drug policy in county hospitals, the basic drug catalogue should be perfected to meet the needs of the counties and the purchase and supply of the drugs should be normalized. The relevant departments should be organized to create favorable conditions to enlarge the pilot and to abolish the compensation system for the medical cost through drug-selling profits in county hospitals by 2013 and in all the public hospitals by 2015.

The policies and measures of the pilot reform of the public county hospitals should be sincerely carried out. The 7 main tasks of the pilot reform of the public county hospitals include: clarifying functions and orientations, reforming the compensation mechanism, reforming the human resource system, establishing the modern hospital management system, elevating the basic medical service ability, strengthening collaboration of departments at different levels and optimizing the supervisory mechanism.

The system that will maintain the public nature, boost the initiative and guarantee the sustainable development of the public county hospitals should be established by reforming the compensatory mechanism. The association of medical insurance, prices and fiscal measures should be made full use of to abolish the compensation system for the medical cost through drug-selling profits. The medical service system and the medical insurance system should be closely linked. The payment models of the new rural cooperative medical care system like paying according to the number of people and the kind of diseases should be pushed forward to realize the full coverage of the payment reform in the pilot county hospitals. The competitive human resource mechanism and the incentive-based distribution system should be established and perfected to mobilize the medical workers. The county hospitals should be managed autonomously and the administration and supervision should be strengthened.

The construction of the talent contingent should be enhanced through the reform to improve the service ability of the county hospitals. Special positions should be set up and subsidies should be provided to attract talents from cities to counties. The treatment and insurance for 20 major diseases should be bettered and the medical service ability of relevant departments should be enhanced as well. The role of the county hospitals as the connecting link should be fully utilized to form the situation where the prevention and treatment will be combined. The construction of the talent contingent should be enhanced. The Project of Thousands Doctors' Support for the Rural Area and the training of the backbone doctors in the county hospitals should be continued. The normalized training of resident doctors and the general practitioner system should be implemented and the information network for telemedicine and tele-consultation should be set up to ensure that all the county hospital reach the level of a First-class Hospital at Grade 2.

The affordability and accessibility to medical service should be realized through the reform and the major diseases will be treated within the counties. The system should be patient-centered with the medical insurance paid immediately and the nursing service bettered to raise the satisfaction of the patients. The clinical paths should be formulated and the county quality control centers should assume their responsibilities to normalize the medical activities and control the medical expenses. The labor division and cooperation mechanism between county hospitals and township hospitals should be established, the coverage of techniques should be enlarged and the training of medical workers and medical tours should be conducted. In addition, the two-way referral system should be set up. Thus, the ability of medical service network that covers the counties, townships and villages will be elevated and the major diseases can be treated without leaving the counties.

The harmonious doctor-patient relationship should be forged through the reform. All the pilot counties should adopt the mechanism of the third-party mediation. Specialized departments and persons should be set up to be in charge of the patients' rights. A specialized government fund should be arranged to buy medical liability insurance for the pilot county hospitals.

III. The leadership should be strengthened and the implementation should be intensified to push forward the comprehensive pilot reform of the public county hospitals actively and steadily

The organization and management of the pilot reform of the public county hospitals should be done well by strengthening the leadership. The Scientific Outlook on Development should be implemented in strengthening the sense of responsibility. The provincial health departments should actively carry out the responsibility of coordination and push forward the establishment of the coordinating mechanism among relevant departments. The policies in price adjustment, human resources management and internal distribution should also be implemented by them with certain autonomy left to the pilot institutions. Ministry of Health and other central departments should trace the pilot reform closely, organize experts to access the pilot areas and strengthen the guidance and support to the pilot work.

The duties of the government should be fulfilled and the policies should be implemented vigorously. The planning and distribution of the health industry within the counties should be done well. The structure and layout of county hospitals should be rational and the guidance and restriction to the development of the county hospitals should be strengthened. Supervision should be intensified to prevent the hospitals from expanding blindly. The financing duty should be fulfilled and the investment for the proper infrastructure construction of the county hospitals should be made. However, the construction with loans borrowed should be prohibited. The ways of solving the long-term debts of the county hospitals should be explored so the county hospitals can develop without burdens.

The health departments at all levels should function well as the administrative bodies with a sense of mission and responsibility. They should do well the initiative work for the comprehensive pilot reform of the public county hospitals. Recently, vice premier Li Keqiang made important instructions. He said, "Over the 3 years, the whole health system and the medical workers have done a lot of work to push forward the health care reform, accomplished all the major tasks and functioned as the main force. According to requirements of the deployments and action plans of the health care reform during the 12th Five-Year Plan, the periodic achievements should be consolidated and efforts should be focused on the difficult problems like the reform of the public hospitals. Thus, the health care reform can be further pushed forward." The health administrative departments at all levels shoul d follow the instructions of Li Keqiang and make efforts to mobilize all the medical workers to conquer difficulties to complete the plans for the 12th Five-Year Plan. The action organization and management should be centered on the weak points in the county hospitals. The manpower problem in the county hospitals should be solved. The construction of the training system of resident doctors and general practitioners should be intensified. Centering on the medical needs within the counties, the development plans for special medical disciplines and the plans for the establishment of special positions should be drawn. The counterpart aid between cities and rural areas and the training of backbone doctors should be intensified and the supervision and inspection should be carried out to ensure the completion of the tasks. The service ability of the county hospitals should be continuously elevated. The service and insurance for the 20 major diseases should be well conducted. The treatment ability of the county hospital for diseases like cervical cancer, breast caner and terminal renal diseases should be elevated to provide adequate service for the patients. The screening of diseases like childhood leukemia and congenital heart disease should be done well and the referral system should be established. The supervision on the medical institutions and medical workers should be earnestly conducted. The professional ethics that represents the essence of the nature of medicine should be cultivated and the impetus against corruption should be formed. The cases in the field of medicine purchase and sale should be firmly handled and the unhealthy practice should be eliminated. Cooperation with the financial departments should be actively carried out and the investment policies of the governments should be conscientiously implemented. The fiscal investments for the reform should be well managed, the supervision on the investments enhanced and the utilization rate of the investments elevated.

The medical workers in the county hospitals should participate in the reform with enthusiasm. The management ability of the hospitals should be elevated by means of the informatization and the clinic path management. The service that is beneficial to the mass people should be conducted to improve their satisfaction with medical service. The income of the medical workers should be increased, the clinical workers should be favored in income distribution and the ratio of the expenditure for medical workers to the operational expenditure should be raised to mobilize the medical workers.

The reform of the public county hospitals is a major task of the health care reform in the 12th Five-Year Plan. We believe that with the strong leadership of the Central

Committee and the State Council, the enthusiastic support of the mass people, the close collaboration of all departments and the pioneering spirits of the pilot areas we will be able to push forward the reform actively and steadily and make more contribution to solving the problem of poor accessibility to medical service for the county residents.

(Qu Yang)

6. Serve the Overall Development and Strive to Make New Progress in the Scientific Development of the Undertaking of the Traditional Chinese Medical Science and Medicines
—Working Report by Wang Guoqiang, Vice Minister of the Ministry of Health and Concurrently Commissioner of the State Administration of Traditional Chinese Medicine (TCM) at the 2012 National Working Conference on Traditional Chinese Medicine (January 10, 2012)

The main task of this year's National Working Conference on Traditional Chinese Medicine is to thoroughly carry through the spirit of the 17th National Congress of the Party, the 5th and 6th Plenary Session of the 17th Central Committee of the Party, the Central Economic Working Conference and the National Health Working Conference, follow the guidance of Deng Xiaoping Theory and the important thought of the Three Representatives, deeply study and practice the Scientific Outlook on Development, profoundly analyze the situation faced with the reform and development of the traditional Chinese medical science and medicines, focus on the major task of promoting the scientific development of the undertaking of the traditional Chinese medical science and medicines, take full implementation of the *Several Opinions* of the State Council in the in-depth medical and health care reform as the underlying guideline, review the work experience in 2011, make deployment for main tasks in 2012, comprehensively implement the *12th Five-Year Plan for the Development of the Undertaking of the Traditional Chinese Medical Science and Medicines*, seize opportunities, serve the overall development and strive to make new progress in the scientific development of the undertaking of the traditional Chinese medical science and medicines.

The State Council attached great importance to the conference and Li Keqiang, member of the Standing Committee of the Political Bureau and Vice Premier, made an important instruction specially, in which he fully affirmed the last year's achievements in the development of the undertaking of traditional Chinese medical science and medicines and put forward ardent hopes and requirements for new year's work. Chen Zhu, Minister of the Ministry of Health, attended the conference and delivered an important speech and will put forward specific requirements for further improvement of the work and fulfillment of new tasks in deepening the medical and health care reform in new situations. We must earnestly learn and fully understand leaders' instructions and implement them comprehensively.

Next, I'm to talk about my opinions on three aspects for your discussion.

I. Review of work in 2011

The year 2011 was a crucial year for fully carrying out the *Several Opinions* of the State Council and also the first year for developing the undertaking of the traditional Chinese medical science and medicines in the 12th Five-Year-Plan period. Under the correct leadership of the Party Central Committee and the State Council and with the high attention paid by the Ministry of Health, staff members of the whole system jointly worked hard, made reform and innovation, did solid work and remarkable progress was achieved in all respects.

(1) The influence of the traditional Chinese medical science and medicines in economic and social development was further improved

While seriously formulating and implementing the *12th Five-Year Plan for the Development of the Undertaking of the Traditional Chinese Medical Science and Medicines*, we made active coordination and made efforts to incorporate the development of the traditional Chinese medical science and medicines into relevant plans so as to further improve the position and role in economic and social development. Firstly, development of the traditional Chinese medical science and medicines was listed as a separate part and as one of the five major tasks for the improvement of the basic medical and health care systems in the *Outline of the 12th Five-Year Plan for National Economic and Social Development of the People's Republic of China* (hereinafter referred to as "the *Outline*"), meanwhile, the traditional Chinese medical science and medicines was also taken as a part in the improvement of foreign trade structure and the maintenance of long-term stability and prosperity in Hong Kong and Macao. Secondly, the traditional Chinese medical science and medicines was taken as an important part in the improvement of science and technology for people's livelihood in national special plans for relevant fields, such as the *National 12th Five-Year Plan for Science & Technology Development,* the *12th Five-Year Plan for Medical Science & Technology Development* and so on. The engineering of cultivating the talents in the inheritance and innovation of the traditional Chinese medical science and medicines was taken as one of the five major ones in the *Medium- and Long-Term Development Program on Medical and Health Talents(2011-2020)*. We actively coordinated with relevant sectors and strived to corporate the traditional Chinese medical science and medicines into plans for other relevant fields. Thirdly, with active support of member units of the Inter-Ministerial Joint Conference on the work of the traditional Chinese medical science and medicines, we fulfilled the formulation of the 12th *Five-Year Plan for the Development of the Undertaking of the Traditional Chinese Medical Science and Medicines*, organized the implementation and put into effect some major projects in the *Plan* such as the construction of service capacity in TCM hospitals (hospitals of ethnic minority medicine). Moreover, we already finished or sped up the formulation of special plans on informatization standardization, scientific and technological innovation, cultural construction and foreign exchange and cooperation. Fourthly, all the localities smoothly formulated and implemented 12th Five-Year plan for the development of the traditional Chinese medical science and medicines and many localities attached more importance to the formulation of the plan and gave greater support to the development of the traditional Chinese medical science and medicines. For example, Shanghai and some other localities incorporated the development of the traditional Chinese medical science and medicines into provincial or municipal special plans for the first time; Inner Mongolia listed the capital construction of all city-level and county-level hospitals of Mongolian medicine and traditional Chinese medicine into the 12th Five-Year Plan of Inner Mongolia Autonomous Region; Liaoning Province allocated 45 million yuan of special funds for supporting the development of the traditional Chinese medical science and medicines and planned to continue the allocation in the 12th Five-Year-Plan period; Hubei Province strengthened the construction of the infrastructure of all the TCM hospitals. Listing the traditional Chinese medical science and medicines as a separate part and as one of the major six tasks for the improvement of the basic medical and health care systems in the *National 12th Five-Year Plan* and incorporating the traditional Chinese medical science and medicines into relevant national special plans not only fully represented the high attention attached by the party and government, but also showed the increasingly important position and role in our country's development strategies and the huge potential and bright prospect for future development. It should be noted that the fulfillment of the survey on the basic status quo of traditional Chinese medicine provided a powerful support for our country and all the localities to accurately understand the development situations and scientifically plan the objectives and tasks.

(2) The role of the traditional Chinese medical science and medicines was brought into further play in the in-depth medical and health care reform

In 2011, the Ministry of Health and the State Administration of Traditional Chinese Medicine jointly issued the *Opinions on Further Playing the Role of Traditional Chinese Medicine in Deepening the Reform of the Medical and Health Care Systems* (hereinafter referred to as *Opinions*) which made comprehensive deployment on how to bring the role of the traditional Chinese medical science and medicines into further play and strengthen the talent cultivation in fulfilling the five major tasks of the in-depth medical and heath care reform. What has been done is a specific action of the Ministry of Health and the State Administration of Traditional Chinese Medicine to carry out the spirits of deepening the medical and health care reform of the Party Central Committee and the *Several Opinions* of the State Council and an important measure to construct our country's basic medical and health care systems.

In the past three years, we continuously promoted the active participation of the traditional Chinese medical science and medicines in the fulfillment of the five major tasks of the in-depth medical and heath care reform and positive progress was gained. Firstly, in the construction of the basic medical security system, more attention was paid to encouraging the offering and use of traditional Chinese medical services. Increase in the subsidiary percentage of the traditional Chinese medical science and medicines required by the new rural cooperative medical care system further stirred up farmers' enthusiasm and they reaped benefits from using them. Henan Province printed and issued the *Notice on Issues concerning the Guidance and Encouragement of the Use of the Services of the Traditional Chinese Medical Science and Medicines by the Basic Medical Insurance for Non-Working Urban Residents*. The number of service items of traditional Chinese medicine and traditional Chinese medicines covered by medical insurance grew unceasingly. 987 Chinese patent drugs were listed in the Drug Catalogs of National Basic Medical Insurance, Industrial Insurance and Birth Insurance (2009 edition), 164 drugs added compared with last edition, and most provinces (autonomous regions, cities) took Chinese herbal preparations of medical institutions into the coverage of medical insurance. Secondly, in the construction of the essential drug system, the principle of putting equal stress on traditional Chinese medicine and western medicine was insisted on and attention was attached to the encouragement of the use of traditional Chinese medicines. 102 Chinese patent drugs and the Chinese traditional medical herbal pieces with issued national standard were listed in the *National Essential Drug List (for provision and use of grassroots medical and health institutions)* and all the localities actively promoted the addition of traditional Chinese medicines to the supplementary list. The added categories outnumbered western medicines in some localities; traditional Chinese medicines increased amounted to nearly 62 % in Guizhou Province and most of the supplemented medicines in Tibet Autonomous Region and some other ethnic minority areas were mainly traditional ethnic medicines. Thirdly, in the work of gradual equalization of the basic public health services, we positively promoted the application of techniques and methods of health prevention and health protection with the traditional Chinese medical science and medicines. In the *National Basic Public Health Service Norms (2011 edition)*, requirements of traditional Chinese medical services for child health care were supplemented and requirements for the health management of patients with hypertension and type II diabetes were made more specific; technical specifications for TCM health management of children, pregnant and puerperal women, old people and patients with hypertension and type II diabetes were formulated; at the same time, pilot work of service items of the traditional Chinese medical science and medicines was initiated in the basic public health services. In Gansu Province, TCM department was established in all the disease prevention and control institutions; "preventive treatment of diseases" in traditional Chinese medicine was taken as a service item in the basic public health services and contents concerning the traditional Chinese medical science and medicines were required to account for no less than 20 % and 30% in residents' health records and health education respectively. 10 yuan of special fund per capita was allocated to people aged over 55 years for the identification of constitution in traditional Chinese medicine in Qingdao, Shandong Province; it was required in Shijiazhuang, Hebei Province, that no less than 10 percent of funds for public health service items should be used for the treatment with the traditional Chinese medical science and medicines; 10 yuan of the total 25 yuan of public health funds was set specially for each person's payment for TCM service items in Gongshu District of Hangzhou, Zhejiang Province. Fourthly, in the construction of urban and rural basic medical and health service systems, we attached importance to the improvement of the accessibility to traditional Chinese medical services. 382 county-level TCM hospitals were reconstructed and standardization was promoted in the construction of the department of traditional Chinese medicine and the dispensary of traditional Chinese medicines in a great number of township and community health care centers. 13 prefecture-level, city-level and above cities including Beijing, Tianjin, Shanghai, Hangzhou and so on and 139 counties (county-level cities, districts) won the honorary title of "Advanced Unit" in the national grassroots (countryside, community) TCM work, which energetically motivated the enthusiasm for support and concern from local governments and the whole society for the development of urban and rural grassroots TCM work. Achievements were gained in the exploration of unified management of county-level, township and village rural work of the traditional Chinese medicine and medicines (ethnic minority medical science and medicines) in provinces of Anhui and Heilongjiang and autonomous regions of Guangxi and Inner Mongolia Autonomous Region. Yunnan Province allocated 12.3 million yuan to the provision of medical equipment for 4,100 village clinics. All the township health care centers in Hubei Province conducted the construction of "*san tang yi shi*"("*san tang*":*guo yi tang*:place for national honored great TCM masters practicing medicine; *ming yi tang*: place for famous TCM doctors practicing medicine;

yang sheng tang: place for people to consult on health preservation; *yi shi*: famous TCM doctors' workroom). In Tianjin, the construction of *"guo yi tang"* was pushed forward comprehensively in community and township health service centers and exploration was made in the patterns of comprehensive services of TCM general practice. 10 prescriptions of Chinese traditional medical herbal pieces and 10 appropriate techniques were formulated and popularized for the treatment of 4 diseases commonly seen at the grassroots level in Ningxia Autonomous Region. What had been done effectively promoted the service capacity of the traditional Chinese medical science and medicines in grassroots medical institutions. Fifthly, we actively conducted the pilot of the reform of public TCM hospitals and paid attention to bringing the characteristics and superiorities into play. All the localities made efforts to explore the investment and compensation mechanisms that were beneficial to bringing the characteristics and superiorities into play. Fully-budgeted management was conducted for the salaries of the staff in public hospitals of traditional Chinese medicine (ethnic minority medicine) in provinces (autonomous regions, cities) of Beijing, Inner Mongolia, Shaanxi and so on. Patients going to TCM outpatient department and inpatient department of government-run hospitals were subsidized 8 yuan each time and 15 yuan each day respectively in Ningbo of Zhejiang Province. Exploration in compensatory mechanisms for traditional Chinese medical services in public TCM hospitals was carried out in Jining of Shandong Province and Pingxiang of Jiangxi Province. A large body of TCM hospitals continuously perfected performance evaluation systems and made active exploration in the incentive mechanisms that encouraged the application of techniques and methods of the traditional Chinese medical science and medicines. The pilot work of comprehensive reform in county-level TCM hospitals was pushed forward in an orderly way and the pilot of the formulation and implementation of clinical pathways of traditional Chinese medicine developed gradually, the total number of TCM clinical pathways being up to 210. The activity of TCM hospital management year with the theme of "taking patients as the center, play of the characteristics and superiorities of the traditional Chinese medical science and medicines as the focus" was carried out more deeply; measures beneficial to the masses were put into effect; the process of diagnosis and treatment was optimized and medical conducts were regulated. The engineering that promoted the application of TCM medical equipment was carried out; small packages of Chinese traditional medical herbal pieces were popularized and used; guidance on the construction and management of clinical departments were intensified and the construction of key specialties was promoted orderly; the connotation construction of TCM hospitals was strengthened and the maintenance and play of the characteristics and superiorities were pushed forward, as a result, patients had a better feeling and environment when seeing doctor. Meanwhile, the work of integrating traditional Chinese medicine with Western medicine and the work of ethnic minority medical science and medicines were intensified continuously. Evaluation and acceptance inspection on 9 hospitals of traditional Chinese medicine and Western medicine of the key construction project were complete and on the basis of summary of the experience, working guidelines for hospitals of traditional Chinese medicine and Western medicine were formulated. The acceptance inspection on 10 hospitals of ethnic minority medicine of the key construction project finished and investigation on the standards of medical qualification examination for the doctors of ethnic minority medicine was conducted. 93 general hospitals were constructed into the exemplary units of traditional Chinese medical work. The State Administration of Traditional Chinese Medicine issued opinions on the intensification of folk medical work in order to further promote the exploration in it.

(3) Policies and measures put forward in the *Several Opinions* were further implemented

In the three year since the issue of the *Several Opinions* of the State Council, we continuously gave priority to "development" and "support and promotion" and carried out all the policies and measures put forward in the *Several Opinions* in an earnest way. The first was to make greater efforts to promote the implementation of the *Several Opinions* in all the localities. All-level party committees and governments attached more importance to the development of the undertaking of the traditional Chinese medical science and medicines, strengthened organization and leadership, rendered more policy support and financial investment and adopted measures to promote solution to difficulties and problems, which forcefully forwarded the development of the undertaking of the traditional Chinese medical science and medicines in each locality. Last year, provinces of Liaoning, Heilongjiang, Hunan, Shaanxi and Hebei issued the implementation opinions on supporting and promoting the development of the traditional Chinese medical science and medicines or the action plans on accelerating the development; Guangxi Zhuang Autonomous Region issued the decisions on accelerating the development of traditional Chinese medical science and medicines and the ethnic minority medical science and medicines, the plans for vitalization of Zhuang and Yao medical science and medicines and the implementation schemes on 10 key projects concerning the development of the traditional Chinese medical science and medicines and the ethnic minority medical science and medicines; Sichuan Province and Xinjiang Uygur Autonomous Region fulfilled the draft of the implementation opinions on carrying out the *Several Opinions* of the State Council and planned to issue the opinions after amendment. Provinces of Jilin, Shaanxi, Hebei, Guizhou and Hunan held conferences on the development of the traditional Chinese medical science and medicines and the industry of traditional Chinese medicines in the name of provincial governments and Tibet Autonomous Region and some other regions also sped up preparation for such conferences. Moreover, principal party and governmental leaders of numerous provinces (autonomous regions, cities) such as Hebei, Shanxi, Jilin, etc. gave instructions and put forward requirements on the acceleration of the development of the traditional Chinese medical science and medicines. Since the issue of the *Several Opinions*, 19 provinces (autonomous regions, cities) issued special documents on the implementation opinions on carrying through and implementing the *Several Opinions* or on the support and promotion of the development of the undertaking of the traditional Chinese medical science and medicines and 11 provinces (autonomous regions, cities) held conferences on the traditional Chinese medical science and medicines and the ethnic minority medical science and medicines in the name of Party committee or government. The second was to strengthen the joint action of all-level administrations in order to make innovation in the working mechanisms that promote the scientific development of the undertaking of the traditional Chinese medical science and medicines. On the basis of the comprehensive reform pilot in Pudong New District in Shanghai and Dongcheng District in Beijing, last year the State Administration of Traditional Chinese Medicine signed an agreement with Gansu Provincial Government on the construction of the demonstrative province of the pilot of comprehensive reform in the development of the traditional Chinese medical science and medicines, a cooperative agreement with Hainan Provincial Government on the promotion of the development of the traditional Chinese medical science and medicines, a cooperative agreement with Chongqing Municipal Government on the promotion of overall-planning urban and rural development of the undertaking of the traditional Chinese medical science and medicines and issued specific opinions on the support to the development of the undertaking of Tibetan medical science and medicines in Tibet Autonomous Region and the leapfrog development of the undertaking of the traditional Chinese medical science and medicines in Xinjiang Production and Construction Corps. The State Administration of Traditional Chinese Medicine incorporated "promotion of the development of the traditional Chinese medical science and medicines" into the agreement signed by the Ministry of Health and Shanghai Municipal Government on further deepening ministerial-municipal cooperation, signed agreements with Jiangsu Provincial Government and Henan Provincial Government respectively on joint construction of Nanjing University of Chinese Medicine and Henan University of Traditional Chinese Medicine and offered support to the China Academy of Chinese Medical Sciences and Qinghai Tibetan Medicine Research Institute for signing the agreement on cooperative promotion of the researches on the inheritance and innovation of Tibetan medical science and medicines. The third was to make efforts to obtain more support and further increase investment in the development of the traditional Chinese medical science and medicines. In 2011, the central government invested nearly 6 billion yuan, of which the newly-added 4.212 billion yuan were invested in the construction of service capacity for 1,814 county-level hospitals of traditional Chinese medicine (hospitals of ethnic minority medicine), 58 prefecture-level and city-level hospitals of ethnic minority medicine and 88 prefecture-level and city-level hospitals of traditional Chinese medicine in the western regions; 1.014 billion yuan were allocated for supporting the construction of 70 county-level hospitals of traditional Chinese medicine; 300 million yuan of newly-added funds were invested in the construction of 88 TCM specialties in the national construction project of key clinical specialties and 412 million yuan were allocated for supporting the construction project of workrooms for inheritance of national veteran TCM doctors' experience and so on. Meanwhile, all-level governments also increased input in the development substantially. In the past three years, the central government invested over 17.3 billion yuan all together, of which 4.53 billion yuan of special funds were arranged for support of the construction of 16 national TCM clinical research bases and 313 prefecture-level, city-level and above key TCM hospitals and the investment task in the *Plan for the Construction and Development of Key Hospitals of Traditional Chinese Medicine* was fulfilled smoothly. 5.67 billion yuan of special funds were allocated for supporting the construction of 382 county-level TCM hospitals and 7.143 billion yuan of special funds were allocated to county-level TCM hospitals for organizing and conducting the construction of the capacity for first-aid treatment in emergency department, the construction of the dispensary of traditional Chinese medicines, the training of TCM general practitioners, the construction of key TCM disciplinary fields and specialties and the popularization of TCM techniques appropriate for common diseases and frequently-encountered diseases at the grassroots level and other projects for the construction of the capacity for traditional Chinese medical services in city-level and county-level TCM hospitals (hospitals of ethnic minority medicine). At the same time, all-level governments also increased investment dramatically. The fourth was to strengthen communication and coordination and make the policies and measures on supporting and promoting the development of the traditional Chinese medical science and medicines more specific. For example, contents concerning the traditional Chinese medical science and medicines were included in the *Guiding Opinions of the State Council on Establishing the System of General Practitioners*, which provided a policy guarantee for TCM general practitioners' standardized training, admittance and employment; the *Guiding Opinions of the General Office of the State Council on further*

Strengthening the Construction of the Contingent of Village Doctors clarified village doctors' responsibilities and requirements for their treatment of rural residents with common diseases and frequently-encountered diseases with the traditional Chinese medical science and medicines. The plan for directional and tuition-free cultivation of rural medical students was worked out last year and 1,093 college students majoring in traditional Chinese medicine were enrolled. The pilot of reform in modes of cultivating TCM clinical talents combining college education with master-disciple education was launched and reform in education and teaching of TCM colleges and universities was promoted. The first selection of "National Honored Great Master of Traditional Chinese Medicine" was conducted; methods for the appraisal of titles of TCM medical staff's professional and technical posts were adjusted and exploration was made in the establishment of incentive mechanisms for TCM talents. The construction of the systems of clinical research on the prevention and treatment of infectious diseases with the traditional Chinese medical science and medicines and the special projects or subjects concerning the traditional Chinese medical science and medicines were set up in 973 Program (Key Project of Chinese National Programs for Fundamental Research and Development), the National Science and Technology Support Program, the special science and technology projects of public-welfare industries and the major special science and technology projects on the prevention and treatment of infectious diseases and the creation and preparation of new medicines. Registration systems for traditional Chinese medicines were perfected and opinions on strengthening the management of Chinese herbal preparations in medical institutions were discussed and worked out. Measures on the intensification of the work of TCM intellectual property were put forward and policies on the promotion of the development of TCM service trade were clarified. Implementation schemes for recent prior work in ethnic minority medical science and medicines were issued to accelerate the promotion of the development. Moreover, in close cooperation with the Health Bureau of the PLA Logistic Department,we actively promoted the integration of military-civil resources of the traditional Chinese medical science and medicines and made the military TCM work fully play the leading role.

(4) New progress was made in the legislation of the *Law of the People's Republic of China on Traditional Chinese Medicine*, the standardization and the informatization

The *Law of the People's Republic of China on Traditional Chinese Medicine (Draft)* (hereinafter referred to as *Draft*) was adopted after examination and approval by the conference of the Ministry of Health and was reported to the State Council by the end of 2011. The general train of thought of the *Draft* included following points: the first was to focus on the legislative purpose of protection, support and promotion of the development of the traditional Chinese medical science and medicines; the second was to obey developmental laws, embody the characteristics of the traditional Chinese medical science and medicines, attach importance to institutional innovation and strive to make breakthroughs; the third was to take traditional Chinese medical services as foundation, highlight the characteristics and superiorities and satisfy people's needs for the services of the traditional Chinese medical science and medicines; the fourth was to highlight focal points, make overall plans and take all factors into consideration and promote the comprehensive, coordinative and sustainable development of the traditional Chinese medical science and medicines. The *Draft* gave priority to the play of the characteristics and role of the traditional Chinese medical science and medicines, the intensification of inheritance, the encouragement of innovation and the promotion of the coordinative development of traditional Chinese medical science and traditional Chinese medicines and made institutional arrangements. Rapid progress in the legislation of the traditional Chinese medical science and medicines in recent years benefited from following respects. First of all, foundation for the legislation was solid. The issue of the *Several Opinions* of the State Council laid a solid foundation of policy and guarantee for the legislation; successful exploration in reform and innovation and practice in all the localities provided a profound basis of practice and masses and the issue and implementation of the *Regulation of the People's Republic of China on Traditional Chinese Medicine* and the local rules and regulations laid a forceful foundation for enforcement. Next, communication and coordination with relevant sectors were more effective. We made efforts to obtain forceful support from the National People's Congress, the Legislative Affairs Office of the State Council and the Ministry of Health, fully played the role of the inter-ministerial coordinative mechanism for traditional Chinese medical work, took suggestions and opinions from all sectors into serious consideration, paid attention to the coordination with relevant departments and administrations of the Ministry of Health and the State Food and Drug Administration, unified ideology and reached a consensus. Lastly, in-depth study was conducted on these major and difficult problems in the legislation and a series of discussions on special subjects were organized, which pooled intelligence and experience inside out and provided a powerful support for the legislation. We shall draw on the experience continuously in following legislative work and use it for reference in other traditional Chinese medical work.

In addition, we also pushed forward the standardization of the traditional Chinese medical science and medicines in an all-round way, conducted thorough strategic researches on the standardization, strengthened top design of the standardized systems, sped up the formulation and revision of the standards of the traditional Chinese medical science and medicines and gave more attention to the construction of the supporting capacity for the work of the standardization. Guangdong Province took the lead in the establishment of the standardization technical committee of traditional Chinese medicine and the standardization technical committee of traditional Chinese medicines and Shenzhen and some other localities promoted local construction of the standardization, too. Basic work for the informatization of the traditional Chinese medical science and medicines was intensified earnestly; informatization construction of TCM hospitals was accelerated; website construction of TCM administrations was intensified and transparency in information on government operations was promoted. Supervision on the traditional Chinese medical science and medicines was further enhanced and great efforts were made to monitor and punish false and illegal TCM medical advertisements.

(5) New prospect was opened for the cultural construction of the traditional Chinese medical science and medicines.

We seriously studied and implemented the spirit of 6th Plenary Session of the 17th Central Committee of the Party,held the National Working Conference on TCM Cultural Construction, at which we comprehensively reviewed the experience and achievements in the cultural construction carried out by the whole system, further clarified the significance , put forward objectives and tasks for development and prosperity and deployed measures on accelerating the cultural construction. The first was to energetically propagandize the core values of the traditional Chinese medical science and medicines and by organizing a series of activities such as Zhang Zhongjing Cultural Festival of Medical Science and Technology, Li Shizhen Medical Festival and especially the First Sun Simiao Cultural Festival of Traditional Chinese Medicine, do researches on the cultural essence and connotation and the core value system of the traditional Chinese medical science and medicines, develop and expand the value of "great masters' super skills and absolute sincerity", inherit cultural spirit, set up good medical ethics and promote harmonious doctor-patient relationship. The second was to make greater efforts to publicize the popular science of the traditional Chinese medical science and medicines with more diversified forms, rich contents and extensive platforms. The activity of "the Traditional Chinese Medical Science and Medicines in China·Entering Villages, Communities, Families" was popular with the masses and programs on health care with the traditional Chinese medical science and medicines organized by some media developed into brands. What I should mention is that the full-length documentary film, *Traditional Chinese Medicine*, produced jointly with the CCTV began shooting and lectures on popular science knowledge of health care with the traditional Chinese medical science and medicines for diplomatic envoys to China also created a positive stir. The third was to make active exploration in the mechanisms that integrated the cultural construction with health protection. Provinces and cities such as Beijing, Guangdong, etc. launched TCM cultural and healthcare tourist demonstrative bases and TCM culture and health preservation with the traditional Chinese medical science and medicines were incorporated into the construction of the international tourist island in Hainan Province. The construction of publicity and education bases of traditional Chinese medical culture was strengthened continuously and the cultural construction of TCM hospitals was also pushed forward unceasingly. The work of news propaganda for the traditional Chinese medical science and medicines was further intensified, which created a sound atmosphere of public opinion for the undertaking.

(6) New achievements were gained in the inheritance and innovation of the traditional Chinese medical science and medicines

Last September, Tu Youyou, a researcher from China Academy of Chinese Medical Sciences, won the 2011 Lasker DeBakey Clinical Medical Research Award for the discovery of artemisinin, a drug therapy for malaria, which fully exhibited Chinese scientists' academic spirit and innovative capacity and showed the huge potential and broad prospects for the development of the traditional Chinese medical science and medicines. This is not only the pride of the whole medical and health care systems, but also the pride of the system of traditional Chinese medical science and medicines. In the scientific and technologic work of the traditional Chinese medical science and medicines, we highlighted the principle of "innovating independently, prioritizing major tasks, working in a more earnest and down-to-earth way, intensifying transformation and integration of systems" and attached more importance to the close integration of inheritance and innovation, the transformation and popularization of scientific achievements and the organization patterns for the integration of resources and the coordinative research. The first was to take the acceleration of the construction of national clinical research bases as the key task, strengthen the construction of clinical scientific and technologic systems, put forward the train of thought that in professional construction of the bases, researches on the key diseases should be taken as the foundation, construction of the sharing systems of the information on clinical scientific research as the principal part and regulation of clinical scientific research and training of backbone talents as the "both wings", formulate guidelines for the construction of information sharing systems and guiding opinions on regulating clinical scientific research, strengthen the training for the backbone of scientific research bases and basically set up the cooperative mechanism with research alliances as the main body. The second was to bring the role of TCM clinical research systems into full play in the treatment of infectious diseases, conduct systematic researches on theories, clinical treatment and medication and positive progress was made in the treatment of influenza and other exogenous diseases, of which the comparative study on the efficacy of oseltamivir and the Chinese traditional prescription of the "ma xing shi gan" (4 kinds of traditional Chinese medicines)–the Lonicerae and Forsythiae Powder on Influenza A (H1N1) proved the effect of the traditional Chinese medical science and medicines and release of the research result drew an extensive concern of the world. The third was to enhance the research on the inheritance of the traditional Chinese medical science and medicines and new achievements were gained in research-based inheritance of famous veteran TCM experts. Achievements such as "comprehensive service platform of famous veteran TCM experts' clinical experience and academic ideology" and "prescription analysis system of traditional Chinese medicine" acted as means of improvement in the efficiency of inheritance research. The third-batch collation of 400 ancient books went on smoothly and the formulation and implementation of the working guidelines for the collation of the literature on the ethnic minority medical science and medicines and the selection of the projects of the popularization of TCM appropriate techniques regulated collation and selection. The fourth was to strengthen the transformation and application of the research achievements in the prevention and treatment of major complicated and difficult diseases and common diseases, the characteristic acupuncture and moxibustion therapies, the technical standards and the key techniques in traditional Chinese medicines in the 11th Five-Year-Plan period, which provided scientific and technologic support for the medical services, the construction of the essential drug system, the popularization of appropriate techniques and the training of grassroots talents. The fifth was, according to unified technical standards and task requirements, to conduct the pilot of survey on natural resources of Chinese medicinal materials orderly and forcefully in 6 provinces (autonomous regions), including Anhui, Sichuan, Xinjiang and so on. We also seriously implemented Vice Premier Li Keqiang's instruction, investigated the causes for the rise in the prices of Chinese medicinal materials and reported the countermeasures and suggestions to the State Council.

(7) New patterns were created for the construction of talent contingent in the traditional Chinese medical science and medicines.

We earnestly carried through and implemented Vice-Premier Li Keqiang's and State Councilor Liu Yandong's instructions on TCM education work and in accordance with the requirements of the *Medium-and Long-Term Development Program on Medical and Health Talents(2011-2020)*, launched the project of "talent engineering of inheritance and innovation of the traditional Chinese medical science and medicines". The first was, for the purpose of cultivation of high-level talents, to steadily promote the projects concerning the inheritance of the academic experience of veteran experts in the traditional Chinese medical science and medicines, the further study of excellent TCM clinical talents, the cultivation of academic pacemakers and so on, strengthen management on the link between master-disciple education and professional degrees, establish 226 workrooms for the inheritance of the academic experience of national famous veteran experts in the traditional Chinese medical science and medicines and explore the experience of the "classes of great TCM masters" in the cultivation of high-level talents. The second was to enhance the cultivation of grassroots talents and train 2,375 county-level clinical technical backbone of traditional Chinese medicine. Cultivation of general practitioners of traditional Chinese medicine and standardized training for resident doctors were forcefully pushed forward. Job-transfer training for general practitioners of traditional Chinese medicine was launched and more than 2,200 TCM personnel from grassroots medical and health institutions took part in the training. Construction of training bases of TCM general practitioners was carried out and the pilot of standardized training for TCM resident doctors was launched. The third was, by joint construction of the Ministry of Health, the State Administration of Traditional Chinese Medicine and each province, to strive to push forward the connotation construction of colleges and universities of traditional Chinese medicine; meanwhile promote reform in education and teaching. Construction of key disciplines was also pushed forward actively and construction programs on 323 key disciplines were made. The fourth was to accelerate the development of occupational education. The National TCM Occupational Education and Teaching Committee was set up and the First National Skill Competition of Occupational Education was organized. The training for teachers evaluating professional skills of 5 types of jobs peculiar to the industry of the traditional Chinese medical science and medicines including pharmacists of traditional Chinese medicines and the appraisal on 3 kinds of professional technical personnel including *gua sha shi* (doctors treating patients' illness by scraping the patient's neck, chest or back) was initiated. The fifth was to intensify continuing education and play the role of continuing education bases of the superior disciplines and the role of the urban community and rural demonstrative training bases of knowledge and skills on the traditional Chinese medical science and medicines. As a result, quality and coverage of the continuing education were improved dramatically.

(8) A new pattern of foreign exchange and cooperation in the traditional Chinese medical science and medicines was formed.

The National Working Conference on Foreign Exchange and Cooperation in the Traditional Chinese Medical Science and Medicines was held at the beginning of last year, which defined the guiding thought and basic principles and proposed key tasks and specific measures for promoting the traditional Chinese medical science and medicines to exert more extensive influence on the world. In the past year, firstly, multilateral platforms were made good use of and big country's role in traditional medical science and medicines was well played. We strived to further implement the

Resolution of Traditional Medicine adopted in the 62nd World Health Assembly, took an active part in the formulation of the part of traditional medicine for ICD of WHO (International Classification of Diseases of the World Health Organization), positively promote WHO Western Pacific Region to formulate and carry out the *Regional Strategy for Traditional Medicine in the Western Pacific Region (2011-2020)* and manage to establish 5 working groups at the second conference of ISO Technical Committee of Traditional Chinese Medicine (tentative name) with Chinese experts being the organizers of 3 groups. Moreover, after examination and approval of the UNESCO, two ancient books—Huang Di Nei Jing (Emperor's Inner Canon) and Ben Cao Gang Mu (Compendium of Materia Medica) were selected into the Asia-Pacific Memory of the World Register. We timely pushed forward China and the European Union to establish mechanisms that promoted the registration of traditional Chinese medicines and further promoted the construction of the high-level China-ASEAN cooperation platform. Secondly, bilateral cooperation was consolidated and developed and with focus on carrying out inter-governmental agreements, fields of cooperation were further expanded. Abundant achievements were gained in the Sino-America Seminar on Traditional Chinese Medicine, the Sino-Russia First Meeting of the Working Group of Traditional Chinese Medicine and the Sino-Korean Cooperation and Coordination Committee for Traditional Medicine and cooperation with Malaysia, Vietnam, New Zealand and Australia was enhanced. Provinces (Autonomous regions) of Heilongjiang, Fujian, Guangxi, Yunnan, etc. brought regional advantages into play and positively developed the service trade of traditional Chinese medical science and medicines. Thirdly, relations of the two sides of the Taiwan Straits, Hong Kong and Macon were closer. The Administration of Traditional Chinese Medicine and Xiamen Municipal Government jointly held the Cross-Strait Forum on Traditional Chinese Medicine and some prominent figures in the field of traditional Chinese medical science and medicines, including some academicians and national honored great masters, went to Taiwan to attend the 3rd Cross-Strait Forum on Herbal Medicine Cooperation & Technological Exchange and other such activities, which had a positive impact inside and outside of Taiwan and their activities were said to be a successful healthy and cultural trip.

(9) New experience was created in the activity of "striving to excel in performances".

According to the requirements of the Party Central Committee's deployment, we earnestly studied and carried through the spirits of the General Secretary Hu Jintao's important speech on July 1, fully implemented the *Several Opinions* in deepening the medical and heath care reform, deeply carried out the activity of "striving to excel in performances" and a great number of advanced collectives and excellent Party members sprang up, including Guang'anmen Hospital of China Academy of Chinese Medical Sciences, Guangdong Hospital of Traditional Chinese Medicine, Chongqing Hospital of Traditional Chinese Medicine and Zhang Boli from Tianjin, Chen Xiangyi from Jilin Province, Lu Youqiang from Shaanxi Province and so on, which created a good atmosphere that every Party member competed in study, work and devotion and also learned from and caught up with each other and tried to be the advanced; therefore, Party members' and cadres' capacity and level of putting the people first and governing for the people were greatly improved. Hospitals of traditional Chinese medicine combined "three good and one satisfaction" (good service, good quality, good medical ethics; masses' satisfaction) with the activity of "striving to excel in performances", the cultural construction, the connotation construction and the construction of mechanisms that promoted the play of the characteristics and superiorities of the traditional Chinese medical science and medicines and created a series of advanced working experience. The Affiliated Hospital of Shanxi Provincial Hospital of Traditional Chinese Medicine put forward "whether patients were rich or poor, saved their life first"; Yanzhou Municipal Hospital of Traditional Chinese Medicine of Shandong Province raised the mode of "rescuing and treating patients before their payment and enabling everyone to get access to green life passage"; Jingde Municipal Hospital of Traditional Chinese Medicine of Jiangxi Province resolved doctor-patient conflicts and constructed harmonious doctor-patient relationship and TCM service vehicles of Fangshan Hospital of Traditional Chinese Medicine travelled through all the villages of Fangshan District of Beijing. What they did forcefully promoted innovation in the carriers of the activity and made the contents and forms richer, which pushed forward the construction of harmonious doctor-patient relationship and the improvement of service quality and was very popular with people.

Comrades, new progress was gained in every respect of the traditional Chinese medical science and medicines in 2011. We owe it to the correct leadership of the Party Central Committee and the State Council, the concern and support of all-level local Party committees and governments, the powerful support of relevant sectors, especially the member units of the Inter-Ministerial Joint Conference on the work of traditional Chinese medical science and medicines, all sectors of the society and mess media, the cooperation and hard working of all-level health administrative departments, TCM administrative departments and broad workers in the system of the traditional Chinese medical science and medicines. On behalf of the State Administration of Traditional Chinese Medicine, I extend my heartfelt thanks and sincere respect to all-level local Party committees and governments, relevant sectors, all sectors of the society and mess media that support the development of the traditional Chinese medical science and medicines, all-level health administrative departments, TCM administrative departments and broad workers in the system of the traditional Chinese medical science and medicines!

At the same time, we shall be keenly aware that we are still faced with many difficulties and problems in traditional Chinese medical work. For example, development of medical treatment, health protection, education, scientific research, culture and industry is not coordinative; effective policies and measures in deepening the medical and heath care reform and tasks for support and promotion of the development of the undertaking of the traditional Chinese medical science and medicines raised in the *Several Opinions* shall be further perfected and implemented; service systems of traditional Chinese medicine , in particular, urban and rural grassroots service networks need further perfection; service of prevention and health protection is in need of immediate intensification; lack in leading talents and medical personnel at the grassroots level is not improved radically; backwardness in academic development is still a prominent problem; governing capacity, administrative level and especially executive power of the administrative departments of the traditional Chinese medical science and medicines shall be further improved. Some of them are long-standing difficulties and problems because of systems and mechanisms; others are newly-emerged in the process of development. There must be some difficulties and problems when developmental laws and characteristics of the traditional Chinese medical science and medicines can't be brought into full play in current systems, which attracted attention and concern from inside and outside the industry. We shall be sober-minded, not only seize opportunities for development, but also have a keen sense of crisis and urgency and with sense of mission and responsibility expected by our ancestors, offspring and broad masses, confront all kinds of difficulties and problems on the way forward, make research and judgment accurately, try to find solutions in advance, make decisions scientifically, spare no effort to solve difficulties and problems and promote the reform and development of the traditional Chinese medical science and medicines unceasingly.

II. Deeply understand new reform and developmental situation, effectively advance academic progress, promote cultural development and prosperity and endeavor to push forward and realize scientific development of the undertaking of the traditional Chinese medical science and medicines

(1) Do search on the situation, serve the overall development and effectively promote the reform and development of the traditional Chinese medical science and medicines.

Reform and development of the traditional Chinese medical science and medicines shall comply with the national overall situation of economic and social development. Our country's economic and social development has sped up since reform and opening up, particularly in the five years in the 11th Five-Year-Plan period, GDP per capita rose to nearly 5,000 USD, up to the level of middle-income countries. In such a period, people pay more and more attention to health, expect more of the improvement of health level and living quality and have more needs for multi-level and diversified medical and health services including services of the traditional Chinese medical science and medicines, which provides more space for the development of the undertaking of the traditional Chinese medical science and medicines. The 12th Five-Year-Plan period is a critical period for our country to build a well-off society in an all-round way, deepen reform and opening up and accelerate the transformation of patterns of economic development and our country attaches more importance to putting the people first and ensuring and improving people's well-being. The *Outline of the 12th Five-Year Plan for National Economic and Social Development of the People's Republic of China* requires that medical and health care systems should be offered to people as a public product and takes the support to the development of the traditional Chinese medical science and medicines as a vital part of the improvement of the basic medical and health care systems, which fully shows the significant position of the development of the traditional Chinese medical science and medicines in the overall development and brings new vigor and vitality into the development of the undertaking. The Central Economic Working Conference takes "making progress while ensuring stability" as a fundamental rule for current economic and social development and demands specially that we should give special attention to continuous focus on scientific development and acceleration of the transformation of economic developmental patterns, fully understand the strategy of expanding domestic demand, pay attention to the solid foundation of development of the real economy, make good use of the strong power of accelerating reform and innovation and firmly keep to the fundamental goal of ensuring and improving people's well-being. The traditional Chinese medical science and medicines are not only important medical and health care resources, but also our country's important economic resources and independent innovative resources; they can play a unique role in promoting the sound development of strategic emerging industries, creating more opportunities of employment, pushing forward residents' health consumption such as medical preservation and health protection, boosting adjustment of agricultural structure and farmers' earning and promoting development of service trade. The transformation of the advantages of resources and knowledge into industrial and economic advantages and the conversion of original innovative potential into independent innovative capacity are of vital importance for the fulfillment of the Party Central Committee's tasks for ensuring steady growth, maintaining price stability, adjusting structure, benefiting people, advancing reform and promoting harmony, the promotion of economic development and change in developmental patterns, the improvement of people's living standards and the construction of socialist harmonious society.

Reform and development of the traditional Chinese medical science and medicines shall comply with the overall national medical and heath care reform and development. Currently, our country's medicine and health have already stepped into a new stage of overall and rapid development. Since the in-depth medical and heath care reform in particular, the coverage of the basic medical security expands significantly; grassroots medical and health service capacity, including that for the services of the traditional Chinese medical science and medicines, improves greatly and the coverage of public health services also increases substantially; the essential drug system is set up; the pilot of reform in public hospitals is pushed forward orderly and people's burden of medical expenses begins to relieve. After three years' practice and exploration in the medical and heath care reform, we are sure of the direction and the train of thought for reform. Now we are in the region of "deep water" of the medical and heath care reform, so we will have more difficulties and problems. Only continue to move forward, can we consolidate and develop the achievements we have already gained. We must further raise our level of understanding for the importance and urgency of deepening the medical and heath care reform and fully realize deepening the medical and heath care reform is a urgent need for ensuring and improving people's well-being, a significant measure for accelerating the transformation of the patterns of economic development and a revolution in our country's economic and social areas. We must stick to the basic ideology that medical and health care systems shall be offered to people as a public product, the fundamental principle of ensuring the basic medical and healthcare systems, strengthening grassroots medical and health institutions and constructing mechanisms and the essential way of making overall arrangement, giving priority to focal points and making gradual progress. Last year's Central Economic Working Conference raised that we should continue to deepen reform in the medical and health care systems, formulate and implement the 12th Five-Year plan for the medical and heath care reform, focus on key problems, give priority to focal and difficult points, establish and perfect the medical and health care systems that covers all the people. The traditional Chinese medical science and medicines are vital medical and health resources of our country with accurate clinic effects, unique advantages in prevention and health protection, flexible patterns of treatment and comparatively low expanses. Making full use of traditional Chinese medical resources, bringing the traditional Chinese medical science and medicines into full play and sufficiently presenting the advantages of the traditional Chinese medical science and medicines are beneficial for establishment and perfection of medical and health care systems that cover all urban and rural areas and blazing an trail for medical and health development that is affordable, sustainable, with focus on prevention and with Chinese characteristics.

We shall fully realize the overall economic and social situation and the new changing situations for health reform and development, firmly seize the rare opportunities for the development of the undertaking of the traditional Chinese medical science and medicines, deeply understand the new demands and tasks under the new circumstances, focus on the fulfillment of the fundamental goal for satisfying people's demands for traditional Chinese medical services, insist on the development of the solid foundation of TCM services including medical treatment, prevention and health protection, take advantage of the powerful driving force from accelerating reform and innovation, adhere to the strategic pattern of the overall coordinative development of "six in one" and strive to promote and realize scientific development of the undertaking of the traditional Chinese medical science and medicines.

(2) Meet challenge, do contribution and rapidly promote the academic development of the traditional Chinese medical science and medicines.

Nowadays economy and society are changing profoundly; science and technology are altering from day to day; modern medicine is advancing by leaps and bounds; therefore, the academic development of traditional Chinese medical science and medicines is confronted with many new situations and problems. Viewed from the external environment, with continuous thorough implementation of the *Several Opinions* of the State Council in the in-depth medical and heath care reform and increasingly more attention to the traditional Chinese medical science and medicines given by all-level governments, policies and environment for the development become better and better and people's expectations are more and more urgent, so requirements for the academic development are much more demanding. The key whether the traditional Chinese medical science and medicines can play an effective role and really earn trust lies in the unceasing improvement of clinic efficacy and the contributions to the maintenance and promotion of people's health. Meanwhile, the international community has a new understanding for the traditional medical science and medicines and makes changes in the attitude. Many countries are taking their advantages in funds and technology to actively research and make use of the traditional Chinese medical science and medicines, which threatens our country's original innovative superiority and resource advantage. We should also see, in contemporary society that modern medicine develops rapidly, we meet severe challenges in traditional advantageous fields of the traditional Chinese medical science and medicines and we have a long way to go to accelerate the exploitation of new service fields. Undoubtedly, all these form a state of "forced development" for the traditional Chinese medical science and medicines.

Considering the self-development of the traditional Chinese medical science and medicines, we have not done well enough in the exploitation of the connotation of original thoughts, the overall inheritance and the innovation in the theories and technological methods based on the original thoughts of the traditional Chinese medical science and medicines. We meet many challenges in abiding by the developmental laws and maintaining the characteristics of the traditional Chinese medical science and medicines, yet we have not done well enough in insisting on the original thoughts and maintaining the essential characteristics while making innovation with modern science and technology. We have neither set up the research and appraisal methods and the standardized systems appropriate to the characteristics of the traditional Chinese medical science and medicines nor the independent innovative systems adapting to the needs of time. At the same time, due to the differences in historical backgrounds, cultural deposits and way of thinking, it is hard for modern society to understand and accept universally the complex phenomena of life and disease in the traditional Chinese medical science and medicines and the scientific connotation expressed in traditional concepts. At present, the issue of slow academic development of the traditional Chinese medical science and medicines has attracted the whole society's attention and worries. If the traditional Chinese medical science and medicines make no new progress in the technology of disease prevention and treatment, no new improvements in clinic efficacy and no new contributions in the maintenance and promotion of people's health, the situation is like going upstream. In that case, formulation of policies will be short of sound grounds; advance of the undertaking will lack powerful support and existence and development will be faced with severe challenges. We can't run away from these problems, so we must bravely face and seriously cope with them, have a keen sense of urgency and crisis, improve predictability and foresightedness and take rapid promotion of the academic development of the traditional Chinese medical science and medicines as a strategic focus for policy support and development of the undertaking.

To accelerate the promotion of academic development, we shall firstly clarify our thoughts, further emancipate our minds, be practical and realistic, have an accurate command of development trend, profoundly analyze the elements restricting the academic advance, precisely locate entry points and areas to make breakthroughs in inheritance and innovation and clearly know the objectives and tasks for the academic progress in the traditional Chinese medical science and medicines.

Secondly, we shall insist on inheritance and innovation. Innovation is an inexhaustible motive force for academic development; acceleration of the academic development of the traditional Chinese medical science and medicines must take independent innovation that is based on inheritance as a strategic foundation; in the process of innovation, we must stick to original thoughts, consistently take them as a premise for theoretical and technologic innovation and strive to gain unceasing achievements from original thoughts and form original advantages. Thirdly, we shall pay attention to actual effects, endeavor to make substantial progress and major breakthroughs in the fundamental and clinical research and the research on traditional Chinese medicines and enable the theoretical innovative achievements to guide clinical practice, the clinical innovative achievements to improve the capacity for disease prevention and treatment, the innovative achievements in traditional Chinese medicines to meet the needs of clinical treatment and production and the innovative achievements in methodology to be used by the traditional Chinese medical science and medicines. To sum up, we shall make people reap the actual benefits from the academic advancement of the traditional Chinese medical science and medicines. Fourthly, we shall innovate mechanisms, deliberate on big projects concerning focal and difficult issues on the academic development of the traditional Chinese medical science and medicines and the most immediate and practical health needs that people are most concerned about, gather advantageous forces from every respect with an open-minded attitude, construct a huge platform, pay attention to the integration of systems so that efforts of different levels of the whole system and people inside and outside the system are joined together and we have a big union. Fifthly, we shall intensify transformation. The goal of the academic development of the traditional Chinese medical science and medicines is to effectively solve the actual problems in clinical practice and improve people's health level, so we shall transform academic achievements into effective and applicable techniques, products, methods and designs or guidelines as soon as possible, and then apply them to practice and make them serve people.

(3) Seize opportunities, make inheritance and innovation and focus on promoting the cultural construction of the traditional Chinese medical science and medicines

The *Decision of the CPC Central Committee on Major Issues Pertaining to Deepening Reform of the Cultural System and Promoting the Great Development and Flourishing of Socialist Culture* (hereinafter referred to as *Decision*) passed at the 6th Plenary Session of the 17th CPC Central Committee lays stress on the construction of the excellent traditional cultural system. We shall understand our country's traditional culture in an all-round way, inherit and pass down Chinese excellent traditional culture, make it compatible with modern society and coordinative with modern civilization and have both national traits and contemporary characters. The *Decision* points out the excellent traditional culture embodies the Chinese nation's spiritual pursuit for unremitting self-improvement and intellectual treasure that has lasting charms and is a solid foundation for the development of advanced socialist culture and a crucial support for the construction of the Chinese nation's common spirit home. The *Decision* requires that we should strengthen the exploitation and exposition of the excellent traditional cultural thoughts, preserve its fundamental elements and enable the excellent traditional culture to become a spiritual power that could encourage people to move forward in the new era.

Traditional Chinese medical science and medicines, including every ethnic minority medicine, are important components and outstanding representatives of our country's excellent traditional culture and medical sciences that are gradually forged and continuously developed and enriched in working people's thousands of years' life practice and production and the struggle with diseases. They contain a wealth of philosophical thoughts and spirit of humanity and combine medicine and culture perfectly. The ideological basis of the unity of heaven and nature, the integrity of man and nature, the harmony of heaven, nature and man and the harmony in diversity, the way of thinking that advocates harmony and pursuit for balance and the moral standard that attaches importance to people's interest and doctors' super skill and absolute sincerity represent profoundly the Chinese nation's cognitive style and value orientation, embody the Chinese nation's rich excellent traditional cultural quintessence and display our country's cultural soft power. Just as what Vice-President Xi Jinping said that the traditional Chinese medical science and medicines have pooled profound philosophical wisdom and the Chinese nation's thousands of years of health preservation theories and experience; it is the gem of ancient Chinese science and also the key to the treasure of Chinese civilization.

Currently, we just have the rare strategic opportunities for the development and flourish of traditional Chinese medical culture, so we must realize and understand the significant importance of strengthening the construction of traditional Chinese medical culture in the overall situation of developing and flourishing the socialist culture and fully realize that intensification of the construction of traditional Chinese medical culture is the fundamental requirements for promoting the great development and flourish of socialist culture and the construction of a powerful socialist cultural country, an important part of the construction of the socialist core value system and the establishment of the Chinese nation's common spiritual home and an effective way to improve cultural soft power and promote Chinese culture to be on the way to the world. We shall realize and understand the significant importance of the intensification of the construction of traditional Chinese medical culture from the overall development situation of the undertaking of the traditional Chinese medical science and medicines and fully realize that traditional Chinese medical culture is the soul and root of the traditional Chinese medical science and medicines, an internal motivation for the sustainable development of the undertaking of the traditional Chinese medical science and medicines, an inexhaustible source for the academic innovation and progress and also an important focus for pooling strength and demonstrating image. Intensification of the construction of traditional Chinese medical culture is an important measure for the scientific development of the undertaking of the traditional Chinese medical science and medicines and an inevitable choice for the satisfaction of people's health and cultural needs. To accelerate the construction of traditional Chinese medical culture, we shall have an accurate understanding of the developmental laws, profoundly understand the connotation and essence, deeply discuss core value ideology such as "great masters' super skill and absolute sincerity", construct the core value system and the medical and health professionalism of the traditional Chinese medical science and medicines with characteristics of the times. We shall also strengthen strategic research on the cultural development, make exploration in the establishment of systems and mechanisms for cultural inheritance, protection and development, inherit the cultural spirit in an all-round way, fully exploit cultural value, innovate dissemination forms and ways, promote the development and utilization of rich cultural resources, intensify the propaganda and population of traditional Chinese medical culture and scientific knowledge, build health culture with the cultural elements of the traditional Chinese medical science and medicines and improve people's health literary. We shall coordinate the relationship between the development of traditional Chinese medical culture and medical treatment, health protection, education, scientific research, industry and that of the movement towards the world, make it a crucial support for the comprehensive and coordinative development of the traditional Chinese medical science and medicines and do contributions to the promotion of the great development and flourish of socialist culture, the improvement of the nation's ideological and cultural quality, the popularization of China's excellent culture, the improvement of the Chinese nation's cohesion and the increase of the Chinese cultural influence on the world.

III. Major tasks in 2012

It is still a focal task for us in traditional Chinese medical work this year to fully carry through the *Several Opinions* of the State Council and actively promote the traditional Chinese medical science and medicines to effectively play the role in deepening the medical and health care reform. Since the main working arrangements have been printed and issued for you to discuss, now I'll give my opinions on the major tasks.

(1) Efforts shall be made to promote the implementation of the 12th Five-Year Plan.

The 12th Five-Year-Plan period is of a vital importance in the achievement of the leapfrog development of the traditional Chinese medical science and medicines and the key in this period is to effectively implement the 12th Five-Year Plan. The first is to fully play the leading role of the 12th Five-Year Plan, work out practical implementing plans in accordance with the major tasks for supporting the development of the undertaking of the traditional Chinese medical science and medicines put forward in the 12th Five-Year Plan and well coordinate the implementation of key projects. The second is to discuses and formulate detailed and practical action plans and working programs for those relevant to the traditional Chinese medical science and medicines that have been incorporated into the specific plans on scientific technology, talents, education, service trade, standardization, in particular, medical and heath care reform, health, medical and pharmaceutical industries and make efforts to initiate and implement those plans and programs. The third is to fully implement the *12th Five-Year Plan for the Development of the Undertaking of the Traditional Chinese Medical Science and Medicines* and the development plans in all the localities, do practical work to fulfill the key tasks in the plans, break down tasks, make action plans more specific and clarify working responsibilities. We shall also seriously implement key major projects such as the standardization construction of county-level TCM hospitals (hospitals of ethnic minority medicine), the construction of key TCM clinical specialties and so on, do well budgeting for the projects, practically accelerate the performance of budget, make good use of the project funds and accomplish the projects. The fourth is to further strengthen communication and coordination with relevant sectors, put the arrangement of the projects into effect, strive to obtain supporting policies and carry out the tasks in an earnest way.

(2) Efforts shall be made to promote the implementation of all the polices and provisions on bringing the role of the traditional Chinese medical science and medicines into full play in the in-depth medical and heath care reform.

This year is a crucial year for continuing to deepen the medical and heath care reform. We should, in accordance with the general requirements and key tasks of the 12th Five-Year-Plan period, seriously carry through and implement the spirit of the National Health Working Conference, take earnestly playing the role of the traditional Chinese medical science and medicines in deepening the medical and heath care reform as focal work, draw on experience, focus on key work, make innovation in mechanisms, comprehensively carry out the *Opinions on Further Playing the Role of Traditional Chinese Medicine in Deepening the Reform of the Medical and Health Care Systems* and give priority to the work in the following five aspects. The first is, with focus on county-level public TCM hospitals, to push forward reform of public TCM hospitals in an all-round way. All the localities shall give priority to maintenance and play of the characteristics and superiorities of the traditional Chinese medical science and medicines, take perfecting investment and compensation mechanisms as a starting point, make active efforts to obtain support from governmental leaders and health administrations and strive to create conditions for implementing relevant policies on the abolishment of "subsidizing doctors' earning with drug-selling profits" and establish mechanisms. Efforts shall also be made to positively push forward the reform in pricing mechanisms for traditional Chinese medical services that embody the characteristics and laws of traditional Chinese medicine, clarify functions and orientation of all-level public TCM hospitals, rationally set distribution plans and establishment standards, explore new developmental patterns, continuously put into effect all kinds of service measures that offer conveniences and benefits to people and further improve scientific management level of TCM hospitals. The second is to further implement policies that encourage the offer and application of the traditional Chinese medical science and medicines in the new rural cooperative medical care system and the basic medical insurance systems for urban employees and non-working urban residents, actively explore and promote reform in payment methods and systems that fit the characteristics of traditional Chinese medical services, promote the making of TCM clinical pathways and the pilot work, strive to explore the payment methods that are beneficial to bringing the characteristics and superiorities into play, such as global budget and quota payment for specific diseases and service units and push forward reform synchronously in payment systems and the abolishment of "subsidizing doctors' earning with drug-selling profits". The third is, in perfection of the essential drug system, to follow the principle of attaching equal importance to Western medicines and traditional Chinese medicines, further improve the work related to the selection of traditional Chinese medicines for the National Essential Medicine List (2012 edition), strengthen guidance and training, promote rational medication, explore ways for the establishment of the systems that fit the characteristics of traditional Chinese medicines, concerning the production and supply, purchase and distribution, provision and application and price formation of Chinese traditional medical herbal pieces and optimize the policies that encourage medical institutions to prepare and apply Chinese herbal preparations. The fourth is, in the work of promoting the equalization of the basic public health service, to take bringing the characteristics and superiorities of prevention and health protection in TCM "preventive treatment of diseases" into full play as a goal, unceasingly carry out and comprehensively summarize the pilot work of TCM service items in the basic public health services, set service items, define service contents, unify service standards and perfect relevant policies. The fifth is, while accelerating the construction of county-level TCM hospitals, to continuously push forward the activity of building TCM grassroots advanced units in all the localities, further enhance the construction of the capacity for characteristic services of the traditional Chinese medical science and medicines in township and community health centers, carry out the projects that improve service capacity at the grassroots level, perfect urban and rural grassroots service networks and increase service capacity.

(3) Efforts shall be made to promote the implementation of all the policies and measures in the *Several Opinions*.

It has been nearly three years since we implemented the *Several Opinions of the State Council on Supporting and Promoting the Development of TCM Undertaking* and positive progress has been made in the work of every respect; while on the whole, we still do not do well enough in understanding the overall situation, summarizing specific experience and conducting systematic evaluation on the overall effects. In order to fully carry through and implement the *Several Opinions*, this year, we shall, on the basis of further promoting all the policies on support of the development of the undertaking of the traditional Chinese medical science and medicines to be more specific and practicable and all the measures to be fully carried out, continue to do a good job in general investigation and supervisory guidance and attach importance to the organization of the evaluation and promotion of the implementation of the *Several Opinions*. The first is to have a suitable evaluating goal and by evaluation, we can review achievements, find out shortcomings, draw on experience and perfect policies and measures so as to further promote the implementation of the *Several Opinions*. The second is to have an elaborate plan for the contents of evaluation and emphatically evaluate which policies have been put into effect, which work has been accomplished and which experience is worth summarizing and popularizing, in addition, which tasks are to be fulfilled and which measures are to be strengthened. The third is to work out an evaluating scheme with focus on appropriate evaluating standards that are scientific, rational, measurable and easy to operate so that we can have systematic, objective and fair results. The fourth is to make great efforts to organize evaluation, strengthen leadership, make overall arrangement and deploy carefully in order for us to take joint actions, cooperate well with relevant sectors, enhance evaluating effects, expand impact and ensure that we have effective results from the evaluation. While summarizing and popularizing successful experience, we shall, by supervising and guiding the evaluation, strengthen service consciousness at grassroots medical institutions and the ideology to offer better TCM service to people, summarize and popularize the working methods and experience created by all the localities in bringing coordinative mechanisms of all the TCM sectors into full play and making all the sectors well coordinate, further perfect polices and measures and put them into effect so as to solve practical difficulties and problems in all the localities.

(4) Efforts shall be made to promote the fulfillment of all the tasks in the construction of traditional Chinese medical culture.

We shall further carry through and implement the Party Central Committee's *Decision* and do well the work in the following respects according to the spirit of the National Working Conference on the Cultural Construction of Traditional Chinese medicine and the objective tasks and working deployment defined by the *Guiding Opinions on Strengthening the Cultural Construction of Traditional Chinese Medicine*. Firstly, we shall deepen the research on the culture of the traditional Chinese medical science and medicines, explore thoroughly the cultural value, enhance the protection and exploitation of intangible cultural heritage, construct core value system, further discover the essence of the culture and enrich the connotation of the traditional Chinese medical science and medicines. Secondly, we shall intensify the construction of the platforms that spread the culture of the traditional Chinese medical science and medicines. While continuing to improve the activity of "the Traditional Chinese Medical Science and Medicines in China", strengthen the construction of cultural publicity and education bases and make TCM hospitals and other traditional Chinese medical institutions fully play the role of "window", we shall also pay more attention to making good use of newspaper, broadcast, television, Internet and other forms of social resources, build public platforms to spread traditional Chinese medical culture and increase the extension of popularity. Thirdly, we shall enrich cultural products of the traditional Chinese medical science and medicines, accelerate the creation of cultural products, launch some excellent products that fully display the ideology of the core value of the traditional Chinese medical science and medicines; at the same time, attach more importance to innovation in product forms and take full advantage of the characteristic superiorities of the Internet and some other new media so as to better satisfy people's different needs and increase the effectiveness of propagation. Fourthly, we shall speed up the construction of medical cultural professional contingent, closely integrate systematic cultivation and training with the construction of propagation platforms and the creation of cultural products, construct a talent contingent with a rational structure of specialties, high level of professional quality and excellent ideological style and bring up a great number of masters in popularizing traditional Chinese medical culture and science who are popular with people and have extensive influence on the society.

(5) Efforts shall be made to improve the capacity for traditional Chinese medical treatment, prevention, health protection and emergency rescue and treatment

In recent years, with focus on the construction of the capacity for traditional Chinese medical service, we have done a great deal of work, take numerous measures and gain some achievements; however, we shall also realize that preventive and healthcare services and emergency rescue and treatment are the weaknesses in all the service areas of the traditional Chinese medical science and medicines, therefore, we shall continue to improve service capacity and at the same time, make special efforts to deal with problems in these weak areas this year. The first is to heighten the level of traditional Chinese medical treatment, promote the construction of national key clinical specialties, do well the State Administration-level 12th Five-Year-Plan projects on key specialties and construct cooperative centers that diagnose and treat diseases with TCM superiorities. Efforts shall be made to strengthen clinical application and management of the techniques of traditional Chinese medicine, organize evaluation on TCM hospitals, consolidate the achievements of "management year", promote connotation construction and manage TCM hospitals scientifically and elaborately. We shall also continue to popularize appropriate technology of traditional Chinese medical science and medicines in grassroots medical institutions, construct advanced units in communities and rural areas, further push forward TCM work in general hospitals and coordinate the work of the integration of Western medicine with traditional Chinese medicine, ethnical minority medicine and folk medicine. The second is to accelerate the development of TCM preventive and healthcare services, deepen our understanding of the strategic significance of the development of TCM preventive and healthcare services, unify our thinking and pool strength. We must carry on the experience gained in the health project of "preventive treatment of diseases", take putting the people first and serving people as purpose and "preventive treatment of diseases" as core, keep on innovation in technology under the guidance of TCM theories, adhere to the principle of governments' guidance, market orientation and multi-sectors' participation, by beginning the work as pilot with high-quality and standardized services, gradually expand service coverage, accelerate standardized construction of TCM preventive and healthcare service platforms in all-level TCM hospitals and other medical and health institutions that have qualified conditions and construct basic systemic frameworks for offering the services. Efforts shall be made to improve service level, further speed up research and development of service techniques and methods and relevant products, enrich service contents, set service norms and items, accelerate the construction of service contingent, effectively improve comprehensive quality and technical capacity, enhance control on service quality and organize evaluation on service quality. The third is to strive to improve the capacity for emergency rescue and treatment with the traditional Chinese medical science and medicines. We shall summarize the achievements and experience in recent years' emergency rescue and treatment in an all-round way and further optimize working mechanisms and technical plans on emergency rescue and treatment with the traditional Chinese medical science and medicines so as to cope with common occurrences in sudden public events. We shall also strengthen contingent construction, build a professional technical contingent with every member having solid basic skills in the traditional Chinese medical science and medicines, rich clinical experience and master of skills in emergency rescue and treatment and in addition, enhance the construction of the bases of emergency rescue treatment.

(6) Efforts shall be made to intensify the construction of talent contingent and the cultivation of special talents of the traditional Chinese medical science and medicines.

Firstly, we shall accelerate the cultivation of grassroots talents and technical backbone in the traditional Chinese medical science and medicines, conduct training for county-level clinical technical backbone and job-transfer training for general practitioners majoring in traditional Chinese medicine and do well the projects on the inheritance of clinical experience of grassroots veteran experts. Secondly, we shall further strengthen the cultivation of high-level talents and do a good job in the inheritance of veteran TCM experts' academic experience, the projects of excellent TCM clinical talents' advanced research and training, the cultivation of academic pacesetters and the construction of workrooms for the inheritance of famous veteran TCM experts' experience and TCM academic schools. Thirdly, we shall enhance negotiation and cooperation with the Ministry of Education, further promote educational and teaching reform in traditional Chinese medical universities and colleges and implement the agreements on joint construction of traditional Chinese medical universities and colleges by provinces, ministries and state administrations. Fourthly, we shall enhance the construction of key disciplines, do a good job in the new round of projects and push forward the construction of sharing management platforms. Fifthly, we shall speed up the development of vocational education, intensify the cultivation of high-quality skilled talents and do well the work of training and appraisal on the professional techniques and skills peculiar to the traditional Chinese medical science and medicines. Sixthly, we shall do exploration in the establishment of standardized training systems for TCM residents, further promote the construction of training bases for TCM general practitioners and accelerate cultivation.

(7) Efforts shall be made to make new achievements in the construction of scientific and technological systems and the implementation of key projects of the traditional Chinese medical science and medicines.

The first is to earnestly construct national clinical research bases, deepen research on key diseases, unceasingly make innovation in technical methods and solve clinical problems and strive to initially build the sharing systems of the information on clinical scientific research in 16 research bases so as to promote further cooperation in clinical treatment and scientific research. We shall also adhere to the rules on management and operation and construct standard systems of clinical scientific research. By way of special training, short-term study, high-level forums and some other ways, we shall cultivate talents and improve the capacity of clinical research teams. Efforts shall be made to promote the construction of the base union and giant scientific research platforms, fully play the role of the China Academy of Chinese Medical Sciences and other institutions and jointly construct the platforms of clinical research methodology, ethic review, etc. We shall discuss and formulate outlines and standard systems for periodical acceptance inspection and evaluation on profession construction of the bases and well review the experience regularly. The second is to promote research and development of preventive and healthcare services of traditional Chinese medicine (preventive treatment of diseases), work out outlines, guide multi-resources, adjust service patterns and the needs for the development of technological products, follow traditional Chinese medical theories, lead and support service development with scientific and technological progress, improve service quality and effect, speed up research and make more achievements in people's health preservation, prevention and control of major serious diseases and rehabilitation. The third is to seriously carry out the pilot of the general survey on natural resources of Chinese medicinal materials, draw up working plans according to unified technical requirements, quicken the pace, guarantee the quality and provide experience for the general survey; at the same time, do practical exploration for the establishment of dynamic monitoring system of natural resources of Chinese medicinal materials. The fourth is to push forward the transformation of scientific and technological achievements, perfect registration system, set up achievement banks, conduct the pilot that ensures the scientific and technological achievements of the 11th Five-year Plan to be popularized and do exploration in the construction of the platforms that transform and popularize achievements. We shall also establish guiding mechanisms to lead scientific research personnel to transform achievements into clinical appropriate techniques and practical productive technology, promote comprehensive reform trial regions to construct transforming bases and explore interactive mechanisms of production, academy, research and application. The fifth is to well organize the implementation of national key scientific and technologic projects on the traditional Chinese medical science and medicines, fully play the role of administrative departments concerned, set up and optimize performance evaluation systems, cultivate a high-level and specialized management team for the projects, improve management level and make it more scientific and standardized. Project bank shall be set up and a good job shall be done in selecting such projects that embody the overall train of thought and the fundamental principle that intensify inheritance and innovation and promote academic progress, the scientific and technological tasks for the traditional Chinese medical science and medicines in all the national plans and the urgent needs for the development of the traditional Chinese medical science and medicines. Construction of expert advisory systems shall be optimized and experts' role in strategic guidance, consultation, supervision and assessment shall be fully played so as to ensure the projects to be democratic, scientific and fair in the process of organization and implementation. Mechanisms for the organization of key scientific research projects of the State Administration of Traditional Chinese Medicine shall be improved and we shall, with focus on solution to special problems hindering development, guide non-governmental resources, explore multi-part investment mechanisms and organization patterns of cooperative research and develop scores of achievements that promote the enterprises to conduct technology research and development and the traditional Chinese medical science and medicines to be popular in the world. The sixth is to further understand the train of thought and the methods concerning the construction and research of the theories of traditional Chinese medicine, solve new problems, explore new laws and accelerate the integration of theoretical construction and research with the fundamental problems in the development of the undertaking of the traditional Chinese medical science and medicines and the academic development.

(8) Efforts shall be made to promote solution to key and difficult issues in the legislative process of the traditional Chinese medical science and medicines.

The *Law of the People's Republic of China on Traditional Chinese Medicine (draft)* has been reported to the State Council and we strive to issue it as early as possible; while we still have much arduous work to do and shall accelerate the pace. The first is to conduct profound research on major and difficult legislative issues. For example, there remain different opinions on such issues as law terms, protection of traditional knowledge on the traditional Chinese medical science and medicines, integration of Western medicine and traditional Chinese medicine and we are short of detailed operating plans on solution to some institutional arrangements put forward in the *Draft*, which requires us to cooperate with relevant departments and conduct thorough research in order to provide basis for pushing forward the legislative process. The second is to carry out investigations on particular subjects. We shall actively cooperate with departments concerned to investigate a series of subjects, review successful exploration and legislative practice in all the localities and draw on experience in the legislation of traditional medicine and even traditional Chinese medicine from other countries and regions so as to use them for reference in the legislation of the traditional Chinese medical science and medicines. The third is to strengthen coordination and strive to obtain support. To certain extent, the process of pushing forward the legislation is a process of coordination, so we shall continuously focus on coordination and make efforts to get more common views. Meanwhile, efforts shall be made to accelerate the construction of law-based administration in the system of traditional Chinese medicine, effectively carry out the *Sixth Five-Year Plan for Popularizing Law*, enhance supervision on the traditional Chinese medical science and medicines and perfect supervisory mechanisms. The fourth is to push forward the standardized work, speed up the construction of the standardized system, give priority to formulation and issue of the diagram of standardized systems and accelerate the formulation and revision of the standards for the traditional Chinese medical science and medicines with focus on the basic and general standards, the standards for diagnosis and treatment of traditional Chinese medicine and the standards for natural resources of Chinese medicinal materials. We shall also strengthen the construction of supporting systems for the standardized work, perfect management systems for the standards of the traditional Chinese medical science and medicines and optimize the systems for organizational leadership and technology management. Construction of research bases of the standards of the traditional Chinese medical science and medicines shall be conducted and research on the theories of the standards and the key technology shall be intensified. Construction of the bases for popularizing the standards shall be promoted also and assessment on the propagation and application of the standards shall be enhanced. The fifth is to rapidly push forward the informatization of the traditional Chinese medical science and medicines. With focus on the construction of information platforms and application systems, we shall promote the sharing and application of information resources, further strengthen the construction of governmental websites of the industry, promote transparency in government operations and safeguard people's rights and interests.

(9) Efforts shall be made to promote the comprehensive implementation of the guidelines on foreign exchange and cooperation in the traditional Chinese medical science and medicines.

In foreign exchange and cooperation in the traditional Chinese medical science and medicines, we shall insist on the principle of "from the domestic to the foreign, from culture to theory, from the non-governmental to the governmental, from the pharmaceutical to the medical, form the easy to the difficult and form the specific to the general", firmly seize favorable historical opportunities, follow the guiding principles, working objectives and key tasks defined in the National Conference on TCM Foreign Exchange and Cooperation, make overall coordination and orderly carry through and implement the *Outline of the Plan for Foreign Exchange and Cooperation in Traditional Chinese Medicine*. The first is to actively carry out governmental cooperative agreements, give priority to the agreements with America, Russia, Malaysia and some other countries, build high-level coordinative mechanisms and cooperative platforms of production, academy and scientific research, direct cooperation and innovate cooperative forms. The second is to strengthen multi-lateral cooperation, make further response to the *Resolution of Traditional Medicine* of WHO, carry through and implement the Regional Strategy for Traditional Medicine in the Western Pacific (2011– 2020), prepare the Forum on World Traditional Medical Science and Medicines, formulate the part of traditional medicine for ICD codes of WHO (International Classification of Diseases of the World Health Organization), make full use of the platform and working mechanisms of the Technical Committee of Traditional Chinese medicine of ISO and create favorable atmosphere and environment for the foreign exchange and cooperation in the traditional Chinese medical science and medicines. The third is to explore ways that can promote the spread of traditional Chinese medical culture in the international community and through overseas Confucius Institutes, China culture exchange centers, the activity of "year of a certain country" organized by and held in both China and foreign countries and other such platforms, spread traditional Chinese medical culture and knowledge to foreign countries. The fourth is to deepen strategic research on service trade, coordinate relevant departments, perfect policies and measures, work out development programs and action plans, explore patterns and methods and promote the development of the service trade of the traditional Chinese medical science and medicines. The fifth is to deepen the contact of four districts of Cross-Straits, bring the advantages of each district into full play and promote practical cooperation in production, academy and scientific research. The sixth is, with focus on the needs for the development of our country, enhance the introduction of foreign talents and intelligence, conduct projects on overseas exchange and training, promote the construction of exchange and cooperation bases, hold training for export-oriented talents and further heighten the level and capacity of foreign exchange and cooperation in the traditional Chinese medical science and medicines. The seventh is to support people-to-people foreign exchange and cooperation in the traditional Chinese medical science and medicines and lead the exchange and cooperation to develop in an orderly way so as to pool forces and jointly improve the international image and influence of the traditional Chinese medical science and medicines.

(10) Efforts shall be made to deeply carry out the activities of "striving to excel in performances" and "three good and one satisfaction" (good service, good quality, good medical ethics; people's satisfaction) and do something practical for people

This year, we shall review and commend the activity of "striving to excel in performances" and make efforts to explore and establish long-term mechanisms for the activity. The first is to closely center on the focal work, deeply carry out the activity, make the activity of "three good and one satisfaction" act as an important carrier and breakthrough for the activity of "serving people and striving to excel in the performances", focus on the major tasks of providing excellent traditional Chinese medical services for people, do well the things that make people reap benefits and feel convenient, improve service conduct and quality, make people more satisfied with their much-loved traditional Chinese medical work and truly feel the changes and benefits brought by the activities. The second is, in accordance with the Party Central Committee's working deployment and requirements, to think out such contents and forms of the activities that are visible, motivating, easy to participate and able to be evaluated and carry out the activities deeply and in an down-to-earth way. The fourth is to further find out, set up and propagate advanced models, make serious summary and commendation and strive to create a sound environment for the activity of "serving people and striving to excel in the performances" in which everyone learns from advanced models, respects advanced models and tries to be and overtake advanced models. The fourth is to take the activity of "striving to excel in performances" as an opportunity, promote the improvement of professional spirits of the industry of the traditional Chinese medical science and medicines, push forward the construction of industrial culture and the ideological and ethic progress and provide a powerful driving force and guarantee for the promotion of the scientific development and the realization of the 12th Five-Year development goals for the undertaking of the traditional Chinese medical science and medicines. The fifth is to continue to strengthen the construction of the systems for the punishment and prevention of corruption in the system of the traditional Chinese medical science and medicines, further carry out the responsibility system for the rectification of malpractice and the evaluation system for medical ethics, strengthen combat against commercial bribery in drug sales and purchase, strictly punish conducts that violate the law and discipline and damage people's interests, intensify the prevention and control of integrity risk in public hospitals and establish systems for the evaluation on whether patients are satisfied.

Comrades, it's a glorious mission to push forward the development of the undertaking of the traditional Chinese medical science and medicines and benefit people's health; while it's also an arduous task and great responsibility. Let's closely unite around the Party Central Committee with Hu Jintao as the General Secretary, deeply carry through and implement the Scientific Outlook on Development, keep in mind the overall situation, proceed with confidence, activate our spirit, work effectively, strive to accomplish every piece of work of 2012 and greet the 18th National Congress of the Communist Party of China with greater achievements.

(Zhao Yinghong)

7. Address at 2012 Work Conference of National Food and Drug Administration —By Shao Mingli, Vice Minister of Health and Commissioner of State Food and Drug Administration (December 20, 2011) (Excerpts)

In the following parts, I'll talk about three aspects on behalf of the State Food and Drug Administration.

I. Summary on administration in 2011 (omitted)

II. The implementation of the 12th-Five-Year-Plan programs

The 12th-Five-Year-Plan period is very crucial for building a prosperous society in China comprehensively, deepening reform and opening-up and speeding up the transformation of the pattern of economic development. It is also very important for the reform and development of food and drug administration, for it means very precious strategic opportunities. The CPC Central Committee and the State Council attach great importance to food and drug administration. On December 7, the Standing Committee of the State Council discussed and approved *National Drug Safety Program (2011-2015)*. The Legislative Affair Office of the State Council is leading the compilation of *National Program for Food Safety Administrative System (2011-2015)*. These two programs are the extended and detailed versions of the national plan for the development of economy and society for food and drug administration, as well as the important guidelines for food and drug administration and the development of the cause. Therefore, we must attach great importance to these two 12th-Five-Year programs, make joint efforts, do our utmost, try to implement them to ensure the effective implementation of the programs and the fulfillment of the working objectives of food and drug administration during the 12th-Five-Year period, so that we will lay a significant foundation for the long-term safety of food and drug. This is the common task and common responsibility facing the whole system. During this process, we must handle several major problems properly.

(1) The implementation of the 12th-Five-Year programs must be based on the overall development of economy and society. In order to safeguard the fundamental interests of the overwhelming majority of the people and achieve the long-term stability of the nation, the CPC Central Committee forcefully propel the social

construction focusing on safeguarding and improving people's livelihood, strengthen and innovate social management and deepen the reform of medical and health care system. At present, food and drug administration is still at the important period of strategic opportunities for the accelerating development. However, there are some new changes in the exterior environment, which can be mainly referred to as "Four Acceleration"

1) the acceleration of transforming the pattern of economic development. Even though the economic structure has been adjusted, industrial concentration has been increased and enterprises have been merged and reorganized frequently, the overall level of industry is not high, the ability of development and initiative innovation is not great and the quality control system is not perfect.

2) the acceleration of adjusting the market pattern. Even though the relationship between demand and supply has changed, the total market has been increasing rapidly and competition has become fiercer, the comprehensive reform on the system of production and circulation is not adequate, the operation of enterprises is not normative and the competition of homogeneity is always leading to the competition of low prices.

3) the acceleration of implementing the policies on medical and health care reform. The reforms on medical and health care system and food and drug administrative system are being deepened, which presents us with a historic opportunity to solve some major problems and makes some higher requirements for us to improve policies, regulations and systems of administration as well.

4) the acceleration of internationalization. International communication and cooperation has been increasingly active in the field of food and drug administration, and the globalization of products and enterprises has been more and more obvious. Therefore, we must undertake the administrative pressure from home and abroad. All in all, the changes mentioned above have brought precious opportunities for development as well as many predictable and unpredictable challenges. All these old and new contradictions, problems and conditions coexist and influence each other and are liable to convert into safety risks for food and drug, and may even cause severe safety accidents, which makes administration more difficult and uncertain. For us, this is both pressure and the motivation for promoting administration and improving our work. Food and drug administrative departments at all levels must further strengthen our sense of responsibility and sense of emergency. We must seize the important opportunity of implementing the 12th-Five-Year programs firmly, integrate ourselves into the overall development of economy and society, and accelerate our own construction to safeguard food and drug safety better and promote administration to a higher level.

(2) The implementation of the 12th -Five-Year programs must be based on the main principle of scientific supervision and administration. The external factors are the conditions and the internal factors are the roots. In order to practically fulfill our duties of supervision and administration and properly tackle the challenges of various risks, we need to unswervingly adhere to scientific supervision and administration, safeguard food and drug safety for the public and promote the harmonious development of economy and society.

1) Efforts will be made to improve the ability of social management with completing the system of responsibility as the key point. Food and drug safety is a major social problem, and therefore, comprehensive social management must be implemented. Just for this reason, the national 12th -Five-Year Plan lists implementing safety responsibility and completing the system of responsibility as an important task. Under the leadership of the Party committees and governments, food and drug administrative departments at all levels will include food and drug safety into the evaluation system of the government and mobilize all the departments and the whole society to promote the innovation of the administrative system and mechanism. We will break the limitation of departments and professions social management to solve the problems and contradictions and achieve consensus by making good use of the methods of.

2) Efforts will be made to improve the ability of technological support with the implementation of major projects as the key point. Efforts will be made to gain support for the implementation of the major projects of the 12th -Five-Year Plan, and the construction of the projects will promote the implementation of the Plan and lead to some breakthroughs. The construction of the projects must strengthen the basis and highlight the construction of the central and local overall ability. The focuses will be on implementing the action plan for improving the national standards, the project of surveillance on adverse drug reaction and the re-evaluation on safety of post-market drugs, the second phase project of the national information system of drug supervision and administration, the project of constructing emergency management system, the project of improving the quality of talent team, and the project of infrastructure construction so that the system of technological support will be further improved.

3) Efforts will be made to improve the capacity of risk prevention and control with improving regulations and mechanisms as the key point. After years of efforts, we have established a complete set of regulations and mechanisms for supervision and administration, but there still exist the problems of not being scientific enough, not being systematic enough and not being effective enough. Therefore, the 12th-Five-Year Programs attach special importance to the construction of supervision

and administration regulations and mechanisms, emphasizing on improving the regulations of whole-process supervision and administration, adopting stricter admission standards, strengthening the re-evaluation on products in markets and improving the level of emergency handling.

4) Efforts will be made to improve the capacity to promote the scientific development of the industry with strengthening the guidance of the policies as the key point. Food and drug industry is a strategic industry concerning people's livelihood and national safety, with great significance to the prosperity and great renaissance of the Chinese People. We have been emphasizing that scientific supervision and administration is the effective insurance for scientific development and scientific development is the important basis for scientific supervision and administration. It is the important duty of the supervisory and administrative departments to promote the scientific development of the industry and protect and promote the advanced productivity on the basis of putting the public's interest first and ensuring food and drug safety. We must adapt to the relations and development trends of international market and domestic market, make full use of the policy adjustments on improving standards, evaluation and approval, experiment and test, examination and authentication, surveillance evaluation, and other technical guidance to promote the restructure of the industry, encourage scientific and technological innovation, change the situations of repeated construction and competition at the low levels, improve the capacity and level of self-supply, support the internationalization of enterprises and improve the competitiveness of "Made in China".

(3) The implementation of the 12th-Five-Year programs must be based on strengthening the systematicness and effectiveness of supervision and administration. Establishing a scientific, fair, open and efficient system of food and drug supervision and administration is a major objective of the 12th-Five-Year programs. Especially when the organizational reform has almost been completed, we must emphasize the systematicness and effectiveness of supervision and administration, which are mainly reflected in the following four aspects:

1) The common goals. To ensure food and drug safety is the aim of supervision and administration and the sole criterion to judge the effects of implementing the programs. The whole system must work on this common goal to improve food and drug safety through our unswerving and effective effort so that the public and the whole society can really feel the noticeable effects of supervision and administration. If any department deviates from this goal, their value of "For Whom to Supervise and Administrate" will distort, their function orientation will dissimilate and local protectionism and crimes may follow. The safety risks and fake and counterfeited commodities produced in the local regions may influence the whole nation through

the grand circulation of food and drug, which will cause severe harm.

2) The complete system. Efforts will be made to complete the food and drug administrative organs at the grassroots, provide them with the adequate manpower and resources to perform their functions so that they can perform their functions by law independently. Efforts will be made to strengthen the connection and cooperation between the administrative supervision and technical supervision and establish a complete set of working regulations to ensure the orderly functioning of supervisory and administrative departments at all levels.

3) The smooth implementation of policies. Consistency is essential for food and drug supervision and administration. The subordinates must obey the orders from the superiors. Countermeasures to the policies or acting in one's own ways must be prohibited. Administration by law must be strictly carried out and supervision on law enforcement must be strengthened to safeguard social fairness and justice. Performance evaluation on supervision and administration must be strengthened. Equal importance will be attached to both deployment and supervision & inspection so that rewards and punishments can be meted out fairly.

4) The efficient functioning. Modern technology will be used to optimize the working procedures and accelerate information sharing. Cooperation and coordination will be enhanced to further strengthen the connection between supervision and administration links and perfect the regional coordination mechanism. Administrative methods, scientific and technological methods, publicity methods and internet methods etc. will be made use of comprehensively to improve the efficiency of supervision and administration.

Talents are of utmost significance to the development of our cause. Food and drug administrative departments at all levels must firmly establish the concept that talent resources are the primary resources. In accordance with the requirements of the CPC Central Committee that "Priority must be given to the development of talent resources, the adjustment of talent structure, the guarantee of talent investment and innovation of talent regulations", food and drug administrative departments at all levels must innovate the systems and mechanisms for the development of talents and create a good environment for the growth of the talents on the basis of their actual situations. While we strengthen training of the staff and improve the overall quality of the whole team, greater efforts will be made to promote the construction of a talent team which consists of high-leveled international talents and professional talents in short supply so as to improve the professionalism of our supervisory and administrative team and hopefully a highly qualified and professional talent team for food and drug supervision and administration can be created. Such a team is the most important talent guarantee and intellectual support for us to perform our function of food and drug supervision and administration and smoothly achieve the goals for the development of our supervision and administration during the 12th-Five-Year period.

The program is just a blueprint, so its key lies in the implementation. The implementation of the 12th-Five-Year program is the common duties of the central government and the local governments. In accordance with the development goals and main tasks set by the program, all the localities must include the work in the major agenda and make overall consideration together with the local programs for the development of economy and society and unified deployments and synchronous implementation will be made with the livelihood projects. With definite goals, definite projects, definite funds and definite measures, the implementation of tasks listed in the programs can be ensured. Food and drug supervisory and administrative departments at all levels must establish scientific and effective mechanisms for the implementation of the programs, strengthen organization and leadership, and research and decide on the major events and prominent problems during the implementation of the programs in time. The tasks in the programs must be divided, leading departments must be specified and the annual working plans and implementation plans must be made so that the work can be carried out orderly without any delay. Mechanisms for the evaluation, examination and adjustment must be established to strengthen dynamic monitoring and inspection and scientifically evaluate the quality and effects of the implementation.

III. Key Work in 2012

The year 2012 is a crucial year for the comprehensive implementation of the 12th-Five-Year programs and also an important year for pushing forward the new round of reform on medical and health care system. The Central Committee conference on economic work held lately emphasized on reforming medical and health care system, strengthening supervision and administration on the key products like food and drug comprehensively and severely cracking down on violations of laws or regulations. Food and drug supervision and administration must be carefully carried out to effectively safeguard the harmony and stability of the society. Therefore, it means great significance and arduous tasks. The whole system must view it from a strategic and overall perspective, further enhance our sense of mission, sense of responsibility and sense of urgency; we must take politics and overall situations into consideration and observe the disciplines rather than be frightened by any risks or disturbed by anything so that we can concentrate on supervision and administration and unswervingly safeguard food and drug safety.

The overall requirements for food and drug supervision and administration in

2012 are: to fully implement the essence of the 17th CPC National Congress, the fifth and the sixth plenary sessions of the 17th CPC National Congress and the Central Economic Work Conference, take the Scientific Outlook on Development as our guide, vigorously apply the concept of scientific supervision and administration, promote the supervision and administration culture, whose core value is "supervision and administration for the people", act on the general ideas of "innovating supervision and administration system and mechanism, improve the ability to supervise and administrate, perfect supervision and administration system and fulfill the responsibility of supervision and administration", strictly regulate supervision and administration, severely crack down on violation of laws or regulations, closely prevent and control any risks for food and drug safety, consolidate the good beginning of the 12th-Five-Year Plan period, accelerate laying a solid foundation for the long-term stability of food and drug safety and welcome the holding the 18th CPC National Congress with our excellent achievements.

The focus will be on the follow work:

(1) Perfect supervision and administration regulations and mechanisms and strengthen the construction of normalization. The construction of normalization is the important guarantee for effectively performing the functions and strengthening administration by law. Compared with the requirements of the supervision and administration tasks and the development of supervision and administration situations, the construction of normalization is faced with the problems such as being lagged behind, disjointed and ill-suited, which have to be solved with great efforts, i.e. to normalize supervision and administration with regulations and improve the efficiency of supervision and administration with normalization. Firstly, strengthen the construction of laws and regulations. We will vigorously assist the Legislative Affair Office of the State Council to promote the promulgation of *Provisions for the Supervision and Administration of Health Food* and *Provisions for the Supervision and Administration of Medical Devices*. We will organize the formulation and revision of some regulations and normative documents including *Measures for the Management of Drug Supply Licenses, Good Supply Practice for Drugs, Provisions for the Management of Drug Standards, Measures for the Management of Health Food Registration* and *Measures for the Management of Licenses of Cosmetic Manufacturers*, etc. Attention will be paid to the connection and coordination between systems. The construction of the connecting mechanisms between administrative law enforcement and criminal law enforcement will be sped up and guiding opinions will be formulated on strengthening transferring suspected criminal cases. The sixth Five-Year of Law Publicizing will be further pushed forward to continuously improve the capability and level of administrating by law. Secondly, strengthen research on policies and theories. Efforts will be made to research on

the major problems concerning food and drug supervision and administration, including the influence of medical reform on drug production and circulation, the accountability system for food and drug safety and performance evaluation, globalization and internationalization of supervision and administration, reform on supervisory and administrative system and the systematicness of supervision and administration etc. so that predicative and targeted countermeasures and suggestions can be proposed from the strategic level and the national level. Thirdly, deepen reform on evaluation and approval mechanisms. Efforts will be made to strictly regulate evaluation and approval by law, optimize the procedures, clarify the power and improve efficiency. Exploration will be made to establish the authorization mechanism for the technical evaluation of drug supplementary application and keep on promoting the authorization of biological products' lot release at the provincial institutes for food and drug control. The quality and efficiency of evaluation and approval will be improved and mechanisms will be established to correct errors and rectify deviations. Pilot on the electronic evaluation of health food will be carried out. Fourthly, accountability will be strictly carried out. Specific normative documents will be formulated; supervision and inspection on evaluation and approval, examination and test, inspection and authentication, monitoring and assessment, and inspection and law enforcement etc., will be enhanced as well as accountability. Supervision on law enforcement will be strengthened, focusing on the severe violations of laws and regulations reflected in law enforcement inspection, administrative review and administrative lawsuits. We will analyze the causes, settle these violations and punish all the people responsible seriously.

(2) Improve the level of scientific supervision and administration and prevent and control risks for food and drug safety. To adapt to the needs of development, we will take modern, professional and social measures comprehensively to prevent and control risks and improve our ability. Firstly, improve the overall standards and the quality control of technical norms. The compilation of *Chinese Pharmacopeia* (2015 Edition) will be carried out comprehensively. Guiding and management on national drug standards will be strengthened and sped up to ensure the quality. Working procedures will be normalized and the formatting mechanism and abolishing mechanism will be improved. The policies will vigorously play the role of guiding to encourage the creation of new drugs, guide the development of drugs for rare diseases and children, support the development of traditional Chinese medicine and ethnical medicine, perfect the regulations for the registration management of technology transfer and relocation to a new place and the technological requirements, and promote the upgrade of the industry and the restructure of products. Work will be done to organize the formulation and revision of standards for medical devices

so as to speed up the construction of standard system for medical devices. The plan to improve the technical requirements for health food will be started. The capacity building of drug and medical device examination and test will be strengthened and the perfection of examination and test system for catering service, health food and cosmetics will be sped up. Secondly, complete quality control system. Quantitative grading management of food safety for catering services will be carried on orderly and the staffing of food safety management for cater service entities will be sped up. Joining hands with the commercial departments, we will select the first group of national demonstrative counties for food safety in the catering services. Pilot on qualified person in health food manufacturers and cosmetic manufacturers will be carried on to strengthen supervision on sub-contract production, implement grading and classified management on manufacturers and establish traceability system for quality safety. The whole process supervision on drug development will be strengthened to perfect and normalize the standards and procedures for on-site verification of drug registration. Taking advantage of the promulgation and enforcement of the new revised drug GSP, we will seriously carry on the authentication and inspection. The system of licensed pharmacists will be perfected faster to strengthen the guiding of licensed pharmacists on the rational drug use by the public. Management on the supply licenses of drugs and medical devices will be strengthened to perfect the market access and withdrawal mechanisms. The construction of drug inspection system will be strengthened. Supervision and administration on blood products, vaccines, special drugs and high-risk medical devices will be strengthened. The re-evaluation on the safety of TCM injections will be carried on. The establishment of demonstrative counties for drug safety will be further carried on. Thirdly, work well on the implementation of the newly revised drug GMP. The newly revised drug GMP is an important measure to protect the advanced productivity, eliminate the backward productivity, promote restructure of the industry and enhance the international competitiveness of our medical and pharmaceutical industry. Food and drug supervisory and administrative departments at all levels must act on the general arrangements of implementing drug GMP step by step, adhere to the time limits and standards, strengthen the supervision and instruction on the enterprises, tighten on-site inspections and guarantee unified standards to ensure the quality and efficiency of authentication. Fourthly, strengthen the construction of informatization. The informatization of food safety supervision for catering services will be carried on. Risk monitoring and pre-warning platform for health food and cosmetics will be established. A management system for drug registration information will be gradually set up, which can integrate all the resources, share the resources and operate efficiently. The management system for auditing business information will be perfected. The implementation of the first phase project for national information system of drug supervision and administration will be sped up to promote the implementation of projects like the supporting platform for electronic administrative information service, business application system, information safety platform and backup centers etc. so that the informatization level for supervision and administration will be further improved.

(3) Crack down on violations of laws and regulations severely, especially for the major and serious criminal cases. Food and drug supervisory and administrative departments at all levels must act initially and promptly to strengthen collaborative action and guarantee implementation. Firstly, work will be carried on to crack down on illegal additives in catering services, health food and cosmetics. Special rectifications will be carried out with the school canteens and tourist areas as the key sites and the purchase of raw materials and the use of food additives as the key links. Special rectifications on illegal adding chemicals to health food and illegal use of prohibited substances in cosmetics will be carried out. Rectifications on health food with the functions of relieving physical fatigue and losing weight and cosmetics with the function of lightening freckles will be even severer. Once illegal additives are detected, relevant permits will be revoked. The intensity of cracking down on counterfeit drugs will be carried on. Joining hands with relevant departments, we will carry on with the joint cracking down, ask the public to supervise the investigation and punishment of some major and serious criminal cases which have much social influence and with which the public are the most dissatisfied. As for the enterprises involved in the cases, we will punish them severely by law without any mercy. If drug manufactures are found to produce or sell counterfeit drugs, all the approval documents will be rescinded. For those who produce counterfeit drugs deliberately, their *Drug Production Licenses* will be revoked. If drug supply enterprises are found to lease or transfer licenses, permits, bills or notes to supply counterfeit drugs, or purchase or sell counterfeit drugs even when the channels are unclear or formalities are incomplete, their *Drug Supply Licenses* will be revoked. The transferring of criminal cases will be carried on well and vigorous efforts will be made to assist the police to investigate them. *Measures for the Management of Drug Supervision and Administration at Medical Institutions (Interim)* will be implemented to strengthen the supervision and inspection on medical institutions and retailer drug stores. The construction of the complaint website "12331" will be sped up, which means greater importance will be attached to clues found from complaining and reporting, supervision and sample inspection and on-site inspection, and the connection between supervision & inspection and checking will be strengthened. Thirdly, drug trade online and information release online will be normalized. The release of drug information

online and the qualification approval of transaction websites will be tightened and the supervision and inspection on the approved websites will be strengthened. Work will be done to assist relevant departments to severely crack down on the illegal action of releasing false drug information or selling drugs on the internet. Fourthly, advertisement censorship will be strengthened. A surveillance network covering broadcast, television and newspaper above the prefectural-level will be set up to strengthen the responsibility of the localization management. The enterprises that release illegal advertisements and their products will be especially monitored and rectified.

(4) Supervision and administration of essential drugs will be tightened to ensure their quality and safety. The quality and safety of essential drugs have great influence on the reform of medical and health care system. Therefore, we must attach great importance to them and consistently work well on them. Firstly, emphasize on the key points of supervision and administration. Sampling inspections on all varieties of essential drugs will be carried on. Closely monitor the quality of the varieties of essential drugs that have won the bids yet with especially low prices, especially the two key aspects, i.e. tracing the source of the raw materials and excipients and the material balance during the production, and severely investigate and punish any deception or fraud. Include some high risk varieties into the national evaluation and sampling testing plan to further optimize sampling tests. A linkage mechanism for drug control, ADR monitoring, on-site supervision and inspection on production and the rise of standards will be established. Inspections on distribution enterprises will be enhanced. Secondly, speed up electronic supervision and administration. By the end of February, 2012, the essential drugs produced by all the enterprises must be assigned a code, and all the distribution enterprises of essential drugs must upload date via the electronic supervising net. No enterprises that cannot enter online drug information about the arrival at and discharge from warehouses will be qualified to distribute essential drugs. By the end of February, 2013, all the supplementary drugs to the essential drug lists in all the provinces will be covered by electronic supervision. Thirdly, improve the capability and level of ADR monitoring. Efforts will be made to implement *Measures on the Management of ADR Reporting and Monitoring*, strengthen the construction of monitoring institutions at the grassroots level and stress on improving the capability of analyzing and evaluating risk signals so as to give full play to its function of risk pre-warning. Great importance will be attached to the research and judgment of safety situations and further research will be conducted into the serious problems revealed to find out the causes and solve them properly.

(5) The construction of the cadres' team and the building of Party's style and a clean government will be strengthened to ensure the fulfillment of supervision tasks.

Conscientious work will be done to analyze the new situations faced by the cadres' team of food and drug administrative system and the building of Party's style and a clean government, go on deepening reform on cadres' personnel system and go on with the campaign of Excellent Service to comprehensively strengthen the construction of cadres' team of the food and drug administrative system. Greater importance will be attached to combating corruption and upholding integrity with stronger leadership and improved measures to construct a system to punish and prevent corruption. The building of Party's style and a clean government will be combined with the construction of the cadres' team. Aiming at such phenomena as great personnel changes, fluctuation of thoughts and being unfamiliar with the situations etc. in some departments or some localities, we will strengthen training, guiding and helping; we will strengthen supervision and punishment on problems such as nonfeasance, disordered feasance, dereliction and neglect of duties etc. and rectify the problems uncompromisingly. The building of Party's style and a clean government will be combined with supervision and administration. The implementation of the deployments on some key work such as supervision and administration on the essential drugs, cracking down on counterfeit drugs and rectifying inferior drugs and the investigation and punishment of criminal cases will be strengthened as well as the supervision and inspection on the key posts and key links. Equal importance will be attached to punishment and prevention, with more emphasis on prevention. We will go on investigating and punishing the criminal cases to severely punish the corruption, but meanwhile, we will put prevention first by establishing a long-term mechanism for the prevention and control for the risks of corruption, which has perfect regulations, rigorous procedures and effective restrictions, so that corruption can be prevented from the source. Political disciplines, organizational disciplines and working disciplines will be tightened to ensure the implementation of the Party's and the government's policies in the food and drug administrative system and the smooth fulfillment of orders in the whole system. The building of working styles will be strengthened to fight against and overcome formalism, bureaucratism, flatulent working styles or being unproductive, etc. solve the problems of mediocrity, laziness and slacking so that we can ensure the implementation of all the tasks for food and drug supervision and administration with a good Party's style and government's working style.

(Zhao Xuemei)

Part II
Policy and Statute

Contents of Health Standards Issued in 2012

1. WS/T 88-2012 For Coal and Soil, Total Fluorine Determination Method, High Temperature Hot Hydrolysis—Ion Selective Electrode

2. WS/T 367-2012 Standardizations of Disinfection Technique for Medical institutions

3. WS/T 368-2012 Management Standardizations of the Air Purification of Hospitals

4. WS 369-2012 Diagnosis of Trichinosis

5. WS 370-2012 Establishment standardizations for the Basic Data Collection of Health Information

6. WS 371-2012 Basic Data of Basic Information: Individual Information

7. WS 372.1-2012 Part 1 of Basic Data Collections of Management of Disease: Management of Hepatitis B Patients

8. WS 372.2-2012 Part 2 of Basic Data Collections of Management of Disease: Health Management for Patients with Hypertension

9. WS 372.3-2012 Part 3 of Basic Data Collections of Management of Disease: Health Management for Patients with Severe Psychosis

10. WS 372.4-2012 Part 4 of Basic Data Collections of Management of Disease: Health Management for the Aged

11. WS 372.5-2012 Part 5 of Basic Data Collections of Management of Disease: Health Management for Patients with Type II Diabetes Mellitus

12. WS 372.6-2012 Part 6 of Basic Data Collections of Management of Disease: Management of Tumor Cases

13. WS 373.1-2012 Part 1 of Basic Data Collections of Medical Service: Abstracts of Outpatient Service

14. WS 373.2-2012 Part 2 of Basic Data Collections of Medical Service: Abstracts of Inpatient Service

15. WS 373.3-2012 Part 3 of Basic Data Collections of Medical Service: Adult Physical Examination

16. WS 374.1-2012 Part 1 of Basic Data Collections of Health Management: Health Supervision, Inspection and Administrative Punishment

17. WS 374.2-2012 Part 2 of Basic Data Collections of Health Management: Administrative Approval and Registration of Health Supervision

18. WS 374.3-2012 Part 3 of Basic Data Collections of Health Management: Surveillance and Evaluation of Health Supervision

19. WS 374.4-2012 Part 4 of Basic Data Collections of Health Management: Institutions and staff of Health Supervision

20. WS 375.1-2012 Part 1 of Basic Data Collections of Disease Control: Comprehensive Prevention and Control of HIV/AIDS

21. WS 375.2-2012 Part 2 of Basic Data Collections of Disease Control: Management for Patients with Schistosomiasis

22. WS 375.3-2012 Part 3 of Basic Data Collections of Disease Control: Management for Patients with Chronic Filariasis

23. WS 375.4-2012 Part 4 of Basic Data Collections of Disease Control: Reports of Occupational Diseases

24. WS 375.5-2012 Part 5 of Basic Data Collections of Disease Control: Occupational Health Surveillance

25. WS 375.6-2012 Part 6 of Basic Data Collections of Disease Control: Reports of Injury Surveillance

26. WS 375.7-2012 Part 7 of Basic Data Collections of Disease Control: Reports of Pesticide Poisoning

27. WS 375.8-2012 Part 8 of Basic Data Collections of Disease Control: Behavioral Risk Factor Surveillance

28. WS 375.9-2012 Part 9 of Basic Data Collections of Disease Control: Medical Certification of Deaths

29. WS 375.10-2012 Part 10 of Basic Data Collections of Disease Control: Reports of Infectious Diseases

30. WS 375.11-2012 Part 11 of Basic Data Collections of Disease Control: Reports of Tuberculosis

31. WS 375.12-2012 Part 12 of Basic Data Collections of Disease Control: Preventive Vaccination

32. WS 379-2012 Diagnosis of Taeniasis

33. WS 380-2012 Diagnosis of Paragonimiasis

34. WS 381-2012 Diagnosis of Cysticercosis

35. WS 382-2012 Diagnosis of Pneumonia

36. WS 383-2012 Diagnosis of Bronchial Asthma

37. WS 384-2012 Diagnosis of Hypertensive Disorder Complicating Pregnancy

38. WS 385-2012 Diagnosis of Congenital Biliary Tract Malformation

39. WS 386-2012 Diagnosis of Colorectal Cancer

40. WS 387.1-2012 Part 1 of Common Operative Technique of Clinical First Aid: Cardiopulmonary Resuscitation (CPR)

41. WS 387.2-2012 Part 2 of Common Operative Technique of Clinical First Aid: Emetic Method, Gastrolavage

42. WS 387.3-2012 Part 3 of Common Operative Technique of Clinical First Aid: Oxygen Therapy and Establishment of Artificial Airway

43. WS 387.4-2012 Part 4 of Common Operative Technique of Clinical First Aid: Extraction of Respiratory Secretions

44. WS 387.5-2012 Part 5 of Common Operative Technique of Clinical First Aid: Emergency Hemostasis, Binding up and Carrying for Trauma Patients

45. WS/T 388-2012 Premature Diagnosis

46. WS/T 389-2012 Medical X-ray Examination Regulations

47. WS/T 390-2012 Standardized Processes of Emergency Department in Hospital

48. WS/T 391-2012 Operation Regulations of CT Examination

49. WS 392-2012 Clinical Application of Ventilator

50. WS/T 393-2012 Formulation and Implementation of Clinical Pathway of Medical Institutions

51. WS 394-2012 Sanitary Specifications for Central Air-conditioning Ventilation System in Public Places

52. WS/T 395-2012 Hygienic Evaluation Specifications of Central Air-conditioning Ventilation System in Public Places

53. WS/T 396-2012 Decontamination and Disinfection Specifications of Central Air-conditioning Ventilation System in Public Places

54. WS 397-2012 Screening and Diagnosis of Diabetes Mellitus

55. WS/T 398-2012 Quality Control of Diagnosis and Treatment for Ischemic Stroke

56. WS 399-2012 Requirements for Blood Storage

57. WS/T 400-2012 Requirements for Blood Transportation

58. WS/T 401-2012 Requirements for the Configuration of Blood Donation Sites

59. WS/T 402-2012 Formulation of Reference Compartments for Testing Items of Clinical Laboratories

60. WS/T 403-2012 Analytical and Quality Indicators of Regular Items for Clinical Biochemistry Test

61. WS/T 404.1-2012 Part 1 of Reference Compartments for Common Clinical Biochemical Tests: Alanine Aminotransferase (ALT), Aspartate Aminotransferase (AST), Alkaline Phosphatase (ALP) and gamma-glutamyltransferase (GGT)

62. WS/T 404.2-2012 Part 2 of Reference Compartments for Common Clinical Biochemical Tests: Total Serum Protein, Serum Albumin

63. WS/T 404.3-2012 Part 3 of Reference Compartments for Common Clinical Biochemical Tests: Serum Potassium, Serum Sodium and Serum Chlorine

64. WS/T 405-2012 Reference Compartment for Blood Cell Analysis

65. WS/T 406-2012 Requirements for Analytical Quality of Regular Items for Clinical Hematology

66. WS/T 407-2012 A Guide to the Comparability Validation of Testing Results Decided within Medical Institutions

67. WS/T 408-2012 A Guide to Linear Evaluation of Clinical Chemistry Equipments

68. GBZ 165-2012 Radiological Protection Requirements for X-ray Computerized Tomography

69. GBZ/T 229.4-2012 Part 4 of Work Classification of Occupational Hazards: Noise

70. GBZ 241-2012 Diagnosis of Radiation-induced Heart Disease

71. GB 7959-2012 Sanitary Requirements for Innocuous Treatment of Faeces

72. GB 9981-2012 Hygienic Specifications for Rural Housing

73. GB 11654.1-2012 Part 1 of Width of Sanitary Protection Zone of Paper-making and Paper Products Industries: Pulp Manufacturing Industry

74. GB 11655.1-2012 Part 1 of Width of Sanitary Protection Zone of Synthetic Materials Manufacturing Industry: polyvinyl chloride (PVC)

75. GB 11655.6-2012 Part 6 of Width of Sanitary Protection Zone of Synthetic Materials Manufacturing Industry: Neoprene Manufacturing Industry

76. GB 11661-2012 Width of Sanitary Protection Zone of Coking Industry

77. GB 11662-2012 Width of Sanitary Protection Zone of Sintering Industry

78. GB 11666.1-2012 Part 1 of Width of Sanitary Protection Zone of Fertilizer Manufacturing Industry: Nitrogenous Fertilizer Manufacturing Industry

79. GB 11666.2-2012 Part 2 of Width of Sanitary Protection Zone of Fertilizer Manufacturing Industry: Phosphatic Fertilizer Manufacturing Industry

80. GB 15982-2012 Sanitary Standards for Hospital Disinfection

81. GB/T 16125-2012 Test Method of Acute Toxicity for Daphnia Magna

82. GB/T 16149-2012 Measurement Estimation Specifications for Chronic Radiation Sickness

83. GB 16361-2012 Specifications of Protection and Quality Control for Clinical Nuclear Medicine Patients

84. GB/T 17216-2012 Environment Sanitation Requirements for the Daily Use of Civil Air Defense Shelters

85. GB/T 17222-2012 Width of Sanitary Protection Zone of Coal Gas Industry

86. GB/T 17223-2012 Hygienic Requirements for a Day of Learning of Primary and Secondary School Students

87. GB 18055-2012 Hygienic Specifications for Planning of Villages and Small Towns

88. GB 18068.1-2012 Part 1 of Width of Sanitary Protection Zone of Non-metallic Mineral Products Industry: Cement Manufacturing Industry

89. GB 18068.2-2012 Part 2 of Width of Sanitary Protection Zone of Non-metallic Mineral Products Industry: Lime Manufacturing Industry

90. GB 18068.3-2012 Part 3 of Width of Sanitary Protection Zone of Non-metallic Mineral Products Industry: Asbestos Manufacturing Industry

91. GB 18068.4-2012 Part 4 of Width of Sanitary Protection Zone of Non-metallic Mineral Products Industry: Graphite and Carbon Manufacturing

92. GB 18071.1-2012 Part 1 of Sanitary Protection Zone of Basic Chemical Raw Materials Manufacturing Industry: Caustic Soda Manufacturing Industry

93. GB 18071.3-2012 Part 3 of Sanitary Protection Zone of Basic Chemical Raw Materials Manufacturing Industry: Sulfuric Acid Manufacturing Industry

94. GB 18071.6-2012 Part 6 of Sanitary Protection Zone of Basic Chemical Raw Materials Manufacturing Industry: Sodium Sulfide Manufacturing

95. GB 18071.7-2012 Part 7 of Sanitary Protection Zone of Basic Chemical Raw Materials Manufacturing Industry: Yellow Phosphorus Manufacturing Industry

96. GB 18071.8-2012 Part 8 of Sanitary Protection Zone of Basic Chemical Raw Materials Manufacturing Industry: Hydrofluoric Acid Manufacturing

97. GB 18075.1-2012 Part 1 of Sanitary Protection Zone of Transport and Communication Facilities Manufacturing Industry: Automobile Manufacturing Industry

98. GB 18078.1-2012 Part 1 of Sanitary Protection Zone of Farm Products and Byproducts Processing Industry: Slaughter and Meat Processing

99. GB 18079-2012 Sanitary Protection Zone of Animal Glue Manufacturing Industry

100. GB 18080.1-2012 Part 1 of Sanitary Protection Zone of Textile Industry: Cotton Textile, Chemical Fiber Textile and Fine Machining of Textile Printing

101. GB 18082.1-2012 Part 1 of Sanitary Protection Zone of Leather, Fur and Their Products: Leather Tanning

102. GB/T 18205-2012 Comprehensive Evaluation of School Health

103. GB 18469-2012 Quality Requirements for Whole Blood and Component Blood

104. GB 19379-2012 Hygienic Specifications for Rural Household Toilets

105. GB 28595-2012 Elimination of Endemic Arsenism Area

106. GB/T 28930-2012 Hygienic Requirements for Students' Use of Computers

107. GB 28931-2012 Safety and Health Standards of Chlorine Dioxide Disinfectant Generators

108. GB 28932-2012 Management Standards of Prevention and Control of Infectious Diseases in Primary and Secondary Schools

109. GB/T 28940-2012 Procedures of Pathogen Sampling of Vector Biological Infection: Murine

110. GB/T 28941-2012 Procedures of Pathogen Sampling of Vector Biological Infection: Mosquito

111. GB/T 28942-2012 Procedures of Pathogen Sampling of Vector Biological Infection: Flea

112. GB/T 28943-2012 Hazard Risk Assessment and Guidelines of Vectors: Murine

113. GB/T 28944-2012 Emergency Surveillance and Control of Vectors: Flood

114. GB/T 29433-201 Guide to Psychological Health Education of Students

(Wang Dian)

Part III
Progress of Work

1. The Progress of Health Work in 2012

The year 2012 is a key year connecting the preceding and the following work of the deepening medical reform. According to the monitoring data of medical reform, 33 projects of tasks led by Ministry of Health were completed smoothly and significant results were obtained in all work.

I. The Focal Point of Work in the Deepening of Medical Reform

The guarantee and the abilities of supervision and management of the new rural cooperative medical care system (NRCMCS) were improved further. The NRCMCS was launched in 2,566 counties (cities and districts) nationwide, the number of the NRCMCS participants was 805,000,000 and the participating rate was above 98%. The annual funding was 248,500,000,000 yuan, and the year-on-year growth was 21.4%. The total expenditure was 240,800,000,000 yuan, the year-on-year growth was 40.8% and the annual accumulative number benefited was 1,745,000,000 persons/times. The payment mode reform by disease, capita, bed and day is continuously promoted. The nationwide NRCMCS information network was generally established, the interconnection and interworking, instant settlement and report, and the interconnection of national information platform with 9 provinces (regions and cities) and the cross-provincial supervision and management were realized in 89% of the whole-planned places. The commercial insurance institutions were entrusted to launch the NRCMCS pilot management, and the new mechanism for management, disposition, the separated supervision and management was explored for establishment.

The basic drug system was constantly extended, which drove the further promotion of the comprehensive reform at grassroots. The basic drug system extended continually from grassroots medical institutions, covering 74.6% village clinics nationwide. The 2012 version of the basic drug catalog was studied and issued. The bidding procurement platforms for drugs at provincial level were generally established, and the online procurement of the basic drugs in grassroots medical institutions operated by governments was realized. Full employment system and job management system were practiced in 97.4% grassroots medical institutions of counties (prefectures and districts) across the country.

The reforms of the management system and the operational mechanism in public hospitals were continuously deepened. There are over 1,000 pilot units of the comprehensive reform in county-level public hospitals of more than 600 counties (including the 311 counties of the first batch determined by the state), undertaking the comprehensive reform of management mechanism, compensation mechanism, personnel allocation, procurement mechanism, price mechanism centering around the key link of abolishing "medicine supplement by drugs". 17 pilot cities with public hospital reform are exploring the institutional mechanism reform on the separation of management from enforcement and public service units from government. The measures of the reserved diagnosis and treatment, service for people's convenience and instant settlement were generally implemented in medical institutions nationwide and the masses of the people feel markedly good in seeking medical treatment.

All work such as standardization construction in grassroots medical institutions and the trainings for grassroots medical staff advanced smoothly. The implementation of the basic and major public health projects were further strengthened so was performance assessment.

II. The Improvement in Medical Health Service Ability and Safety Quality

Health service ability in rural and west areas was rapidly improved by means of construction of national clinical key specialty, urban doctors rendering aid to the rural health and hospitals of the third grade in the east areas offering help to county-level hospitals in the west areas. 309 construction projects of national clinical key specialty were selected, covering 130 hospitals, of which 15 hospitals were chosen for the ones of national clinical nursing specialty. The clinical path for 100 diseases was formulated in the whole year (The clinical path and sub-path for 431 diseases have been formulated since 2009) The nursing service of high quality was promoted according to the principle of "mode change, focus on clinics and mechanism construction", and launched in all hospitals of the third grade nationwide and 4,817 hospitals of the second grade. The management of special projects of hospital infection, pharmaceutical affairs and antimicrobial application was widely practiced and the behaviors of diagnosis and treatment were further standardized. The creation of "peace hospital" was carried out, the security administration in medical institutions was enhanced and the order of diagnosis and treatment was improved. The organizations for dispute mediation at prefecture level were generally established, the successful rate of mediation is up to 85% and the satisfaction rate was 93%.

III. Major Disease Prevention and Control, Health Emergency, and Women and Children's Health Work

There is no major epidemic outbreak across the country, and the overall situation of infectious diseases of Class I and Class II and the emerging infectious diseases was stable. The coverage of HIV/AIDS, tuberculosis detection and comprehensive intervention was greatly enhanced and case fatality rate decreased obviously. The prevention and control of measles and malaria was effective and the numbers of the cases fell by 53% and 42% respectively. WHO confirmed that China restored to polio-free status. Hepatitis B surface antigen carrying rate of children under 5 was below 1%, which shows that the planning objectives of hepatitis B control in West Pacific Region were realized. Chronic disease prevention and control was more valued, the activities of healthy lifestyle were carried out in 55% of the counties nationwide and the demonstration areas of comprehensive prevention and control of chronic disease continued to expand. Direct network reports on epidemic situation of infectious diseases and emergent events of public health were realized in 100% of institutions of disease prevention and control, 98% of the medical institutions at or above county level and 94% of town and township health centers, and the rate of timely report and the rate of timely review were both more than 99%.

Women's and children's health situation continued to be improved, and the goal of eliminating neonatal tetanus was achieved. The capability of health emergency security was continuously strengthened and the layout tasks of national area within national health emergency power were entirely completed by establishing 34 national health emergency teams of 4 kinds. Network connectivity of emergency command system was realized in 25 provinces, the tracking monitoring of diseases and health emergency rescue were orderly carried out, and national major events were safeguarded by effective health emergency security. Accumulatively, 153 national sanitary cities, 32 national sanitary regions and 456 national sanitary villages and towns (county towns) were named.

IV. Supervision and Management of Food and Drug Safety, and Health Supervision and Law Enforcement

Food safety standards and risk monitoring plans were continuously improved. 117 national food safety standards were formulated and published. Monitoring coverage of chemical contaminants and food borne pathogenic microorganism involved all provinces and 90% prefectures nationwide. The remarkable effects of comprehensive control of drug quality and safety aimed at key areas, key breeds and key links were achieved. Electronic supervision and management of all enterprises, all varieties and the entire process of the basic drugs was realized, and the sampling percent of pass was 98.7%.

Consistency evaluation of generic drugs was initiated.

Health supervision and law enforcement increased significantly. Monitoring sentinels for drinking water were all over the country and monitoring sentinels for key occupational diseases, medical radiation protection and health of primary and secondary schools were gradually increased. National survey of occupational health was finished. Health supervision and assistant management was carried out in more than 80% of the counties and districts, more timely and effective supervision was achieved.

V. Work of Traditional Chinese Medical Science and Medicines

The advantages of traditional Chinese medical science and medicines were constantly playing a role in medical reform. Proper service projects of traditional Chinese medical science and medicines, standard expenditure per capita and service process were explored in the basic public health service. The guidance of outfit and the use of traditional Chinese medicines in the basic drug catalog were strengthened. The promotion project of grassroots capability of traditional Chinese medical science and medicines and the construction of transmission system were organized for implementation. Pilot resource censors of traditional Chinese medical science and medicines were carried out in 22 provinces. And the activities of the patrol popularization of culture and popular science benefited hundreds of millions of families and the masses.

VI. Information on Talent, Science and Education

The standardized trainings for general practitioners and resident doctors were actively promoted. Major projects of science and technology were smoothly implemented. Appropriate technology at the grassroots level was widely promoted in provinces of west areas. Health informatization played the role in convenience of service for the public, supervision and management by giving out resident health cards and establishing the systems of electronic monitoring of drugs in medical institutions and electronic medical records.

In 2012, the Central Finance invested 24,300,000,000 yuan to improve the construction of medical health service system. Health system launched extensively the investigation, supervision and management of infrastructure and financial affairs, supervision and examination of funds for special projects, and price management of medical service to ensure the standardized use of the funds. Health professional spirit got wider and deeper support of the people by means of the activities of creating the first and striving for excellence, "three goods and one satisfaction", and discussion of the core values of socialism. Governance of business bribery in the field of pharmaceutical sales was intensified, and prevention and control of integrity and risk was enhanced. International cooperation and communication was carried out extensively to improve China's influence on global health affairs. 2012 Strategy Research Report of "Healthy China" and White Paper of *China's Medical Health Undertaking* were issued, and *Law of Mental Health* was issued to promote evidence-based decision-making and administration according to law. Effects of news propaganda, publication of government affairs and health petition letter were achieved, and the society's understanding and support of health was improved.

(Ji Chenglian)

2. Work Progress of the Related Affairs of WTO in Health Field

Ministry of Health actively cooperated with Ministry of Commerce to national strategy of free trade zone and attended market access negotiations of medical service trade involved in Sino-Switzerland, Sino-Australia, and China-Iceland free trade zone negotiations, and timely adjusted price strategy according to the unified deployment of the State Council and the new situation in negotiations. Report and review should be continuously done well in accordance with WTO requirements for transparency. In 2012, Ministry of Health circulated 24 national food safety standards to WTO/SPS committees, 1 standard to WTO/TBT committees and organized experts to study and answer more than 30 review opinions. Review opinions on the limited quantity of aflatoxin in food (Singapore), of ochracin in fragrance materials (European Union) and cadmium in sea algae (South Korea) were put forward. Ministry of Health substantively participated in activities under WTO framework to safeguard the interests of the state, took an active part in the 53rd to 55th regular meetings of WTO/SPS committees, involved in the serious discussion of the related rules, reasonably responded to the attention to China's food safety standards from WTO members and other members, explained and clarified the relevant issues and successfully completed meeting participation and bilateral consultations. Ministry of Health cooperated with Ministry of Commerce to pass smoothly the 4th WTO trade policy review on China. The explanation and clarification of 23 problems from 11 American and European member countries was organized and the retort to false questions was done. The study of "private standards" was carried out, private standards both at home and abroad were analyzed and the counter strategies were put forward.

(Ji Chenglian)

Chapter I Disease Prevention and Control

1. Disease Prevention and Control in 2012

I. To Carry out the Work of Disease Prevention and Control Related to Medical Reform

The guidance of institution of disease prevention and control carrying out the basic public health service to the grassroots was strengthened and policy related to disease prevention and control was promoted for introduction. Ministry of Health and Ministry of Commerce agreed to adjust free AIDS drug directory for antiviral treatment and increase drug varieties, include AIDS opportunistic infections treatment and multi-drug resistant tuberculosis into the pilot protection of the NRCMS major diseases, involve rapid diagnostic techniques of multi-drug resistant tuberculosis into *Specifications for National Health Service Price Project (2010 version)*, and explore to bring major cancers like lung cancer into guarantee of serious diseases and the pilot rescues. Single-disease payment for major diseases like tuberculosis was promoted, and national TB training of clinical pathway was launched and extended. The projects of the basic public health service were sturdily promoted and the supervision and examination of disease prevention and control in 10 provinces, especially public health service related to disease prevention and control at county level was done.

II. To Strengthen the Construction of Disease Prevention and Control System

The 29th meeting of the 11th National People's Congress Standing Committee passed *Law of Mental Health*, which filled the legal blank in China's mental health field. *Methods for Venereal Disease Prevention and Control* was formulated. The revision and formulation of laws and regulations such as *Regulations on Administration of Vaccine Circulation and Vaccination, Regulations on Administration of Iodine Deficiency Elimination with Salt Iodization, Implementation Measures for Law on Infectious Disease Prevention and Control*, and department regulations like *Administration Methods for Tuberculosis (TB) Prevention and Control* were sturdily promoted. The amendment of *Provisions for the Management in Institutions of Disease Prevention and Control* and *Guiding Opinions on Post Setting and Management in Institutions of Disease Prevention and Control* were completed. The research on core ability construction of the centers for disease control and prevention at province level was carried out to improve the ability of disease prevention and control. Ministry of Health, together with Ministry of Human

Resources and Department of Social Security, launched the selection of the advanced collectives and the advanced individuals in national AIDS prevention and treatment. Cultural construction seminar of national disease prevention and control system was held to promote cultural construction of disease prevention and control. *Standards for Performance Evaluation of Disease Prevention and Control (2012 version)* was revised. The planning and study of the construction of institutions of disease prevention and control in the period of the "Twelfth Five-year Plan" was organized and the revision of laboratory equipment in institutions of disease prevention and control was made. Ministry of Health actively communicated and coordinated with the relevant departments, and launched previous preparations for the series of commemorative activities of the 60th anniversary of disease prevention and control, organized and initiated the work of assisting Tibet and Xinjiang in disease prevention and control, the enforcement regulations for the cooperative projects was determined, the oriented assisting projects given by oriented assisting provincial health ministries to oriented assisted health bureaus were coordinated and the talent problems troubling disease prevention and control in Tibet were solved.

III. To Promote Steadily Major Disease Prevention and Control

In 2012, the State Council and the relevant departments issued the "Twelfth Five-year" planning for the development of China's aging undertaking, planning for vaccine supply system construction and the long and medium terms of national animal epidemic disease prevention and control. Marked achievements were scored in the prevention and control of infectious diseases, national epidemic situation was stable as a whole and there was not a major epidemic outbreak of infectious diseases. Regularly reported epidemic situation of infectious diseases was published and news release and risk communication of key infectious diseases was done together with the relevant departments. Departmental coordination was promoted, and the prevention and treatment of infectious diseases among focal groups of people in schools and kindergarten units was strengthened. The prevention and control of key infectious diseases such as influenza, cholera, hand-foot-and-mouth disease, brucellosis and anthrax were promoted, prevention of the new type of coronary virus outbreaks was done well, and malignant pustule and outbreak of dengue fever were effectively handled. The compilations of *Operation Instructions for Field Investigation and Disposal of Infectious Disease Epidemic Situation* and *Manual for Infectious Disease Prevention and Control*, and planning of laboratory network construction of infectious disease prevention and control were launched. *Implementation Program for the Planning of National Elimination of Leprosy Hazards* was printed and distributed and the guiding for elimination of leprosy hazards was strengthened by focusing on provinces with high prevalence.

Polio due to the input of disease in Xinjiang Uygur Autonomous Region was properly responded. By Oct. 9, 2012, no more new case of wild poliovirus has been detected in the 12 months since the last reported case of wild poliovirus. From Nov. 26-30, 2012, the 18th meeting of Committee for Confirmation of Polio Eradication in WHO West Pacific Region gave the final assessment and certification of China's continual maintenance of polio-free status and spoke highly of the fact that "China created record by successfully blocking polio outbreak due to input in the shortest time and gave a brilliant example for the world". Substantial progress has been achieved in measles elimination, national commission for confirmation of measles elimination was established and the construction of measles monitoring and network laboratory was strengthened.

AIDS testing was intensified. In 2012, 100,000,000 persons/times were tested, 82,000 newly infected persons and patients were detected, which increased 20.3% and 10.6% than those of last year. Comprehensive intervention coverage was gradually expanding. The proportion of the newly infected drugsters participating in community methadone drug maintenance treatment was 0.21%, which decreased 35% than that of last year. The coverage of antiviral treatment was expanding. There were 3,496 institutions of antiviral therapy nationwide and 168,000 persons were under treatment, which means another 44,000 persons were covered in the treatment, the proportion between the infected persons conforming to the treatment standards and patients under antiviral therapy was 87.3% and the fatality rate of the patients under antiviral therapy reduced significantly.

TB prevention and treatment was continuously promoted. 894,000 patients were detected and given treatment, of which the curing rate of the patients with new smear-positive pulmonary tuberculosis was above 90%. Standardized diagnosis and treatment of multi-drug resistant tuberculosis was expanded to 91 prefectures (cities). Comprehensive schistosomiasis treatment focusing on infectious source control was promoted vigorously, national schistosomiasis epidemics was in a low level and there were only 13 cases reports on acute schistosomiasis in 2012.

Examination and evaluation of malaria elimination reaching the standards was carried out, and national malaria elimination was steadily promoted. There were 2,451 reports on malaria across the country, which decreased 40%. Investigation on echinococcosis epidemiology was launched, and national competition of microscopy skills for parasitic diseases was held. Monitoring system and control effect evaluation system for endemic diseases were further improved, monitoring schemes for national iodine deficiency disorders, endemic fluorosis, and endemic arsenism were revised, printed and distributed, monitoring scheme for waterborne areas with high iodine was formulated, and professional and technical standards for inspection and acceptance of iodine deficiency disorder elimination, Kaschin-Beck and Keshan disease control and elimination were compiled. All-level examinations of laboratory quality control was carried out, laboratory management standardized and quality control intensified. The schemes for Kaschin-beck disease prevention and treatment in Qinghai-Tibet plateau were formulated to further strengthen the prevention and treatment. The security of original iodine import and supply was ensured in a coordinated way for the smooth implementation of the prevention and treatment of iodine deficiency disorders with salt iodization. Edible salt iodine content standards were promoted for the implementation. The pilots for new standards of iodized salt were set up in 3 provinces of Anhui, Fujian and Shandong. 6,133 patients with Kaschin-Beck disease and 402 patients with Keshan disease suitable for treatment were effectively treated, and 880,000 key groups of people in high-risk IDD areas were given emergency repair iodine.

IV. To Promote Steadily the Comprehensive Prevention and Control of Chronic Diseases

In 2012, 101 counties and districts nationwide were awarded the title of state-level demonstration zones of comprehensive prevention and control of chronic diseases, national action for healthy lifestyle continued to deepen. National action for healthy lifestyle was carried out in 1,870 counties and districts, accounting for 62.6% of all counties and districts across the country, 9,091 demonstrated creations (demonstrated units, communities, cafeterias/canteens, supermarkets and others) were done, 5,212 supportive environments of theme parks, health trails, health blocks for outdoor health were built for the reaching of the objectives of chronic disease prevention and treatment. Intervention and patient management of high risk group was started to promote the early diagnosis and the early treatment of the key cancers. 142 pilots in all rural areas, 22 pilots in Huai River Basin and 9 urban pilots were set up and nearly 370,000 persons underwent screening. 1,440,000 people in high risk of stroke were screened. Monitoring of resident nutritional status and the monitoring of chronic disease risk factors of mobile people were completed. Core information on chronic disease prevention and treatment, core information on healthy lifestyle and expert consensus of chronic disease prevention and treatment were published. Dental hygiene was promoted. Comprehensive intervention for children's oral diseases was carried out in 709 counties and districts across the country, and 14 pilots of demonstration community of "Healthy Mouth and Happy Family" were established.

V. To Promote the Management of Special Groups of People

Work Specifications of Severe Mental Disease Management and Treatment (2012 version) was Implemented and the network for severe mental disease prevention and treatment was improved. By the end of 2012, severe mental disease management and treatment covers 221 cities and 1, 578 counties in 30 provinces (autonomous regions and municipalities directly under the central government) and 3,377,000 home patients were given regular follow-up management and rehabilitation. The service mode of hotline pilot cities of psychological assistance was innovated and convenient platform for public psychological consultation and psychological crisis intervention was established.

(Ji Chenglian)

2. Hepatitis B Prevention and Treatment throughout the Country

In 2012, Ministry of Health continuously implemented the comprehensive strategies for hepatitis B control centering around "vaccination" and launched various forms of propaganda activities on "7·28" World Hepatitis Day. The Central Finance for the first time included hepatitis B monitoring into the central subsidies for local basic public health project funding. 198 pilot counties (districts) of hepatitis B monitoring were established in 31 provinces (regions and cities) and Xinjiang Production and Construction Corps around the country. China CDC formulated, printed and issued *2012 Technical Scheme for Hepatitis B Monitoring Program* and changed the reporting requirements for hepatitis B cases in the "system of disease monitoring report information management" and the "information management system of public health emergency report" with the information on hepatitis B cases report on the "attached card". In May, 2012, the office of WHO in West Pacific Region confirmed that the carrying rate of the children under 5 with surface antigen of chronic hepatitis B decreased to lower than 2% in China.

(Ji Chenglian)

3. Progress in AIDS Prevention and Treatment

According to the national information system for the comprehensive prevention and treatment of AIDS/STD, 385,817 living persons with AIDS virus infection and AIDS patients, and 114,787 cases of deaths had been reported by the end of Dec. 31, 2012. In 2012, the newly detected persons with AIDS virus infection was 58,399, the number of AIDS patients was 240,358 and 17,894 former persons with AIDS virus infection became AIDS patients. In 2012, the Central Finance further increased the investment in AIDS prevention and treatment and 2,390,000,000 yuan for special local AIDS funds was subsidized. Ministry of Health printed and distributed *Circulation of the Implementation of the "Twelfth Five-year" Action Plan for China's AIDS Containment and AIDS Prevention and Treatment*, which includes the opportunistic infection of AIDS into the NRCMS pilot protection of major diseases and the corresponding drug varieties were added into *National Catalog of the Basic Drugs*. In 2012, the number of monitoring sentinels for AIDS/STD/hepatitis C was 1,971, and the numbers of screening laboratory and confirmation laboratory were 17,083 and 377, which means that all provinces have the testing capacity of CD_4 and viral load, and the testing network continued to the grassroots. In 2012, 101 million persons/times were given tests of HIV antibody, which was 20.3% more than that in 2011, and the newly detected cases were over 10.6% more than that in 2011. By the end of 2012, accumulatively, 211,000 patients had been treated, 56,000 more than that in 2011, and the growing rate was 21.8%. 168,000 patients were under treatment, of whom 3,542 children patients with AIDS were accumulatively treated and 2,818 children were under treatment. The proportions of those who are still alive after 12-month treatment, of follow-up visit, CD_4 testing and viral load testing were improved and the treatment was significantly standardized. By the end of 2012, there have been 756 methadone maintenance treatment clinics (including 30 mobile vehicles for medicine taking), and 384,000 drug addicts were accumulatively treated, which was 11.6% more than that in 2011. In Dec. 2012, 208,000 people were under treatment, which was 48.6% more than that in 2011. The newly detected AIDS infecting rate of drug addict groups participating in community drug maintenance therapy was 0.2%, 35% decrease compared with that of 2011. The monthly average number of people dealing with needle exchange was about 47,000. 620,000 prostitutes were given average monthly intervention and the average monthly intervention coverage was 87.0%, 20% rise compared with that in 2011. 252,000 MSM groups were given average monthly intervention and the average monthly intervention coverage was 78.5%, 31.5% rise compared with that in 2011. In 2012, 11,600,000 pregnant and puerperal women were given HIV antibody detection in areas of national prevention of mother-to-child AIDS transmission, of whom 5,700 were detected the carries of AIDS virus and the antiviral drug application proportion of the pregnant and puerperal women infected by AIDS virus was 79.6%. By the end of 2012, the rate of HIV mother-to-child transmission has decreased from 34.8% before intervention to 7.1%.

(**Ji Chenglian**)

4. Launching Ceremony for Theme Activities of 2012 World Tuberculosis Day and TB Knowledge Dissemination by Millions of Volunteers Held in Beijing

March 24, 2012 is the 17th World Tuberculosis Day and China's publicity theme is "You and I Participate in TB Elimination". On March 22, the launching ceremony for Theme Activities of 2012 World Tuberculosis Day and TB Knowledge Dissemination by Millions of Volunteers was held in Beijing. Vice Minister of Ministry of Health, Yin Li and Senior Health Advisor of WHO China's Office, Pei Lei attended the activities and delivered speeches. Official micro-blogs of central and provincial TB prevention and treatment institutions and the public homepage of China TB prevention and treatment were opened at the launching ceremony. The on-site experts at TB prevention answered the questions from net friends. Propaganda ambassador of China TB prevention and treatment, Tan Jing read out the action initiative of TB knowledge dissemination by millions of volunteers. The representatives of the first batch of volunteers said that they would actively participate in knowledge dissemination of TB prevention and treatment. Yin Li, Pei Lei, Tan Jing and others jointly started "Actions of TB Knowledge Dissemination by Millions of Volunteers".

(Ji Chenglian)

5. International Experts Spoke Highly of China's Multidrug-resistant TB Prevention and Treatment

On September 16 to 19, 2012, international experts from Green Light Committee, and Global Fund carried out the supervision of multidrug-resistant tuberculosis prevention and treatment in Liaoning Province and Human Province. Green Light Committee is an authority organization responsible for global technology of multidrug-resistant tuberculosis prevention and treatment and played an important part in promoting WHO strategies for multidrug-resistant tuberculosis control. In this supervision, Green Light Committee acted as the core, and made comprehensive investigation of multi-drug resistant tuberculosis prevention and treatment in China. The body of the experts listened to the reports from all places, visited institutions for TB prevention and treatment and grassroots medical health institutions, communicated with administrators from departments of health administration, professional staff for tuberculosis prevention and treatment and TB patients, and made the comprehensive evaluation on multidrug-resistant tuberculosis prevention and treatment. On September 21, international experts reported the supervision to Ministry of Health. The body of the experts gave full affirmation of China's efforts for TB prevention and treatment and spoke highly of the security policy of a serious illness by reducing the burden of multidrug-resistant TB patients, cooperation mechanisms of medical prevention and the relevant technical measures for patient diagnosis, treatment and management, and proposed opinions on multidrug-resistant tuberculosis prevention and treatment in the future. Michael O'Leary, WHO representative in China, and Catharina, consultant of TB containment in West Pacific Region and the relevant China CDC experts attended the meeting.

(Ji Chenglian)

6. The Second Round Cooperation Projects of TB Prevention and Treatment was Launched by Ministry of Health and Foundation Mérieux

On October 30, 2012, the initiation meeting on the Second Round Cooperation Projects of TB Prevention and Treatment was held in Hubei, Wuhan, at which the implementation plan for the second round cooperation projects of TB prevention and treatment was discussed and passed, and the representatives from the two project areas of Guangxi and Xinjiang gave the speeches of communication. The implementation of the period for the second round cooperation projects of TB prevention and treatment lasts from 2012 to 2017, and the fund of the project is 1,000,000 euros to support multidrug-resistant tuberculosis prevention and treatment in Kashi, Xinjiang and Liuzhou, Guangxi by providing configuration facility and trainings.

(Ji Chenglian)

7. Ministry of Health and 15 Ministries and Committees Jointly Printed and Distributed *China's Planning for Chronic Disease Prevention and Treatment (2012 - 2015)*

In May, 2012, Ministry of Health and 15 Ministries and Committees of National Development and Reform Commission and Ministry of Finance jointly printed and distributed *China's Planning for Chronic Disease Prevention and Treatment (2012 - 2015) (hereinafter referred to as the Planning)*. The *Planning* aims at health core of "1 year older per capita in life expectancy", strives to build service system for chronic disease prevention and treatment covering the whole country, constructs working mechanism for chronic disease prevention and treatment, and clarifies the specific targets, strategies and measures in the period of the "Twelfth Five-year Plan" for chronic disease prevention and treatment. The contents of the *Planning* highlights four characteristics: The first one is to build the mechanism of government leading, coordination between departments and the inter-departmental coordination, clarify the responsibilities of the governments and the relevant departments in chronic disease prevention and treatment and propose development strategies for the incorporation of health into various public policies. The second one is to improve the professional system for chronic disease prevention and treatment and build mechanisms for division of labor with individual responsibility and level-to-level management in institutions for disease prevention and control, hospitals, institutions for specific disease prevention and treatment and grassroots medical health institutions of chronic disease prevention and treatment and realize gradually the sharing of resources and information. The third one is to put forward effective measures for prevention and treatment aiming at all groups of people, people at high risk and patients with chronic diseases in accordance with the third-level preventive strategies and reflect the fundamental principle of prevention first, combination of prevention and treatment, strategic pass moving forward, and the sinking of gravity center. The fourth one is to carry out the construction of demonstration area, jointly establish with provinces and ministries the platform of comprehensive prevention and treatment of chronic diseases, stress the key point, give different guidance and improve the ability and level of comprehensive prevention and control of chronic diseases by leveraging the creation of sanitary cities and towns, and healthy cities and towns.

(Ji Chenglian)

8. The Introduction of *Law of Mental Health*

On October 26, 2012, the *Law of Mental Health of the People's Republic of China* was revised and passed at the 29th Meeting of the Standing Committee of the 11th National People's Congress, which shall be effective from May 1, 2013. *Law of Mental Health* contains 7 chapters and 85 articles, which stipulates explicitly policies, principles, management mechanism for mental health, mental health promotion, mental disorder prevention, diagnosis and treatment of mental disorders, recovery of mental disorders, safeguard measures of mental health, and protection of the legitimate rights and interests the patients with mental disorders.

(Ji Chenglian)

Section 1   Progress in China Center for Disease Prevention and Control

1. Progress of National Major Projects of Science and Technology

China CDC's major projects of science and technology of "prevention and treatment of major infectious diseases such as AIDS and viral hepatitis" passed the audit, check and acceptance of national "Eleventh Five-year Plan" subjects, of which 12 major special projects were included in the "Twelfth Five-year Plan" rolling support and the fund was 330,889,800 yuan. 12 major researches of the first batch on pathogen, the research leading and participating units included in the projects of "Platform for Infectious Disease Monitoring Technology" were determined, and the research programs and working mechanism were made. *Research Program for Infectious Disease Syndrome Pathogens Variation (2012 version)* was formulated and the functions of information system were improved. Early warning research based on the etiology of infectious diseases was further promoted and monitoring data on febrile respiratory syndrome and meningitis encephalitis syndrome in 2009-2011 were analyzed. The major special subject research on "New formulations for TB treatment" was completed and the curative effects, security and biological effects of TB fixed compound dose preparation were observed. The major special project of "multidimensional information integration analysis software for pestilence" in the "Eleventh Five-year Plan" was upgraded and rebuilt. The subjects of "immunological therapy for China's AIDS patients" and "screening system for unknown pathogens and detection technology for rare pathogens" passed the acceptance and sample test by Ministry of Science and Technology.

(Ji Chenglian)

2. West Nile Vims was Isolated and Identified for the First Time in Our Country

In August, China CDC isolated and identified for the first time West Nile Vims in culex pipiens specimen collected in Kashi, Xinjiang, gave retrospective testing of some cases of serological specimen in the unexplained fever outbreaks in Kashi, Xinjiang in 2004, found west Nile virus IgM antibody positive in the acute serum specimens, and that West Nile Vims in the cases of double serum specimens and antibody increased at more than four times, which indicates that human infections probably exist in China. After that, China CDC made an urgent deployment to the south of Xinjiang, especially Yili Prefecture, Kashi Prefecture and the north of Xinjiang to collect mosquito samples and serum specimens of clinical patients for the relevant investigation and research.

(Ji Chenglian)

3. The First Issue of the Cooperation Projects of TB Prevention and Treatment Involved in Ministry of Health - the Gates Foundation were Completed Smoothly and the Second Issue was Launched

The first issue of the cooperation projects of TB prevention and treatment involved in Ministry of Health - the Gates Foundation was launched in 6 provinces (cities) in China in April, 2009 and 4 subprojects came to an end at the end of December, 2012, and the others were at the final stage of summarization. Based on the achievements and contributions of the first issue, the projects of the second issue were successfully approved and officially launched on January 1, 2012. 3 pilot spots of Zhenjiang, Jiangsu, Yichang, Hubei and Hanzhong, Shaanxi were ready by means of selection.

(Ji Chenglian)

4. Regional Targets of Hepatitis B Prevention and Treatment were Realized around the Country

In 2012, the Central Finance included hepatitis B monitoring into the central subsidies for local basic public health project funding and 198 points of hepatitis B monitoring were set up in 31 provinces (autonomous regions and municipalities directly under the central government) and Xinjiang Production and Construction Corps. 1,087,086 cases of hepatitis B were reported by China information system of disease prevention and control, the reported morbidity was 80.68/100,000, and the onset number and morbidity dropped 0.57% and 1.05% respectively. Office of WHO West Pacific Region verified that the regional target of less than 2% drop in chronic HBV infection of the children under the age of five was realized in China by means of examination and verification, and expert committee's argumentation.

(Ji Chenglian)

5. Assist Cambodia in Hand-foot-and-mouth Disease Prevention and Control

On July 5, 2012, after the unexplained disease broke out in Cambodia, China CDC organized the experts for the discussion all at once, and prepared the related personnel and equipment. After receiving Ministry of Health order of sending the personnel to the scene, China CDC quickly sent the working group of three experts and clinical experts to Cambodia, started emergency operation, formulated *Group Work Plan for China CDC Emergency Operations of Technical Assistance in Cambodia*, and set up the leading group and emergency operation group. With the hard work and support of all emergency operation groups, the frontier expert group completed technical guidance for dealing with the local epidemics. After the expert group returned Beijing from Cambodia, emergency center and the experts made the post evaluation on health emergency.

(Ji Chenglian)

6. Projects of Sino-Australian Health and AIDS "Websites for Smoke Quitting and 12320 Hotline for Smoke Quitting"

"Websites for Smoke Quitting and 12320 Service for Smoke Quitting" was subsidized by Sino-Australian Health and AIDS projects, China CDC cooperated closely with Victoria Cancer Institute, Australia in developing Australian QuitCoach for Smoke Quitting in Chinese version with Chinese culture and the characteristics of smoking group. By now, the internal testing is under way. In addition, 12320 public health hotline of counseling service system for smoke quitting was open in Beijing and Shanghai to provide a convenient way for the smokers in seeking help to quit smoking. *Work Book of 12320 Hotline (one-volume edition)* was distributed and the effects of 12320 hotline of counseling service for smoke quitting in Beijing and Shanghai was evaluated.

(Ji Chenglian)

7. The Impact Factor of *Biomedical and Environmental Sciences (BES)* Hit a Historical High

A good momentum of development of *Biomedical and Environmental Sciences (BES)* hosted by China CDC and included in SCI is obvious, 6 issues are published in a year, the page number increases from 80 to 128 and the impact factor in SCI is 1.345, hitting another historical high. In 2012, "China Most International Influence Academic Periodical" was given to BES by Tsinghua University Library, China Academic Journal Electronic Magazine and China Scientific Literature Evaluation Center, and BES ranked the 29th in the comprehensive ranking of the 175 award-winners of natural science journals.

(Ji Chenglian)

Chapter II   Patriotic Health Campaign

National Patriotic Health Campaign in 2012

In 2012, national patriotic health campaign, directed by outlook of scientific development, fully implemented the spirits of the 6th Plenary Session of the 17th CPC Central Committee, of the 11th CPC National Congress and the requirements of national health conference, made the overall planning and the focal points centering around the key health work in 2012, and every task was well done. Series of activities commemorating the 60th anniversary of patriotic health campaign were launched, and the advanced collectives and the advanced individuals were selected and awarded. Minister of Ministry of Health, Chen Zhu and Secretary of the Party Group, Zhang Mao published signed articles in People's Daily to carry forward the spirit of patriotic health campaign. Standards and management measures for national sanitary cities were amended, the long-term mechanism was improved, and the achievements in creating national sanitary cities and towns were consolidated and constantly expanded. Accumulatively, 153 national sanitary cities, 32 national sanitary townships (counties) were named nationwide. Based on the summary and development of healthy cities and counties and the achievements of creating sanitary cities and towns, the guiding opinions on construction healthy (health) cities were compiled and the construction of healthy cities and counties was promoted further, combined with the work related closely to people's livelihood, such as national chronic disease prevention and control and food safety. Delegates to National People's Congress were organized to investigate and research patriotic sanitation work. Investigation on the basic information on administrative agencies of national health was started. The jointly formulated *Planning for National Rural Drinking Water Safety Project (2011-2015)* was carried out. The health monitoring on the water quality in 50,000 projects of the centralized water supply and the rural environment in 14,000 points of 700 counties were implemented. Vector prevention and control was well practiced to guide the removal of vector biological breeding grounds and reduce the density of vector. According to the statistics, and the targets in *Action Plan for National Urban and Rural Environmental Sanitation in 2010-2012*, hazard-free toilets of 18,000,000 rural households were established in 3 years, the comprehensive improvement of the environment was made in 260,000 villages, the qualified rate of rural drinking water quality increased significantly, and the "dirty, disorderly and bad" environmental phenomena was improved obviously.

(Ji Chenglian)

Chapter III   Health Emergency Response

1. Health Emergency Response in 2012

In 2012, health emergency response adhered to the principles of putting prevention first and combining prevention with emergency response and took completing regulations, strengthening preparation and improving capacity as the focuses. Solid foundation was laid for the work to improve the capacity of handling emergencies; the construction of health emergency response system was pushed forward to scientifically prevent and effectively handle various public health emergencies. New progress was made in all aspects of work.

I. The construction of the basis for health emergency response was strengthened. Firstly, the legislations, systems and mechanisms for health emergency response were consolidated and perfected. The construction of legislation system for the management of health emergency response was strengthened and laws related to health emergency response were conscientiously implemented such as *Laws on Emergency Response, Laws on the Prevention and Treatment of Infectious Diseases* and *International Health Regulations (2005)* etc. All the localities were instructed to strengthen the construction of health emergency response management organs and detailed the functions of health emergency management. The coordinative mechanism of health emergency response between the army and the Ministry of Health was perfected with the Operation Department of General Staff Department of PLA and Health Department of General Logistics Department of PLA and coordination was made with General Administration of Quality Supervision, Inspection and Quarantine and Civil Aviation Administration of China to solve the problems of transporting infectious substances by air. Secondly, the normalization and institutionalization of health emergency response management were improved. The revision of two special preparednesses was promoted, i.e. *National Preparedness of Response to Public Health Emergencies and National Preparedness of Response to Medical Rescue on Public Emergencies* and departmental preparednesses were formulated or revised like *MOH Preparedness of Response to Food Safety Incidents. National Work Norms on Health Emergency Response at Health Institutions* was implemented and norms on health emergency response were formulated for various institutions. *Work Norms for Provincial Poisoning Rescuing Bases (for pilot draft)* and its evaluation standards were compiled. Thirdly, the construction of commanding and decision-making platform was promoted vigorously. The construction of commanding and decision-making platforms at prefectural level nationwide for response to public health emergency was promoted and coordination was made to connect the commanding system to the extranet of the e-government. So far, the e-connection has been achieved in 25 provinces, which means the commanding and decision-making platforms at the national, provincial and prefectural levels have been established. Fourthly, the capabilities of monitoring and pre-warning and risk assessment on public health emergencies were improved. Emphasis was laid on improving the level of on-line reporting of public health emergencies. Risk assessment of public health emergencies was vigorously propelled and national risk assessment mechanism was perfected. So far, most provinces nationwide have formulated their respective regional measures for risk assessment, established working mechanisms and expert teams, and monthly risk assessments have been conducted, which means the awareness of risk prevention have been greatly improved in all the localities.

II. The construction of core capabilities of health emergency response was strengthened. Firstly, the construction of national health emergency response teams was propelled. The construction of 34 national health emergency response teams was propelled steadily and the supervision and acceptance inspection of 11 national health emergency response teams which were sponsored by the central finance were completed. For the health emergency response teams established, they have achieved the goals of motorization of the teams, the portability of equipment, the hospitals on-board and self security. The layouts of national force of handing heath emergencies have been generally completed nationwide through the establishment of 34 national health emergency response teams of four categories. Secondly, training and drills on health emergency response were strengthened. In light of the requirements of uniform planning, uniform syllabus, uniform textbooks and uniform teaching staff, a series of textbooks on health emergency response were compiled including textbooks on the management of health emergency response, preparation for emergency response, risk communication, emergency medical rescue, the prevention and control of emergent acute infectious diseases, the control of poisoning incidents and the control of radiation incidents etc. Training classes were held including the training class for eight provinces (autonomous regions) of risk communication on health emergency response to public emergencies, the training class for eleven provinces (autonomous regions) of the prevention and control of emergent acute infectious diseases in border areas, the training class for twenty-five provinces (autonomous regions) of teachers and key employees for emergency response to poisoning incidents, the eighth training class for the cadres of mainland, Hong Kong and Macao for the emergency response management and the training class of health emergency response to nuclear and radiation emergencies. A large-scaled cross-provincial and cross-departmental comprehensive drill was held in Zhengzhou, Henan Province, on health emergency response on the background of an imported new outbreak of epidemic. Thirdly, the construction of emergent medical rescue bases for emergencies was propelled. Such contents as "strengthening the construction of national and provincial emergent medical rescue capacity" were included in *The 12th Five-Year Plan for the Development of Healthcare Service* and *The 12th Five-Year Plan for the Construction of National Emergency Response System*. Surveys were conducted on capacity of the emergent medical rescue to emergencies at the provincial and prefectural comprehensive hospitals. Experts were organized to make analysis and demonstration and plans and project plans were primarily proposed for constructing regional emergent medical rescue bases at the national and provincial levels on the basis of the present medical resources. Fourthly, the support capacity of health emergency response was strengthened. Work was done on the material support for health emergency response. Pilot on integrating the storage of the central and local emergency response materials was conducted, which provided the basis for further working well on the material support for health emergency response; the list for the storage of emergency response materials was developed; and material storage of some urgently needed drugs like antivenin was strengthened. Work on scientific research was forcefully pressed forward to improve the technical support, and two biennial projects were launched, i.e. The Research and Spread of the Key Technology on the Preparation and Handling of Health Emergency Response to Emergencies and The Research and Application of New Technology on the Epidemiology of Plague. Efforts were made to coordinate with the department of science and education to approve the special project of health industry in 2013-The Applicable Research on the Key Technology and Procedure Norms for the On-site Rescue of Health Emergency Response to Public Emergencies. Fifthly, the core capacity of health emergency response at the grassroots level was improved. Work was done to instruct all the localities to construct national health emergency response demonstrative counties (cities, districts). The procedures of evaluating the demonstrative counties were normalized by perfecting plans and strengthening management and experts were organized to re-evaluate the national health emergency response demonstrative counties (cities, districts) in 2012 in 58 counties recommended by 20 provinces nationwide. Preparation was made for the evaluation of the core capacity of health emergency response, *Guidelines on the Evaluation of Health Emergency Response Capacity* and *Standards for the Evaluation of Health Emergency Response Capacity* were formulated and pre-evaluation was carried out and perfected, which laid a foundation for launching the evaluation on the core capacity of health emergency response.

III. Timely and effective efforts were made to prevent and handle various kinds of emergencies. Concentrated efforts were made to properly handle the epidemic of human-infected with highly pathogenic avian influenza in Guizhou, the purported

SARS case in PLA 252 Hospital in Baoding, Hebei, the outbreak of bubonic plague in Litang County in Ganzi, Sichuan and the massive unexplained deaths in Dayao County in Chuxiong, Yunnan. Proactive efforts were made to prevent the import of new corona virus outbreak. A leading group for the emergency response to the new corona virus outbreak was established by the MOH; a coordinative mechanism was founded to jointly respond to the new corona virus outbreak with 13 ministries and departments and the health and religious departments in five key provinces with Muslim pilgrimage; and surveillance on public opinions, risk assessment and the monitoring on unexplained pneumonia with the port cities as the keys were strengthened. At the request of the Ministry of Foreign Affairs, experts were sent to Cambodia to assist on relevant work. Prevention and preparation were made to respond to the imported epidemics such as H3N2 influenza in the USA, the outbreak of Lassa fever in Nigeria, new type of AIDS in America, the massive unexplained deaths in the middle cities in Vietnam, the large-scaled unexplained eye disease in Mid-Japan, Ebola hemorrhagic fever, and West Nile fever etc. Remarkable achievements were made on the emergent medical rescue for the 9.7 earthquake on the boarder of Yunnan and Guizhou. Timely and effective emergency response was made for the disasters and accidents such as the 6.24 earthquake on the boarder of Sichuan and Yunnan, 7.10 mudslides in Min County, Gansu, 7.21 torrential rains in Beijing, 8.29 mine accident at Xiaojiawan Mine, Panzhihua, the traffic accident at Wuqing along the Jingjintang Express Highway and the traffic accident at Shandong along the Qingyin Express Highway etc. Health safeguarding was fulfilled successfully for the major events and important festivals such as the 18th CPC National Congress, the 2nd China-Eurasia Expo, pilgrims, 2012 Spring Festival and the National Day etc. which meant that the social influence and social harm of pubic emergencies were greatly reduced.

IV. The construction of professionalism for health emergency response was strengthened. The construction of the system for punishing and preventing corruption was pressed forward. The power for health emergency response was organized and potential risks for a clean government were troubleshot, the flow chart was made for the operation of emergency response power, and the monitoring on the key links of the operation of emergency response power was strengthened. The values for the health emergency response were forcefully propagated, i.e. be loyal to our missions, be united and dedicatory, be legal and scientific and be orderly and efficient.

(Zhao Xuemei)

2. 2012 International Seminar on the Management of Emergency Response Held

From November 24 to 25, 2012, 2012 International Seminar on the Management of Emergency Response was held in Beijing, jointly hosted by National School of Administration, the Ministry of Public Security, the Ministry of Civil Affairs, the Ministry of Health, State Administration of Work Safety and State-owned Assets Supervision and Administration Commission of the State Council. The theme of the seminar was "Strengthening the construction of emergency response capacity: innovation and cooperation", and present at the seminar were leaders from relevant ministries and commissions of the central government, emergency response organizations in some provinces and municipalities, large and middle enterprises and manufacturers of emergency response products, experts and scholars on the management of emergency response from the school of administration, relevant universities and research institutes as well as over 400 representatives from over 20 countries and international organizations. Vice Minister of Health, Xu Ke, attended the opening ceremony of the seminar and delivered a theme address entitled "Innovating Management, Strengthening Cooperation, and Promoting the Scientific Development of China's Health Emergency Response Service".

(Zhao Xuemei)

3. *International Health Regulations (2005)* **were Implemented**

In March 2012, the Ministry of Health, the Ministry of Environmental Protection, the Ministry of Agriculture and General Administration of Quality Supervision, Inspection and Quarantine jointly carried out the annual assessment on the construction of the core capacity of *International Health Regulations (2005)*; the assessment was conducted on thirteen aspects, i.e. eight core capacities (national legislation, policy and financing, coordination and NFP communication, surveillance, response, preparedness, risk communication, human resources and laboratory), capacity at ports of entry and exit and capacities to handle four kind of risk factors (zoonosis, food safety incidents, chemical incidents and nuclear and radioactive incidents). The outcome of the assessment showed that China had met the capacity requirements for laboratory, points of entry/exit, prevention of zoonosis events, prevention of food safety events and prevention of chemical events etc. In June, 2012, in line with the procedures regulated by *International Health Regulations (2005)*, Ministry of Health, the national focal point of IHR, submitted the request to WHO for the extension of two years, i.e. to June, 2014, in order to establish all core capacities. It is reported that by the end of 2012, 110 State Parties had submitted the requests to WHO for the extension of two years.

(Zhao Xuemei)

4. First Group of National Emergency Response Teams was Established

In 2012, the Ministry of Health established four categories of eleven national emergency response teams by means of transfer payment projects; besides, another five emergency response teams established by Shanghai, Jiangsu, the Health Department of PLA General Logistic Department and the Health Department of Logistic Department of Chinese People's Armed Police Forces with their own funds had passed the acceptance inspections and been recognized as the first group of national emergency response teams. The first group of national teams has the following features: Firstly, the organization was complete and the investment was increased. Both the building contractors and the building entities attached great importance to the teams and leading or working groups were established with specific persons taking charge of the building; in Shanghai, Jiangsu, Guangdong, Sichuan and Shanxi, etc. more financial investment was obtained to improve the standards of allocation and the hardware for handling the emergencies. Secondly, efforts were made to act in accordance with the local conditions and innovate the management. In Sichuan and Xinjiang, equipment was allocated which was suitable to the complicated environments of high altitude hypoxia and mountainous areas so that the capability of health emergency response in harsh environment was improved; in Guangdong, Beijing and the People's Armed Police Force, the mechanism of management was innovated, the management methods of "fixed personnel, fixed material, fixed vehicles and fixed positions" were adopted to improve the mobile ability, handling ability and supporting ability. Thirdly, drills were strengthened and publicity was made in time. Beijing, Shanxi, Guangdong and Xinjiang conducted in time run-in between the people and the equipment and field drills and invited media such as CCTV, local TV stations and Health Daily etc. to make timely reports, which helped to expand the social influence of the national health emergency response. Fourthly, the radiating and driving effects were obvious. Acting on the model of the national teams to get fiscal support, Shanxi, Beijing, Shanghai, Yunnan, Jiangxi and Chongqing launched the building of the local teams.

(Zhao Xuemei)

Chapter IV   Food Safety, Health Supervision and Law Enforcement

1. Comprehensive Coordination for Food Safety and Health Supervision in 2012

In 2012, all the health laws and regulations were further implemented and carried out such as *Food Safety Law* and *Laws on the Prevention of Occupational Diseases* etc. with strengthening the capacity building as the basis and food safety, the prevention of occupational diseases and drinking water safety as the focuses. Efforts were made to effectively strengthen the supervision and administration on public health and severely crack down on medical practice without license and illegal blood collection. All the tasks in 2012 were fulfilled pretty well.

Food Safety

Stable transition with the Food Safety Office of the State Council was achieved, the State Commission Office for Public Sector Reform approved the change of the name of Nation Center for Health Inspection and Supervision and the adjustment of duties, and the Party Group of the Ministry of Health approved the plan for the adjustment of the bureaus and staff within the National Center for Health Inspection and Supervision. In order to implement *Decision on Strengthening Work on Food Safety* and *National 12th Five-Year Plan for the Supervisory System of Food Safety of the State Council*, a plan for the division of work within the Ministry of Health was formulated. Ministry of Health's Implementing *Plan for Food Safety Law, 12th Five-Year Plan for the National Food Safety Standards* and *Technical Guidance on the Epidemiological Investigation of Food Safety Events (2012 Edition)* were printed and issued; *Work Procedure Manual, Norms for Tracking Assessment* and *Guidance on Risk Communication of Food Safety* of national food safety standards were drafted, *Measures for the Management of New Source Food* was revised, and *Anthology of Food Safety Laws and Regulations, Anthology of Cases of Epidemiological Investigation of Food Safety Events* and material for technical training such as the syllabus for training and technical guidance on simulate drills were compiled. Nearly 5,000 food standards were rectified, 117 national food safety standards were formulated and announced and standards for food additives were further revised and perfected. 2012 national monitoring plan for food safety risks was carried out and 1,488 surveillance spots were set nationwide on food contaminant and harmful factors in food, with the number of counties and districts covered increasing from 25% in 2010 to 52%; surveillance on food-borne diseases was further strengthened, with the number of sentinel hospitals increasing from 465 to 950.

Altogether 165,000 food samples were surveyed, and 979,000 surveillance data were collected. The active surveillance system for food-borne diseases and eight national reference laboratories for the surveillance of food safety risks were primarily built. The management on the compilation and issuing of *Food Safety Information* was regulated and twenty-four issues of food safety information of the Ministry of Health were compiled. The daily surveillance system for public opinions on food safety was established and *2011 National Report on the General Situation of Food Safety* was finished. *Training Syllabus for Health Sector's Surveillance Staff for Food Safety* was formulated and three national training workshops were held on risk communication of food safety.

Health supervision

Firstly, the construction of health supervisory system was pushed forward vigorously. Efforts were made to assist the National Development and Reform Commission to start the central investment 4.021 billion yuan, which was mainly used to strengthen the building of houses for over 2,400 health supervisory institutions at the county level, and presently 52% of the projects had started. Over 80% of the counties and districts nationwide carried out health supervision and coordination, employing over 170,000 supervisors and coordinators. *National Investigation System for Health Supervision* was revised. Work was vigorously carried out to aid Tibet and Xinjiang and offer partner assistance to Luliang Mountain Areas on food safety and health supervision. Secondly, the management of the health supervisory team was strengthened. Over 270,000 health supervisors were trained in all the localities. *Measures on Duty-Classified Management for Health Supervisors (Interim)* and related documents were formulated and the pilot on the duty-classified management was launched. National training workshop for health supervision and inspection & communication meeting on inspection was held. Norms for *Document for Administrative Law Enforcement on Health* was revised and issued, which came into force on December 1, 2012. The revised norms include four chapters, i.e. 51 articles of general principles, requirements for writing, management of law enforcement documents and appendix, altogether 37 kinds of documents concerning law enforcement activities such as supervision and inspection, supervision and sample inspection, administrative enforcement, and administrative punishment etc. Thirdly, good work was done on vocational health. There were 486 more inspecting institutions for vocational health and 22 more diagnosing institutions for vocational diseases nationwide, so that there are 3,077 inspecting institutions for vocational health and 562 diagnosing institutions for vocational diseases in total by now. National surveys on vocational health were preliminarily finished. Surveillance was conducted in 120 sentinel stations on key vocational diseases nationwide and the national summary on the surveillance at the sentinel stations on key vocational diseases from 2009 to 2010 was completed. Fourthly, good work was done on radiological health. *Measures on the Management of Technical Service Institutions for Radiological Health, Regulations on the Management of Health Examination of Construction Projects for Radiological Health Diagnosis and Treatment* and *Measures on the Management of Expert Banks for Radiological Health* were printed and issued. A national working model of surveillance network system for the protection of medical radiation was primarily established. Nine pilot entities were selected in Beijing and Shanghai to conduct sentinel surveillance on radiological vocational diseases. National capacity assessment for the technical service institutions on radiological health were conducted and assessments were made on surveillance capacities on the surveillance of individual dosages and γ spectrometry analysis. The national training workshops for key supervisors on radiological health were conducted. Surveillance was conducted on the radiological materials in food and drinking water in eight provinces, including Liaoning and Jiangsu etc., with nuclear power plants completed or under construction. Fifthly, good work was done on environmental health. *Hygiene Standards for Domestic Drinking Water* was fully implemented and 28,000 surveillance stations were established by the national surveillance network for the hygiene of domestic drinking water, which covered all the provinces, 100% of the municipalities and prefectures and 30% of the counties, with nearly 60,000 samples of water surveyed. The number of disease control institutes nationwide, which had the capacity to test 106 indicators for water quality, increased from 10 in 2011 to 25 at present. *Detailed Rules for the Implementation of Regulations on the Management of Public Place Hygiene* was implemented and greater efforts were made to strengthen the supervision on the hygiene in public places. Good work was done on the licenses of disinfection products and water related products as well as the supervision and sampling inspection. Work was done to assist the Ministry of Environment Protection to make pilot surveys on the environment and health in the key areas and the pilot surveys in eight provinces were almost completed. Sixthly, good work was done on the supervision on the prevention and treatment of infectious diseases and the supervision on school hygiene. With the focus on the disposal of medical wastes and the reports of epidemic outbreaks, we strengthened the supervision and inspection on the prevention and treatment of infectious diseases at the medical institutions. From January to November in 2012, virtually 370,800 institutions were supervised, regular health supervision was conducted on 616,700 institutions and 6,314 cases on the prevention and treatment of infectious diseases were investigated and punished by law. Pilot on the graded and classified supervision on the disposal of medical wastes was launched in Zhejiang Province and Anhui

Province. Supervision on school hygiene was pressed forward in all aspects. Form January to November in 2012, actually 126,800 schools were supervised, regular health supervision was conducted on 208,400 schools and 109 cases on school hygiene were investigated and punished by law. Pilot was launched in Beijing and other six provinces (regions, municipalities) to perfect the coordinative working mechanism and establish the supervision surveillance network for school hygiene and the platform for analyzing data and information. The setting up of supervision institutions for school hygiene was strengthened and by now the number of school hygiene department in the provincial health supervisory institutions had increased from six to fourteen. Seventhly, severer punishments were made to crack down on medical practices without licenses and illegal collection and supply of blood. Eighthly, the first national contest of health supervision skills was organized.

(Zhao Xuemei)

2. The 44th Session of Codex Committee on Food Additives was Hosted

From March 12 to 16, 2012, the Ministry of Health hosted the 44th Session of Codex Committee on Food Additives (CCFA) in Hangzhou, which was the sixth time that China had hosted sessions of Codex Committee on Food Additives since we became the hosting country of Codex Committee on Food Additives. The session was chaired by the Chairman of Codex Committee on Food Additives Academician, Chen Junshi (National Center for Food Safety Risk Assessment) and attended by 211 delegates from WHO, FAO, Codex Committee on Food Additives, 51 member countries and 29 international organizations. Discussed at the session were provisions for food additives in many categories of food in *General Standard for Food Additives* (GSFA), provision for aluminum containing food additives, food additive provisions in the standard for infant formulas, international numbering system for food additives and database on processing aids etc. In accordance with the proposals at the 43rd Session of Codex Committee on Food Additives (CCFA), China undertook the construction of the database on processing aids. At this session, we introduced the search module of the database model on processing aids, the main module of the material information for processing aids, the module of renewed application and the module of communication and other reference information. The Chinese delegation, which was composed of 15 members from the Ministry of Health, the Food Safety Office of the State Council, the Ministry of Commerce, the Ministry of Industry and Information Technology, the Ministry of Agriculture, General Administration of Quality Supervision, Inspection and Quarantine, State Food and Drug Administration etc. attended the session, where we expressed our standpoints on the provisions for food additives and actively pushed forward the discussion on relevant topics.

(Zhao Xuemei)

Section 1 Progress of Work on National Center for Food Safety Risk Assessment

International Consultant Committee Established

On September 26, 2012, a meeting was held by the National Center for Food Safety Risk Assessment to celebrate the establishment of the international consultant committee. The main tasks of the international consultant committee are: firstly, to introduce the beneficial experience on food safety to China and give us comments and suggestions on our work from the international perspectives; secondly, to give full play to the role of technological guidance, actively participate in food safety in China and serve as advisers and think tank for the improvement of food safety in China and the development of the National Center for Food Safety Risk Assessment; thirdly, to cultivate some excellent professionals for the National Center for Food Safety Risk Assessment; fourthly, to bridge the gap between other countries for communication and us.

(Zhao Xuemei)

Chapter V   Frontier Health Inspection and Quarantine

1. Inspection and Quarantine at Ports were Tightened

In 2012, all the ports nationwide conducted quarantine inspection on entry/exit persons 437 million person times and 122,085 person times were detected with symptoms of infectious diseases, among whom 17,980 persons were detected with symptoms of infectious diseases by means of infrared thermometry, accounting for 81.4% of the total; 2,929 persons were detected by means of medical quarantine, accounting for 13.26%; 1,176 persons by means of initiative notification, accounting for 5.32%. 2,381 persons with 22 kinds of infectious diseases were confirmed cases, the number detected increased greatly, the number of persons with the symptoms of infectious diseases increased by 50.34% compared with that in 2011, and the number of confirmed cases of infectious diseases increased by 201.77% compared with that in 2011, among which 2,051 cases were influenza, (including 152 cases of H1N1 influenza), increased by 203.4%, as well as other diseases including parainfluenza, malaria, infectious diarrhea, respiratory syncytial virus infection, respiratory adenovirus infection, syphilis, dengue fever, open tuberculosis, HIV infection, and Chikungunya etc. 1,373 person times of on-site rapid tests at the ports were conducted, 11,107 person times were confirmed by laboratory tests, and the number of cases confirmed by laboratory tests increased by 100.73% compared with that in 2011. Altogether 1.187 million person times of entry-exit infectious disease surveillance were conducted, with 7,141 cases detected, including AIDS, open tuberculosis, malaria, influenza, dengue fever, dysentery, venereal disease, and virus hepatitis etc. and 1,128,600 person times were vaccinated. Altogether 1,920 cases of exceeding nuclear and radiation were reported and 1,692 cases were discharged after inspection, 126 cases were returned, one was disposed of by the public security department, 85 cases were disposed of by the department of environmental protection, and 16 cases were disposed of by other departments.

(Zhao Xuemei)

2. Anti-terrorism at Ports was Effectively Enhanced

General Administration of Quality Supervision, Inspection and Quarantine revised *Preparedness for the Emergency Response to Nuclear and Radiation Terrorism Attack at Ports*, *Preparedness for the Emergency Response to Biological Terrorism Attack at Ports*, *Preparedness for the Emergency Response to Nuclear and Radiation Terrorism Attack at*

Ports, and *Preparedness for the Emergency Response to Nuclear, Biological and Chemical Radiation Terrorism Attacks at Ports,* and re-deployed work on information reporting, preparedness, and emergency response etc. In accordance with the requirements of the national anti-terrorism office, *Working Plan on the Supervision and Inspection of Anti-terrorism at Ports* was formulated, supervision and inspection of anti-terrorism at ports were conducted and the working system for the supervision and inspection of anti-terrorism at ports was further improved.

(Zhao Xuemei)

Chapter VI   Rural Health

Work of Rural Health in 2011

In 2012, efforts were made to accomplish all the focal tasks in deepening the reform of the medical and health care systems, further consolidate and perfect the new rural cooperative medical system, push forward reform and development of rural health service systems, promote the equalization of basic public health services and new progress was made in the work of rural health.

I. The new rural cooperative medical system was further consolidated and farmers participating in the system reaped more benefits

In 2012, there were 2,566 counties (county-level cities, districts) throughout the country launching the new rural cooperative medical care and the number of farmers participating in the new rural cooperative medical system amounted to 805 million, a participating rate of 98.26%, of whom184 million, 353 million and 268 million were in the eastern, middle and western regions respectively and the respective participating rate was 99.30%, 98.16% and 97.68% in each region. The subsidies for the new rural cooperative medical care were well arranged by all the localities. In 2102, the total amount of funds raised was 248.471 billion yuan and actual subsidy per person was 308.54 yuan, which was 62.33 yuan higher than that in 2011. The subsidies in Beijing and Shanghai were 1,232.47 yuan and 707.29 yuan respectively. The standard for average personal payment throughout the country was 55.36 yuan, while that in the eastern and the middle and western region was 72.04 yuan and 50.42 yuan respectively. In 2012, farmers reaped the benefits of the new rural cooperative medical care for 1.745 billion person-times and on average, every farmer had 2.17 times, 84.5354 million person-times of hospitalization compensation, 1.415 billion person-times of outpatient overall-planning compensation, 127 million person-times of outpatient family-account compensation, 4.7685 million person-times of inpatient normal-parturition compensation, 14.4587 million person-times of outpatient large-sum compensation for the treatment of special diseases, 21.5967 million person-times of physical-examination compensation and 78.2871 million person-times of other kinds of compensation. In comparison with that in 2011, beneficial person-times throughout the country increased by 32.70% and that of hospitalization compensation increased by 20.21%.

The work of medical security for rural residents' major serious diseases was actively promoted and 20 diseases, including childhood leukemia, congenital heart disease, end-stage renal disease, hemophilia and carcinoma of the lungs were brought into the coverage of the pilot. By the end of 2012, 990,000 people nationwide got the compensation for the treatment of major serious diseases, whose medical expenses totaled 9.5 billion yuan and accumulated compensation amounted to 6.2 billion yuan with the actual compensatory rate of 65.4% (the actual compensation rate for the first 8 diseases was 70% and that for the newly-added 12 diseases was 60%). Organized by each province, the work of medical security for childhood leukemia and congenital heart disease was carried out throughout the country. 25 provinces conducted the pilot work of medical security for 6 diseases, including end-stage renal disease and AIDS opportunistic infections, in all parts or most regions of the provinces. Hubei and other 22 provinces conducted the pilot work of medical security for 12 newly-added diseases, such as carcinoma of the lungs, hemophilia and so on.

Supervisory management on the funds of the new rural cooperative medical care was strengthened and reform in payment forms was promoted actively. In cooperation with the National Audit Office, the Ministry of Health made special audit on the funds of the new rural cooperative medical care and issued the *Notice of the Ministry of Health on Effectively Conducting Audit Rectification on the Funds of the New Rural Cooperative Medical Care (No101〔2012〕of the Department of Rural Health Management of the General Office of the Ministry of Health)*. The Ministry of Health, the State Development and Reform Commission and the Ministry of Finance jointly printed and issued the *Guiding Opinions on Promoting Reform in Payment Forms of the New Rural Cooperative Medical Care (No 28,〔2012〕of the Department of Rural Health Management of the Ministry of Health)*.The Ministry of Health held the video and telephone conference on reform in payment forms and required all the localities to orderly reform payment forms such as quota payment for specific diseases,global budget and so on and promote grassroots medical and health institutions to transform their operation mechanisms. By the end of 2012, the pilot of reform in various payment forms was conducted in over 80% of the overall-planned areas throughout the country.

Participation of commercial insurance institutions in handling of services for the new rural cooperative medical care was actively pushed forward. The Ministry of Health, the China Insurance Regulatory Commission, the Ministry of Finance and the Office of the Leading Group of the State Council for Deepening the Reform of the Medical and Health Care System jointly printed and issued the *Guiding Opinions of the Office of the Leading Group for Deepening Reform of the Medical and Health Care System, the China Insurance Regulatory Commission, the Ministry of Finance, and the State Council Concerning Commercial Insurance Institutions Participating in Handling of Services for New Rural Cooperative Medical Care*. In August, the Ministry of Health and the China

Insurance Regulatory Commission jointly held on-the-spot working conference in Zhengzhou of Henan Province and by the end of 2012, 10% counties (county-level cities, districts) nationwide entrusted commercial insurance institutions with handling the services of the new rural cooperative medical care.

The construction of the capacity for the management of the new rural cooperative medical care was enhanced. From July to October, the Ministry of Health successively organized training classes for submission of the information on the pilot of medical security for major serious diseases, the compilation and report of budgeting social insurance funds and the statistical survey on the new rural cooperative medical care and strengthened the training for the administrative personnel in all the localities. All the localities also took active measures to improve the administrative capacity. Such training projects were conducted in the middle and western regions, too. 46.36 million yuan from the central government and 14.13 million yuan from local governments of Anhui, Hunan, Jiangxi, Heilongjiang, Yunnan, Guizhou and Shaanxi were allocated for the training of the capacity for administration of the new rural cooperative medical care in the middle and western regions. In 2012, 1,711 and 1,966 terms of training classes were held for reform in payment forms and in outpatient overall planning respectively and 344,258 persons were trained, of whom 105,597 were administrative personnel (35,528 persons from county-level institutions, 68,541 persons from township institutions) and 24,289 persons were medical workers of designated medical institutions (80,731 persons from county-level designated medical institutions, 158,406 persons from township designated medical institutions).

The construction of national information platforms for the new rural cooperative medical care was pushed forward smoothly in 2012. In September, the General Office of the Ministry of Health printed and issued the *Notice of the General Office of the Ministry of Health on Promoting the Construction of Information Platforms of the New Rural Cooperative Medical Care*, which reviewed the experience of the first batch of the pilot liaisons, designated 26 hospitals as the second batch of the pilot liaisons, including Peking Union Medical College Hospital and some other hospitals in Beijing, Inner Mongolia Autonomous Region and 5 other provinces (autonomous regions, cities) and expanded the liaison of the national information platforms of the new rural cooperative medical care and the pilot units to 29 medical institutions in 9 provinces.

II. Comprehensive reform in rural grassroots medical and health institutions was promoted and rural health service system was further perfected

Integrated management of rural health services was pushed forward. By the end of November 2012, 91.1% of township health care centers and 77.9% of village clinics conducted the integrated management.

The construction of village doctors was enhanced and the pilot of the responsibility system of initial-attending physician in rural medical and health institutions was explored. Compensatory policies were unceasingly optimized and all the localities tried every means to promote the policies on compensating rural doctors to be put into effect so as to ensure they were fairly treated and took various measures to solve the problems after their retirement. The Ministry of Health encouraged the localities that gained achievements in the integrated management of rural health services to make exploration. The central government invested 281 million yuan in the training for rural health personnel in 22 provinces (autonomous regions, cities) in the middle and western regions and the Production and Construction Corps in Xinjiang Uygur Autonomous Region and 570,000 rural professional health personnel were planned to be trained. By the end of 2012, 590,000 persons were trained and the training task was over-fulfilled.

The project of partner assistance from Grade II and above medical and health institutions to township health care centers was conducted. The central government allocated 219 million yuan for the project of the partner assistance in the poverty-stricken areas of 21 provinces (autonomous regions, cities excluding Tibet) in the middle and western regions and 3,644 township health care centers were assisted and 10,932 medical workers were dispatched.

Special subsidies were allocated to village clinics for carrying out the essential drug system. The central government arranged 2.115 billion yuan to specially subsidize the village clinics that carried out the essential drug system in accordance with the standard of 5 yuan per capita, 80% in the western region, 60% in the middle region and differentiated percentage in the eastern region.

III. Implementation of the project of rural basic public health services was promoted

In 2012, the Ministry of Health continuously promoted the implementation of the project of the basic public health services in rural areas. On the basis of the first 6 liaison counties for rural basic public health services, another 6 counties including Laizhou in Shandong Province, Wuzhi in Henan Province, Qianjiang in Hubei Province, Luoding in Guangdong Province, Luzhai in Guangxi Zhuang Autonomous Region and Huining in Gansu Province were designated as the second batch of liaison counties. Through the on-site observation, the introduction to model experience at conferences and the compilation and issue of news in brief and special issues, the Ministry of Health organized the liaison counties to learn from the regions with outstanding performances so that they could take the lead in promoting the basic public health services in an effective and scientific way. The Ministry of Health forcefully pushed forward the project by holding symposiums on rural basic public health services and working conferences of the liaison counties. Training classes were held in Lhasa of Tibet Autonomous Region and Linfen of Shanxi Province in August and October respectively so as to improve the level of rural basic public health services in agricultural and pastoral areas in Tibet Autonomous Region and in concentrated destitute areas.

(Zhao Yinghong)

Chapter VII   Maternal and Child Health Care and Community Health

Section 1   Maternal and Child Health Care

Work of Maternal and Child Health Care in 2012

In 2012, under the guidance of the *Outline Program for the Development of Chinese Women (2011-2020)* and the *Outline Program for the Development of Chinese Children (2011-2020)*, the work of maternal and child health care closely centered on *"one Law* and two *Programs"* and the major tasks for deepening reform in medical and health care systems and with taking the guarantee of maternal and child safety, the comprehensive prevention and treatment of birth defects, the prevention and treatment of women's and children's diseases and the construction of maternal and child health care systems as focal tasks, efforts were made to comprehensively strengthen the work of maternal and child health care and continuously improve the equality and accessibility of maternal and child health care services in order to effectively safeguard the health rights and interests of women and children. In 2012, the mortality rate of pregnant and puerperal women, infants and the children under 5 decreased to 24.5/100,000, 10.3‰ and 13.2‰ respectively. The first was to formulate and implement development programs for maternal and child health in the new era, establish the Leading Group of the Ministry of Health for carrying out the "two *programs"*, print and issue the *Implementation Plans of the Ministry of Health on Carrying out the Outline Programs for the Development of Chinese Women and Children (2011-2020)* and hold the National Working Conference on Maternal and Child Health. The second was to continuously perfect systems for the management of maternal and child health, organize the drafting of the *Administrative Measures for the Screening of Women's Common Diseases* and the working rules, strengthen administration on the screening of women's common diseases, revise and optimize the *Measures for the Administration of Breast-milk Substitutes (Draft for Soliciting Opinions)*, print and issue the *Working Rules for Healthcare at Nurseries and Kindergartens*, the guidelines on the visits to new-born babies, the child medical examination and the child feeding and nutrition and the technical rules on the administration of children's nutritional diseases. Standards concerning to the screening of new-born babies' inherited metabolic diseases were formulated and methods for intensification of the rescue and treatment of the positive babies were explored. Efforts were made to enhance the management on the print and issue of the "three certificates of mother and infant" and the medical certificate of birth, organize the compilation and print of the *Guiding Book on the Administration of Medical Certificate of Birth* and initiate the fourth-time revision of the medical certificate of birth. The third was to further strengthen the construction of maternal and child health system, fulfill the project of constructing county-level maternal and child healthcare institutions in the middle and western regions, formulate the *Plan and Standards for the Construction of Maternal and Child Healthcare Institutions*, intensify the research on the functions and operating mechanisms of maternal and child healthcare institutions, conduct surveys on service resources of maternal and child health, promote the construction pilot of maternal and child healthcare institutions, organize county-level maternal and child healthcare institutions to conduct performance evaluation and work review and enhance training for administrative and professional personnel in grassroots maternal and child health institutions. Efforts were also made to conduct the advanced learning support in obstetrics and the personnel training project on the examination of rural women's cervical cancer and breast cancer and the prevention of mother-to-child transmission of AIDS, syphilis and B hepatitis, explore the service modes in pregnant and puer-peral period for key groups such as ethnic minorities, mobile population and so on., research major health issues that affected children's health, strengthen the work of the information on maternal and child health and accomplish the revision of statistical survey systems for maternal and child health. The fourth was to extensively carry out maternal and child health interventions and continue the project of "reduction and elimination" (the reduction of the mortality of pregnant and puerperal women and the elimination of neonatal tetanus) and other major public health service projects, including the subsidies for rural women's hospital delivery, the supplement of folic acid for neural tube defect prevention, the examination of "two cancers" for rural women and the prevention of mother-to-child transmission of AIDS, syphilis and B hepatitis. To solve the major health problems of children in the middle and western regions, the pilot project on improving child nutrition in poverty-stricken areas and the key liaison work of comprehensive child health interventions in Nujiang Prefecture in Yunnan Province were launched. In cooperation with the departments concerned, the Ministry of Health carried out the activity of "the elimination of infant anemia", unceasingly strengthened the prevention and treatment of birth defects and held on-the-spot meetings to exchange experience on comprehensive prevention and treatment of birth defects. Screening of infant diseases was subsidized in the rural areas in the western region and the pilot project of the prevention and control of thalassaemia was also launched. International cooperation in maternal and child health was conducted so as to solve the problems concerning family violence, mobile population and other vulnerable spots and key groups and regions such as teen-agers and ethnical minority regions. Phased achievements were gained in the elimination of neonatal tetanus. The World Health Organization (WHO) confirmed China's elimination of neonatal tetanus and China achieved its goal in the elimination of neonatal tetanus.

(Zhao Yinghong)

Section 2　Community Health

Progress in National Urban Community Health Work in 2012

In 2012, the work in community health reform and development was promoted steadily and positive progress was made in the construction of service systems, the perfection of service functions, the reform in operation mechanisms and so on. Firstly, the construction of service systems was enhanced continuously and the number of service institutions and personnel was on the steady increase. By the end of 2012, there were 8, 137 community health service centers, 26,000 community health service stations and about 448,000 community health personnel. Compared with the last year, the growth in the number of community health service institutions and personnel was 786 and 15,000 respectively. The Ministry of Health continued the construction of model community health service centers and 164 centers were up to the standards of the national model community health service centers. Secondly, service functions were further perfected and service capacity was continuously improved. In accordance with local residents' needs, community health service institutions in all the localities provided appropriate basic medical and public health services; 80% of community health service centers and 48% of community health service stations were able to provide services of the traditional Chinese medical science and medicines. 646,000 community health service personnel received various forms of on-the-job training. Thirdly, reform in operation mechanisms was deepened ceaselessly. General Practitioners' signing agreements on health service with community residents was carried out in Beijing and Shanghai; various forms of cooperation were established between community health service institutions and hospitals in Wuhan of Hubei Province and Hangzhou of Zhejiang Province and the system was implemented in Dongguan of Guangdong Province that community residents should go to designated hospitals for medical treatment, community health service institutions should be the initial choice and patients should be transferred level by level. Meanwhile, all the localities made active exploration in the reform of the financing, the modes of payment and the personnel and distribution systems, preserved the non-profit property of community health service institutions and aroused medical personnel's enthusiasm. Fourthly, community health service institutions were more popular with the residents. In 2012, patients of the out-patient department of community health service institutions were 620 million, accounting for 9% of the total; compared with the last year, the total number of the outpatients increased by 13.6% and the percentage increased by 0.3%.

(Zhao Yinghong)

Chapter VIII   Medical Administration

1. Work of Medical Administration in 2012

Work on medical administration in 2012 centered around the general deployments of deepening reform of medical and healthcare system and the national key deployments of health work in 2012, focusing on perfecting medical service system, strengthening capacity building, innovating management methods, bettering service and continuously improving quality.

I. Forcefully press forward work on deepening reform of medical and healthcare system and alleviate the difficult access to medical service for the public

(1) The management of medical institutions and the construction of medical service system were strengthened. Firstly, *Guiding Principles for the Setting and Planning of Medical Institutions* was revised to explore building regional medical centers and plan building national, provincial, municipal and prefectural medical centers. Secondly, *Guiding Opinions on Rehabilitation during the 12th Five-Year Plan Period* was printed and issued, the requirements and deployments on the construction of rehabilitation system during the 12th Five-Year Plan period were clarified and the service models of separated treatment of acute diseases and chronic diseases and dual referral were gradually established. Thirdly, the construction of national key specialties was strengthened. In 2012, 309 projects of national key clinical specialties were chosen, which covered 130 hospitals, 15 of which were selected as the project hospitals for the specialty constriction of clinical nursing. Since the start of the construction projects of national key clinical specialties in 2010, the project evaluation of 30 specialties had been finished, covering 265 hospitals in 31 provinces, (autonomous regions, municipalities) and Xinjiang Production and Construction Corps. Fourthly, the capacity building of some weak specialties like, emergency and pathology, was strengthened. 100 construction projects were carried out in the municipal children's hospitals and the pediatrics departments in the general hospitals, which alleviated the insufficiency in pediatrics service. Fifthly, social capitals were encouraged to invest into hospitals, which pressed forward the diversified forms of running hospitals. Regulations were clarified on the determination and change of the nature of running hospitals with social capitals and the determination of grades, guiding the social capitals into the field of medical service and strengthening the management. Pilot was launched on private clinics run by qualified professionals by law in Beijing and

Tianjin. Support was given to Shanghai, Hainan and Henan etc. to plan and set up medical zones scientifically to explore diversified forms of running hospitals. The pilot scope of hospitals run by Hong Kong and Macao capitals was expanded and the policies for the examination and approval of the setting up were adjusted to simplify the procedures for examination and approval.

(2) Management of clinical pathways and informatization construction were pressed forward. In 2012, the clinical pathways for 100 kinds of diseases were printed and issued (from April, 2009, to the end of November, 2012, the clinical pathways and sub-pathways for 431 kinds of diseases were formulated). By the end of November, 2012, 4,628 medical institutions and 33,498 departments nationwide had carried out the management of clinical pathways, increasing by 33.5% and 31.3% respectively compared with those in the same period in 2011; altogether 3,437,500 cases participated in the management of clinical pathways, accounting for 3.4% of the discharged patients, increasing by 143% compared with that in the same period last year. The average length of stay in hospitals with the clinical pathways was 10.36 days, decreasing by 7.1% and the average expense of hospitalization was 7,725 yuan, decreasing by 5.5% (price rising not included). *Guiding Opinions of the Ministry of Health on Pressing forward the Management of Clinical Pathways during the 12th Five-Year Plan Period* was printed and issued. The pilot on the informatization construction of hospitals with the electronic medical records as the core was pressed forward. By the end of June, 2012, 41.7% of second-leveled and above public hospitals had established the system of electronic medical records. By the end of 2012, altogether 905 tertiary hospitals had participated in the grading evaluation of the system of electronic medical records.

(3) Excellent nursing services were forcefully promoted and reform on nursing services was deepened. *2012 Working Plan for Promoting Excellent Nursing Services* was printed and issued, which clarified the principles of "changing the models, focusing on clinical work, establishing mechanisms" to promote excellent nursing services. By the end of November, all the tertiary hospitals nationwide had launched the campaign of excellent nursing services and 692 tertiary first class hospitals realized the excellent nursing services in the whole hospital, accounting for 75.9% of all the tertiary first class hospitals nationwide; and 4,817 secondary hospitals had launched the campaign of excellent nursing services, accounting for 80.6% of all the secondary hospitals nationwide. 23 hospitals were selected for the pilot of management of nursing positions. *Guiding Opinions of the Ministry of Health on Implementing Management of Nursing Positions* was printed and issued.

(4) Special rectification on the clinical use of antibacterial drugs was deepened. *Measures on the Management of Antibacterial Drugs at Medical Institutions* was

promulgated and implemented. Inspection was made on the special rectification on the clinical use of antibacterial drugs in 241 secondary and above specialized hospitals, including obstetrics and gynecology hospitals, children's hospitals, tumor hospitals, stomatological hospitals and municipal general hospitals.

(5) The treatment of catastrophic diseases for the residents was further ensured. Clinical pathways for some catastrophic diseases were formulated such as holergasia, opportunistic infection of AIDS and MDR-TB etc. In 2012, 4,136 children with leukemia, over 14,000 children with congenital heart disease and over 50,000 psychotics were treated with good results. The information system for hemophiliacs was perfected and over 12,000 hemophiliacs had their information registered nationwide.

(6) The Project of Sight Restoration for Millions of Cataract Patients in Poverty during the 12th Five-Year Plan period was launched. The management plan for the project, the basic standards for the designated operation hospitals as well as the norms for the operation of cataract the standards for the quality control were printed and issued, and the national expert group for technical guiding of the project was founded. By the end of November, altogether 296,000 operations for the project were completed, which meant we had over-fulfilled the task of 250,000 operations in 2012 ahead of schedule.

(7) A series of measures were taken to improve medical services. Firstly, the measure of "treating first, and settling accounts later" was steadily pushed forward. According to incomplete statistics, by the end of September, about 1,020,000 patients benefited from the model of "treating first, and settling accounts later" at the medical institutions everyday, accounting for 30% of the outpatient cases everyday. Patients using the traditional registration method had to wait in line 3.5 times on average, the average waiting time being 11 minutes; while after using the model of "treating first, and settling accounts later", the patients only needed to wait in line 2.2 times, the average waiting time being 7.3 minutes. Secondly, the social work by the hospitals and the voluntary work were pressed forward. According to incomplete statistics, by the end of September, various medical institutions nationwide recruited nearly 530,000 medical volunteers and about 75,000 social volunteers, providing 5,870,000 person hours of voluntary services every year. Thirdly, the mutual recognition of check-up results among the medical institutions at the same level was pressed forward. By the end of June, 83.3% of the secondary and above public hospitals had participated in the mutual recognition of check-up results among medical institutions at the same level. Fourthly, the evaluation on the third group of demonstrative hospitals for making hospital affairs public was made, which aimed to guide the grassroots medical and health institutions to make hospital affairs public.

II. The campaigns of "Three Excellent and One Satisfactory" and "Long March of Medical Quality" were pressed forward.

National Medical and Health System 2012 Working Plan for the Campaign of "Three Excellent and One Satisfactory" was printed and issued, the national teleconference and five sub-working conferences were held, supervision and inspection were conducted and experience and deficiency were summarized to press forward the development of the campaign. Inspection was conducted on the campaign of "Three Excellent and One Satisfactory" in 121 secondary and above specialized hospitals nationwide, including obstetrics and gynecology hospitals, children's hospitals, tumor hospitals, and stomatological hospitals etc.

III. Medical quality management and control were strengthened to improve service quality and level.

(1) The system of medical quality management and control was established and improved. *Measures for Medical Quality Management* was drafted and the construction of MOH center for medical quality control and the provincial and municipal centers for medical quality control of clinical specialties were pressed forward. By the end of 2012, 14 centers for quality control had been established for specialties like neurology and emergency department etc. Quality control index for the tertiary specialized hospitals and the key departments in the hospitals were formulated to conduct quality control over single diseases by information means.

(2) Standardized diagnosis and treatment for catastrophic diseases was conducted. Guidelines for diagnosis and treatment as well as technical norms were formulated for the catastrophic diseases like tumor, cardiovascular and cerebrovascular diseases and chronic renal failure etc. The quality control indexes for the diagnosis and treatment of colorectal cancer, primary lung cancer and breast cancer were formulated, the registration system for medical record information was established and training on standardized diagnosis and treatment was conducted.

(3) Management of medical techniques was further improved and perfected. *Measures for the Management of Clinical Application of Medical Techniques* and the directory for the third type of medical techniques were revised and *Measures for Graded Management of Operation at Medical Institutions (for Trial Implementation)* was printed and issued. The management and quality control of some key medical techniques were strengthened such as implantation of artificial joints, endoscopic diagnosis and treatment and interventional diagnosis and treatment etc. Norms for the management of such diagnosis and treatment techniques were formulated.

(4) Good work was done on the pharmaceutical administration at medical institutions. *Chinese National Formulary for Children, Measures for the Management of Clinical Use of Antibacterial Agents, National Guidelines on Antimicrobials* and other relevant technical norms were formulated and revised. The coverage of Chinese Monitoring Network for Rational Use of Drugs, MOH National Antimicrobial Resistance Investigation Net and MOH Center for Antibacterial Surveillance were expanded, covering over 1,300 medical institutions. 1,349 secondary and above hospitals were determined as the national monitoring units for MOH Center for Antibacterial Surveillance and MOH National Antimicrobial Resistance Investigation Net.

(5) *Regulations on Nurses and The Outline for Developing Nursing Care in China (2011-2015)* were implemented. Standards for nursing industry were formulated and bettered to standardize nursing behavior; studies and pilot on continuing nursing were carried out. A national health system's contest on innovating skills for nurses was jointly held by MOH and All China Federation of Trade Unions. As the results of the contest, three nurses were granted National May 1 Labor Medal and National May 1 Women's Medal, thirty nurses were granted the title of National May 1 Women's Model and over 100 nurses were granted provincial May 1 Labor Medal.

(6) The management of hospital infection was strengthened. *Action Plan for Preventing and Controlling Hospital Infection (2012-2015)* was printed and issued. The main objectives and tasks for the prevention and control of hospital infection during the 12th Five-Year Plan period were clarified. The capacity building was strengthened for the provincial centers for management and quality control of hospital infection. And inspections on the management of hospital infection were conducted.

(7) The prevention and treatment of blindness and the management of drug rehabilitation were pressed forward. *National Program for the Prevention and Treatment of Blindness (2012-2015)* was printed and issued. General deployments were made on the prevention and treatment of blindness nationwide. Phrase III of the project of Vision First-China in Action was launched and implemented. *Opinions of National Health System on the Management of Drug Rehabilitation* was printed and issued, and sample inspections were made on the management of drug rehabilitation in twelve provinces (autonomous regions and municipalities directly under the central government). *Guidelines on the Diagnosis and Treatment of Ketamine Dependence* was printed and issued, which regulated the diagnosis and treatment of new synthetic drugs.

IV. Programs for the training of health talents were implemented and the building of health talent team was strengthened

Doctors' qualification examination in 2012 was held. The construction of examination system for the admission of cardiovascular physicians was launched, 350 cardiovascular professors and nearly 400 examination administrators worked as examiners and examination officials and nearly 1,500 examinees took the examination. *Measures for the Management of Specialists* was drafted to perfect the system of specialists. The training program for ten thousand nursing talents was implemented, and 3,233 nursing administrators from the tertiary hospitals and county hospitals and specialist key nurses from the county hospitals were trained, covering over 300 hospitals nationwide; altogether 2,441 clinical specialist nurses were trained nationwide. In 2012, 1,691 grassroots medical and health technicians were trained with the help of the project of Spark Plan; 2.148 grassroots clinical inspectors were trained with the help of the project of Bud Plan; 3,352 management staff on the clinical use of antimicrobial were trained with the help of the project of Flame Plan; and 10,660 medical staff were trained with the help of the project of Special Drugs. The national training project of rehabilitative therapists was started, training syllabus and standards for diagnosis and treatment were printed and issued and 1,200 rehabilitative therapists were trained.

V. The management of blood was strengthened and blood safety was ensured.

According to incomplete statistics, by November, 2012, approximately 10,674,500 people donated about 3,582.5 tons of blood, which roughly met the need of blood for clinical use. The donation of blood was included as an important index for the evaluation standards for the patriotic hygiene city, the evaluation of the government work and the construction of spiritual civilization, which promoted blood donation. A campaign call Opening Blood Stations Month was launched. MOH, Red Cross Society of China and PLA Health Department of the General Logistic Department jointly organized the 2010-2011 national awarding conference for blood donation. *Guiding Principles for the Setting up and Planning of Blood Stations* was revised and preparation for the construction of national blood safety center was started. *Technical Operation Procedures for Blood Station (2012Edition)* and some other technical standards were improved and some industry standards such as the requirements for the storage and transportation of blood were printed and issued. Nucleic acid testing was pushed forward and 45 blood stations (21 blood centers, 24 central blood stations) in 24 provinces nationwide conducted nucleic acid testing. *Ministry of Health Statistic*

Indexes for Blood Collecting and Supplying Information (for Blood Stations, 2011 Edition) was printed and issued and the situation of blood collection nationwide was reported regularly. The system for opening information at blood stations was established and demonstrative stations were set for opening information at blood stations to enable the public to understand and supervise the supply of blood. *Measures for the Management of Clinical Blood Use at Medical Institutions* was printed and issued to promote the management of rational clinical blood use; work on the diagnosis and treatment of hemophilia and the management of plasma collection stations were carried out with an overall plan.

(Zhao Xuemei)

2. Regulations on the Registration of Physicians Who Have Acquired the Citizenship of Hong Kong or Foreign Countries were Perfected

In accordance with the *Reply of Ministry of Health on the Registration of Physicians Who have Acquired Citizenship of Hong Kong or Foreign Countries (MOH Health Administration [2012] No. 277)*, after the mainland's physicians have acquired the citizenship of Hong Kong, they can hold their Doctor Qualification Certificates and practice in the mainland; however, if the mainland's physicians have acquired the citizenship of other countries, they will not be allowed to practice medicine in the mainland even though they can still hold the Doctor Qualification Certificates; the mainland's physicians, if willing to act as the legal representatives of the mainland's medical institutions after acquiring the citizenship of Hong Kong or the citizenship of other countries, should act in conformity with relevant regulations of the local administrative departments on the registration of legal representatives.

(Zhao Xuemei)

Chapter IX   Medical Service Supervision and Management

1. Work on Medical Service Supervision and Management in 2012

In 2012, the reform of public hospitals and medical service supervision and management were pressed forward effectively and remarkable achievements were made in the reform of public hospitals, supervision on the quality and safety of medical service, harmonious relationship between doctors and patients, partner assistance between urban hospitals and rural hospitals and the evaluation and appraisal of hospitals etc.

I. The reform of public hospitals was pressed forward vigorously. In 2012, the General Office of the State Council printed and issued *Opinions on the Pilot of Comprehensive Reform of County-Level Public Hospitals (No. 33 [2012] General Office of State Council)* and the Ministry of Health and other four ministries jointly issued *Circular on Working Well on Reform of Public Hospitals in 2012 (No. 53 [2012] Ministry of Health).* The Ministry of Health strengthened the contact with 17 national contact pilot cities for the reform of public hospitals and 311 contact counties for the comprehensive reform of county-level public hospitals to grasp the latest progress in all the localities and 93 issues of *Briefing on Pilot of Public Hospital Reform* to summarize experience and lessons. In July, 2012, the Ministry of Health held a symposium on cost control for public hospitals, requiring all the localities to take into account the local development of economy and the society as well as the demand of the public for medical service, formulate the standards of cost control scientifically and establish a long-term mechanism for the surveillance and supervision of medical costs in public hospitals. Meanwhile, *Bulletin on Strengthening Medical Cost Control by All the Localities in 2012 (No. 127[2012] Ministry of Health)* was printed and issued. Exterior supervision was strengthened and the operators of the hospitals were required to include cost control into the performance management of public hospitals. A supervisory mechanism for cost control was established with universal participation of the whole society, and the system for the announcement of medical information was improved, which announced the changes of outpatient costs and average hospitalization costs etc. Clinical appointment service was further pushed forward, *Standards for the Evaluation of Clinical Appointment Service (2012-2013)* was printed and issued and 37 tertiary first class hospitals in 15 provinces (autonomous regions, municipalities directly under the State Council) were inspected from May to September, 2012. By the end of November, 2012, 1,505 tertiary hospitals registered in the information management system for clinical appointment service. Except those in Tibet, 1,232 tertiary hospitals registered were able to provide clinical appointment service by three or more means. Of all the registered hospitals, 1,391 hospitals provided appointment by telephone, 1,112 hospitals provided appointment at the information desks, 1,043 hospitals provided appointment on the internet and 219 hospitals provided appointment on the outpatient appointment machines. Tele-medicine was further pressed forward in tertiary hospitals and county-level hospitals, and a management system for tele-medicine information was established.

II. The campaign of Safe Hospital was carried on and efforts were made to create harmonious doctor-patient relationship. In 2012, the Ministry of Health and other ministries jointly printed and issued *Circular on Adjusting Members of National Working Group and Office for Creating Safe Hospital (No. 157 [2011] Ministry of Health*, which meant that, on the basis of the original seven members, three more members were supplemented as members of the working group for creating Safe Hospital, namely, the Supreme People's Procuratorate, the Ministry of Justice, and China Insurance Regulatory Commission. In June and August, 2012, the Ministry of Health held the conferences of the national working group's office for creating Safe Hospital in Tianjin and Kashgar, Xinjiang, respectively. To counter the several criminal cases involving the medical institutions in different places, a teleconference was held urgently attended by the provincial health administrative departments and large medical institutions, *Circular on Effectively Safeguarding Public Security and Order in Medical Institutions (No. 5[2012] Ministry of Health)* was printed and issued, *Announcement on Safeguarding Public Security and Order in Medical Institutions (No. 7[2012] Ministry of Health)* was printed and issued together with the Ministry of Public Security, which clarified that seven kinds of acts happened in medical institutions, such as burning ghost money for the dead, setting up a mourning hall, laying out wreaths, laying out corpse against the regulations and mobbing etc. shall be subject to security punishments or even to criminal liabilities by the public security organs in accordance with *Public Security Administration Punishments Law*. Progresses were made in people's mediation of medical disputes and medical liability insurance. By October, 2012, 1,853 people's mediation organizations were set up in 31 provinces (autonomous regions, municipalities directly under the State Council), covering all the prefectural-level and above cities. There were 14,318 people's mediators for medical disputes and 42,443 members of the expert bank. From January to October, 2012, people's mediation organizations accepted 33,726 medical disputes, with 29,304 cases mediated successfully, the success rate being 85.3% and satisfaction rate being 93.2%. Except in Tibet, work on medical liability insurance had started in 30 provinces (autonomous regions, municipalities directly under the State Council) and Xinjiang Production and Construction Corp, in 809 cities (autonomous prefectures, leagues) and counties (districts) directly under provinces (autonomous regions, municipalities directly under the State Council) and 5,211 county-level and above medical institutions had participated in medical liability insurance.

III. Partner assistance between urban and rural hospitals was pressed forward. The Project of Ten Thousand Doctors Supporting Rural Health and Training Programs for the Key Doctors in County-Level Hospitals were carried on. In September, 2012, the Ministry of Health held a national teleconference on the Project of Ten Thousand Doctors Supporting Rural Health, which summarized the work in the previous phase, analyzed and studied the existing problems and deployed work in the next phase. Partner assistance between the hospitals in the east and west provinces was organized, agreements on partner assistance between hospitals were signed by the provinces in the east and the west and long-term and stable partner assistance was established. The national medical team was organized to provide tour medical service and eight tour teams were founded by six hospitals, including China-Japan Friendship Hospital and Peking Union Medical College Hospital, to provide tour medical service in Yulin City, Shanxi Province, Linfen City, Shanxi Province, Luliang City, Shandong Province, Yizhou City, Shanxi Province, Yunnan Province, Xinjiang Uygur Autonomous Region and Tibet Autonomous Region. The training programs for the key doctors at the county-level hospitals were carried on, with 6,000 key doctors at the county-level hospitals trained. The program of Getting to the West for training health talents was carried on, with over 12,000 key doctors and management staff at county-lever hospitals trained nationwide.

IV. Supervision and management on medical service and medical institutions were strengthened. Firstly, the reporting system for medical quality and safety accidents was carried out. *Regulation on the Handling of Medical Malpractices and Interim Provisions on the Reporting of Medical Quality and Safety Accidents* were strictly implemented, on-line reporting was conducted by means of the reporting system for medical quality and safety accidents, and meanwhile the serious medical safety accidents were reported in time. Great efforts were made to achieve prevention in advance, proper handling in the process and summary of experience afterward so that medical quality and safety accidents could be effectively prevented. Secondly, the warning talking system for medical quality and safety accidents was implemented. The serious medical quality and safety accidents being the entry points, warning talking was given to the directors of the medical institutions where serious major medical quality and safety accidents occurred or hidden problems of medical quality and safety accidents existed just because the directors didn't implement the core systems, didn't have adequate sense of responsibility or didn't acquire adequate basic theories, knowledge, skills, high demands, rigorous attitudes or serious working styles or just wouldn't interfere even though they were aware of the problems. The medical institutions would be severely punished in accordance with relevant regulations if they couldn't rectify well enough after the warning talking. Thirdly, rational drug use and concentrated prescription comment were pressed forward. In 2012, the surveillance network for prescription comment was established, consisting of 119 hospitals, and the surveillance network for the information of rational drug use was established, consisting of 33 hospitals. Regular communication was made by some domestic hospitals on the experience on prescription comment and discussions were made on the comment standards of outpatient and emergency descriptions, which provided reference for macro decision-making, pre-warned drug risks and intervening irrational drug use. Fourthly, the system for doctors' routine assessment was improved and good work was done on the evaluation of doctors' morality. The Ministry of Health established the management office for the doctors' routine assessment at the Chinese Medical Doctor Association. The management system was established for the registration of MOH doctors' routine assessment information to implement the system of doctors' routine assessment and the system of doctors' morality evaluation by means of information technology so that the information management had made achievements in the registration, application, verification, examination, result announcement and the informing of the doctors' routine assessments and by now 23 provinces (regions, municipalities) had carried out doctors' routine assessments with this system. By the end of October, 2012, 143,424 medical institutions had registered in the system. Of all the 1,520,489 doctors, 1,126,592 had completed the assessment in this cycle, with 1,125,330 doctors passing and 1,262 doctors failing, the passing rate being 99.88%. Fifthly, the supervision and management of human organ transplantation was strengthened. The national coordination mechanism for human organ donation was established and a scientific donating and assisting mechanism was established. Entrusted by the MOH, Xuanwu Hospital Capital Medical University established the quality control evaluation center for brain injury to conduct the evaluation on brain injuries and training on the techniques for judging cerebral death at proper time and in regular manners. From February to May, 2012, 18 hospitals with organ transplantation in Shandong Province, Gansu Province and Chongqing were inspected and suggestions were proposed on how to rectify. Sixthly, tour inspections for large hospitals were pressed forward steadily. In May, 2012, the tour inspection group conducted phase-II tour inspection for 11 hospitals directly under MOH including Xiangya Hospital of Central South University and Qilu Hospital of Shandong University etc. and inspections were made on six aspects of work, i.e. the non-profit nature of hospitals, the construction and development of the hospitals, medical services, safety in hospitals, economic management and industry working style etc.

V. Evaluation on hospitals was conducted. In 2012, the Ministry of Health printed and issued *Detailed Rules on Implementing Examination Criteria for Tertiary Comprehensive Hospitals (2012 Edition)(No, 57[2012] Ministry of Health)*, examination criteria for tertiary cardiovascular hospitals (2011 edition) and the detailed rules on implementing it and examination criteria for tertiary infectious hospitals (2011 edition). *Circular of the General Office of the Ministry of Health on Regulating the Examination of Hospitals (No. 574[2012] General Office of the Ministry of Health)* was printed and issued, which required that all the secondary and above (including secondary) hospitals that had passed the examination before January 1, 2011, be re-examined and the newly approved tertiary hospitals that had passed the examination after December 31, 2010, be re-examined. Meanwhile, in accordance with the new standards and methods for examination, special supervision and inspection on the examination of hospital classification were conducted in provinces with a large number of newly approved tertiary hospitals. In order to further regulate the examination of hospitals, National Institute of Hospital Administration was entrusted to set up the office for the project of hospital examination and evaluation in March, 2012, which was in charge of the check and formulation of examination standards, research on examination methods, and the monitoring of medical service information etc. Training on the new examination criteria was carried out to train key examination experts in all the localities and experts were trained in different provinces and then they made pilot examination for hospitals in some provinces.

VI. The campaign of Three Excellent and One Satisfactory was actively pressed forward. In May, 2012, the Ministry of Health printed and issued *Circular concerning Work Plan for Supervision and Inspection of the Campaign of Three Excellent and One Satisfactory for Medical and Health Sector Nationwide* and the work plan for the supervision and inspection of the campaign of Three Excellent and One Satisfactory for medical and health sector nationwide was formulated. From August to September, supervision groups made the first round of supervision and inspection on the progress of the campaign of Three Excellent and One Satisfactory in Jiangsu Province, Hunan Province, Guangdong Province, Guizhou Province, Gansu Province and Xinjiang. Through the supervision and inspection, guidance on the campaign of Three Excellent and One Satisfactory in all the localities was strengthened, and good methods, experience and innovative measures found in all the localities were summarized; efforts were made to look for and analyze the weak links and problems in our work and effective measures were adopted to rectify in good time.

(Zhao Xuemei)

2. Professional Organization was Founded for Human Organ Donation

On July 6, 2012, State Commission Office of Public Sectors Reform printed and issued *Official Reply on Founding China Management Center for Organ Donation (No. 151 [2012] State Commission Office of Public Sectors Reform)*, which replied to China Red Cross Society to approve the founding of China Management Center for Organ Donation, which would be in charge of the mobilization of human organ donation, signing up and registration, donation witness, fair allocation, aiding incentive, memoriam, the construction of information platform and relevant work. The center was granted 16 posts of public institution with financial subsidy.

(Zhao Xuemei)

Chapter X   Drug Policy and Essential Drug System

Drug Policy and Essential Drug System in 2012

The year 2012 was a key year for consolidating and perfecting the essential drug system. Work on drug policy and essential drug system took safeguarding and improving people's health as the goal, adhered to the basic principles of ensuring the basis, strengthening the grassroots, and constructing the mechanisms, and took consolidating and perfecting the essential drug system as the core. We strengthened the ideological construction, based our work on constructing systems and mechanisms, broadened our mind and innovated our thoughts. As a result, all the tasks for the year were fulfilled.

I. The essential drug system was consolidate and perfected

(1) The implementation scope of the essential drug system was enlarged continuously. Acting on the requirements of the State Council's 12th - Five-Year Plan for medical and heath care reform and by means of special symposiums and research and investigations, we made timely summary and guide on the work of implementing the essential drug system at the village clinics and non-governmental medical institutions at the grassroots level in all the provinces (autonomous regions and cities directly under the State Council). All the localities, on the basis of continuously consolidating the implementation of the essential drug system comprehensively at the governmental medical institutions at the grassroots level, pushed forward the implementation of the essential drug system in village clinics in an orderly way.

(2) The 2012 Essential Drug List was formulated and local supplementary varieties of essential drugs were normalized. Firstly, the dosages and specifications of the essential drugs were normalized. On the basis of conducting relevant research on essential drugs for children, evidence-based medicine and pharmacoeconomics for essential drugs, we made calculations on the paying capability of the New Rural Cooperative Medical Scheme for the essential drugs and proposed the essential drugs. A report was formed on the list of drugs reimbursed by the New Rural Cooperative Medical Scheme and the evaluation on the diseases covered by the basic medical and health service package. By conducting relevant investigations and studies, we primarily formed the standard dosages and specification rules for the essential drugs. Secondly, the work plan for the adjustment of selecting 2012 Essential Drug List was formulated. In accordance with the requirements of *Measures for the Management of*

National Essential Drug List (Interim), the Ministry of Health formulated the work plan and instructions for the adjustment of selecting the 2012 Essential Drug List. In early July, the conference of the National Essential Drug Working Committee was held, at which the working plan for the formulation of the List was approved. Thirdly, a communicating mechanism was established among two ministries and two administrations (i.e. the Ministry of Health, the Ministry of Human Resource and Social Security, State Food and Drug Administration and State Administration of Traditional Chinese Medicine) and the consultant panel was established according to the selecting procedures and many conferences were held. On August 8, evaluations on 2012 Essential Drug List (Draft) were conducted respectively in the east, the middle and the west simultaneously by nearly 1,800 experts on clinical medicine, pharmacy and pharmacoeconomics. Meanwhile, evidence-based medical and phamacoeconomic evaluations were explored to optimize the selection of drug varieties, dosages and specifications. Fourthly, preparations for the promulgation of 2012 Essential Drug List were made. Working plans for the printing of the list and the publicity of its promulgation were made, and expert panels for its publicity were established to form a unified pattern for answering questions from the media. Fifthly, the local supplement of essential drugs was normalized. On the basis of first including into the 2012 Essential Drug List the supplemented varieties with high overlap ratio in all the provinces, *Opinions on Normalizing Local Supplemented Varieties of Essential Drugs (for soliciting opinions)* was drafted, which would be promulgated as the auxiliary document after soliciting opinions from relevant departments.

(3) The procurement mechanism for essential drugs was stabilized to ensure the supply of the essential drugs. Efforts were made to act on the requirements of *Guiding Opinions on Establishing and Normalizing the Procurement Mechanism of Essential Drugs at the Governmental Medical Institutions at the Grassroots Levels* (General Office of the State Council [2010] No. 56) and adhere to the purchasing policies for essential drugs. Firstly, in accordance with the requirements of the 12th - Five-Year Plan for medical and health care reform by the State Council, and on the basis of guiding all the localities to ensure the supply of the essential drugs timely and effectively, we printed and issued *Implementation Plan for Pilot of Designated Production of Essential Drugs that are in Small Demand of yet Indispensable Clinically* (Ministry of Industry and Information [2012] No. 512) together with the General Office of the Ministry of Industry and Information, and *Circular on Further Intensifying the Guiding Opinions on the Construction of Credit System for Drug Safety* (the Commission of Development and Reform [2012] No.2829) together with the Commission of Development and Reform and other departments. Secondly, the implementation of supply policies for essential drugs was pushed forward. In late February, a symposium on ensuring the

supply of essential drugs was held in Hangzhou, Zhejiang province, jointly with other bureaus and departments, at which the Minister of Health, Chen Zhu, attended and delivered an important address, requiring that the safety of quality and supply of essential drugs be ensured. At the end of October, Symposium of Ensuring Supply of Essential Drugs that are in Short Supply & Tracing Handling of Key Proposals by the NPC Representatives was held in Qinhuangdao, Hebei province, at which the attendants introduced the achievements and experience in all the localities in ensuring the supply of essential drugs. By combining ensuring the supply of essential drugs in short supply with handling proposals by the NPC representatives, we established the ensuring system for the supply of drugs based on the essential drug system more effectively and promptly. Thirdly, vigorous efforts were made to assist the handling of medicinal capsules with excessive level of chromium. In accordance with the instructions of relevant ministerial leaders, experts were assembled to discuss and collect relevant information from all the localities and industries to research on and judge the progress of the event. Consequently, notices were printed and issued in time to require all the localities to replace the selected essential drugs using the medicinal capsules with excessive level of chromium. A work conference was jointly held with the administrative department of health on responding to the medicinal capsules with excessive level of chromium. Minister Chen Zhu and Vice Minister Yin Li attended and addressed the conference, which played an important role in responding promptly to the event of medicinal capsules with excessive level of chromium.

(4) Policies for using essential drugs were perfected to promote the rational use of essential drugs. In January 2012, the Ministry of Health solicited openly the opinions on 2009 guidance on the clinical application and formulary of essential drugs via the MOH website, collecting 327 pieces of valid opinions. Research was conducted on the drug use at the medical institutions to carry on the research into and formulation of the management methods on the use of essential drugs. Data on the use of essential drugs at nearly 300 medical institutions at the grassroots levels in over ten provinces and municipalities and information on the demand were collected, which constituted *Investigation Report on the Use of Drug at Medical Institutions at the Grassroots Level*.

(5) The clinical comprehensive evaluations on the essential drugs were carried out. Some first class tertiary hospitals in and outside Beijing were entrusted to study and demonstrate the bases for the clinical comprehensive evaluations on the essential drugs, whose research report was submitted to relevant ministerial leaders.

(6) The first national work conference on pharmaceutical administration was held. In July, 2012, the national work conference on drug policy and the essential drug system was held in Beijing. Over 120 people from relevant ministries, bureaus and all the provinces nationwide (autonomous regions, municipalities directly under the

State Council) attended the conference. Yin Li attended and addressed the conference.

(7) Vigorous efforts were made to participate in work on deepening reform of medical and health care system. In order to assist work on medical insurance for serious diseases for the rural residents, the Ministry of Health selected the essential drugs needed for treating the serious diseases scientifically, included them into the management of the essential drug list; classified management for the essential drugs were implemented in accordance with their respective situations to achieve "one policy for one drug" so that the supply of the essential drugs was ensured. Assisting the Medical and Health Care Reform Office of the State Council vigorously, we participated in the research on and formulation of relevant documents like *Opinions on Consolidating and Perfecting the Essential Drug System* and *Operating Mechanism at the Grassroots Level* and *Several Opinions on Promoting Reforms on Drug Circulation* etc.

II. All the auxiliary policies were implemented to promote the sustainable development of pharmaceutical administration

(1) The construction of electronic supervision system for drugs (vaccines) at medical and health institutions was pushed forward vigorously. Circulars were printed and issued on speeding up the construction of electronic supervision system for drugs (vaccines) at medical and health institutions and training personnel, training textbooks were compiled and several training workshops were held participated by the pharmaceutical administrative departments of the provincial health administrations. Comprehensive promotion was combined with model demonstration, with Jiangsu, Jiangxi, Sichuan and Qinghai as the model provinces for key contact and guidance, and the demonstration system was set up at Yuetan Community Health Center in Beijing; meanwhile, a column was opened on the website of MOH to report the new local development, and many other measures were taken to promote the construction of the system in all the localities in an orderly manner.

(2) The construction of pharmaceutical talent team was strengthened. With the help of the central finance, training projects for pharmacists at the township health centers were conducted in twenty-two provinces (autonomous regions, municipalities directly under the State Council) in the middle and west regions and Xinjiang Production and Construction Corps, with 30,500 people trained, which further improved the service ability and promoted the rational use of essential drugs at the grassroots level. In mid December, a training workshop was held for the pharmaceutical personnel at the grassroots level in Ganzhou, Jiangxi, which was attended by the pharmaceutical administrators for the health administrations in twenty-two provinces (autonomous regions, municipalities directly under the State

Council) in the middle and west regions and Xinjiang Production and Construction Corps.

(3) Study and research on national drug policies and the essential drug system were conducted. In mid May, 2012, the Ministry of Health and the Ministry of Commerce, the Ministry of Information Technology, State Food and Drug Administration and State Administration of Traditional Chinese Medicine jointly listened to the special report by the National Health Development Research Center. It was suggested at the conference that the present policies should be sorted out at regular intervals by means of white paper for drug policies; a normalized and institutionalized working mechanism would be gradually set up in the field of drug policy by releasing white paper for drug policy at regular intervals and finally unified and coordinated national drug policies would be formed at the level of the central government. Work on entrusted research projects in 2012 was done: altogether twelve projects were put up for tender via the website of MOH and Health News, including the regulation framework for the management of essential drugs and the dosages and specifications of essential drugs for children etc. Relevant experts were invited to make primary tender assessments on over 140 tenderers and, by holding tender reviews for the shortlisted projects, decided on twenty-three tenderers to undertake the research projects. Mid-term assessment was made on the research project and the research groups were required to further normalize the use of entrusted funds.

(Zhao Xuemei)

Chapter XI   Food and Drug Administration

1. Supervision on the Import and Export of Special Drugs were Intensified

In 2012, State Food and Drug Administration worked well on the supervision on the import and export of special drugs. SFDA issued 156 import permits for narcotic drugs, 21 export permits for narcotic drugs, 258 import permits for psychotropic drugs, 1929 export permits for psychotropic drugs, 1169 import permits for anabolic steroids and peptide hormone, 66 import and export permits for radioactive drugs and 42 certifications for carrying narcotic drugs and psychotropic drugs. SFDA took control on the varieties imported to the sensitive regions, and meanwhile continuously intensified checks with relevant international organizations and countries. In 2012, altogether 16 international check letters were sent out.

(Zhao Xuemei)

2. Safety Event Involved in French PIP Implants was Handled

In late 2011, after French PIP was revealed to have used unauthorized silicon in its breast implants, SFDA immediately investigated the sales of the implants by PIP's agency in China and contacted relevant regulatory departments in France and WHO to collect relevant information and follow up the progress of the event. A risk assessment conference on PIP breast implants was held attended by experts on plastic surgery, biomaterials and medical tests etc. Decisive measures were taken to control the agency in China and the implants and monitor adverse reaction to the implants; we asked the French authority for reports on relevant events to trace the sale of every single implant in China; we made rapid tests for the implants and released three information reports.

(Zhao Xuemei)

3. US Pharmacopeia Convention (USP) and Chinese Pharmacopeia Commission (ChP) Signed a New Memorandum of Understanding

Upon the invitation of Roger Williams, Chief Executive Officer of the United States Pharmacopeia (USP), Wang Lifeng, Secretary General of Chinese Pharmacopeia Commission (ChP), led a delegation to visit the headquarters of USP from May 15 to 20, 2012, for high-leveled meetings and communications between USP and ChP and a new round of Memorandum of Understanding was signed. During this visit, both parties discussed and exchanged views on the new fields and contents of cooperation, and elaborated every article of the draft of the new round of Memorandum of Understanding. After discussion, both parties reached consensus on the contents of the talk. On behalf of the two parties, Wang Lifeng and Roger L Williams signed a new Memorandum of Understanding on Cooperation between USP and ChP. In accordance with the new round of Memorandum of Understanding, both parties would go on with standard cooperation, working relationships and the translation of pharmacopeias etc. Besides the existent cooperation, both parties agreed: firstly, to extend standard cooperation beyond the scope of pharmacopeias. Both parties would explore on the cooperative development of reference standards to break the restrictions and limits of the present legislations. Secondly, to further enhance cooperation on the standards of auxiliary materials, bio-products and TCM between the two parties. By selecting varieties that would interest both parties, both parties would develop and establish reference standards to further improve drug quality in both countries. Thirdly, to keep on with the system of regular high-leveled meetings between the two parties and go on with Sino-American Pharmacopeia Forum, sales of each other's pharmacopeias, exchange of publications and the project of training and communication etc. Fourthly, to organize staff to assist the translation and updating of American Pharmacopeia so as to consolidate and promote the cooperation and friendship between the two parties. Fifthly, to vigorously explore the verification of joint standards for Chinese and American pharmacopeias.

                                                                      (Zhao Xuemei)

Chapter XII Management of the Undertaking of the Traditional Chinese Medical Science and Medicines

1. Work of Traditional Chinese Medical Science and Medicines in 2012

In 2012, under the leadership of the Party Central Committee and the State Council and with the high attention paid by the Ministry of Health, the whole system of the traditional Chinese medical science and medicines conducted reform and innovation, worked effectively and made remarkable progress in every piece of work.

I. *The Several Opinions of the State Council on Further Supporting and Promoting the Development of the Undertaking of the Traditional Chinese Medical Science and Medicines* **was carried through and implemented**

The *12th Five-Year Plan for the Development of the Undertaking of the Traditional Chinese Medical Science and Medicines (hereinafter referred to as the Plan)* and the *Several Opinions of the of the State Council on Supporting and Promoting the Development of the Undertaking of the Traditional Chinese Medical Science and Medicines* (hereinafter referred to as the *Several Opinions*) were issued and implemented and key tasks and projects were formulated in the light of the conditions of deepening the medical and health care reform. In 2012, with focus on grassroots medical and healthcare institutions and the capacity construction, the central government invested 3.346 billion yuan in support of further expanding the areas and local governments also increased their investment. The State Administration of Traditional Chinese Medicine issued opinions on supporting and promoting the development of the undertaking of the traditional Chinese medical science and medicines and ethnical minority medical science and medicines in Guizhou Province and Xinjiang Uygur Autonomous Region and signed agreements on such contents with Ningxia Hui Autonomous Region and Jiangsu Province. Efforts were made to push forward the construction of experimental regions of the comprehensive reform. Shijiazhuang in Hebei Province was newly added to the experimental cities and the experimental regions such as Dongcheng District in Beijing, Pudong District in Shanghai and Gansu Province actively explored new ways, measures, experience and mechanisms.

II. **The role of the traditional Chinese medical science and medicines was brought into full play in the medical and health care reform**

Efforts were made to take active part in the pilot reform in public hospitals and perfect compensatory mechanisms for the traditional Chinese medical science and medicines. Service items of traditional Chinese medicine increased from 124 to 337 in the National Norms for Prices and Items of Medical Services (2012 Edition) and the "syndrome-differentiation treatment" in traditional Chinese medicine characterized by TCM service techniques was also incorporated into service items. Guidance on the provision and application of traditional Chinese medicines in the *National Essential Drug List* was intensified and grassroots medical personnel's application of Chinese patent drugs was more scientific and reasonable. Ways and patterns for the participation of the traditional Chinese medical science and medicines in the basic public health services were explored. As a separate part, TCM health management was listed into national basic public health service items and "application of traditional Chinese medical science and medicines" was also taken as an important index for evaluating national basic public health service items.

III. The construction of the capacity for grassroots traditional Chinese medical services was pushed forward

In 2012, the State Administration of Traditional Chinese Medicine, the Ministry of Health, the State Food and Drug Administration and the Health Bureau of the PLA Logistic Department jointly began to carry out the project on the improvement of grassroots capacity for traditional Chinese medical services, issued policies and documents concerned, formulated objectives and tasks and put forward ways for carrying out the project. The central government arranged 1.871 billion yuan of special funds for supporting the infrastructure construction of 111 county-level hospitals of traditional Chinese medicine (hospitals of ethnic minority medicine) and 1.475 billion yuan of special funds for public health were almost entirely for supporting the construction of grassroots capacity for traditional Chinese medical services. Service quality of traditional Chinese medical science and medicines improved dramatically and in recent years, the annual increase in the number of patients and the number of discharged patients in TCM hospitals was up to 10% and 15% respectively. All the localities actively explored the new mechanisms for grassroots traditional Chinese medical work. The role of the traditional Chinese medical science and medicines in emergency response rescue and treatment was brought into full play and the working conference on emergency response rescue and treatment with the traditional Chinese medical science and medicines was held for the first time since the founding of new China, at which experience was reviewed and objectives and tasks were clarified.

IV. The inheritance and innovation of the traditional Chinese medical science and medicines was promoted

The construction of national TCM clinical research bases was accelerated and new progress was made. Facilities supporting the construction were basically funded and manning quotas for scientific research were arranged initially; mechanisms were optimized gradually and the capacity for clinical research on major diseases and the diseases concerned was improved continuously. The pilot work of the general survey on resources of Chinese medicinal materials was pushed forward steadily, which was conducted in 655 counties of 22 provinces (autonomous regions, municipalities directly under the central government) attached high attention by all the localities. Transformation and popularization of scientific research achievements in the traditional Chinese medical science and medicines were actively promoted and the bases for transforming and popularizing scientific research achievements were set up in Shanghai and Ningxia.

V. The mechanisms for the cultivation of the talents in the traditional Chinese medical science and medicines were promoted

The fourth batch of inheritance work was fulfilled with the characteristic of linking master-disciple education with the degree in clinical medicine and the forms of the cultivation of high-level TCM talents were innovated that integrated master-disciple education with school education. The national projects of advanced research and training for excellent TCM clinical talents were continued; new achievements were gained in the construction of the workrooms for the inheritance of the academic experience of national famous veteran experts in the traditional Chinese medical science and medicines and the construction of the workrooms for the inheritance of TCM academic schools was also initiated. The State Administration of Traditional Chinese Medicine signed an agreement with Henan Province on joint construction of Henan University of Traditional Chinese Medicine and together with Jiangsu Provincial Government, initiated the project on joint construction of Nanjing University of Traditional Chinese Medicine. The construction of key disciplines was strengthened unceasingly. Efforts were made to support directional and tuition-free cultivation of rural students majoring in traditional Chinese Medicine, enhance post-graduate education and continuing education, promote standardized training for TCM residents and general practitioners, strengthen vocational education and successfully hold 2012 National Vocational Students Skills Competition.

VI. The construction of traditional Chinese medical culture was promoted

Together with the State Administration of Press, the State Administration of Traditional Chinese Medicine recommended the first batch of popular science books on traditional Chinese medical culture, deeply pushed forward the activity of "the Traditional Chinese Medical Science and Medicines in China·Entering Villages, Communities, Families", organized and carried out the "Tour of Lectures on Popular Science Knowledge on the Traditional Chinese Medical Science and Medicines"; nearly 1 million people reaped the benefits of these activities directly. The State Administration of Traditional Chinese Medicine and the CCTV jointly produced the full-length documentary film *Traditional Chinese Medicine,* started the *China Medical Weekly* in cooperation with Beijing Business Today and together with the Chinese Academy of Medical Sciences and many TV stations, continuously improved the quality and level of the propagation and popularization of the knowledge on the traditional Chinese medical science and medicines. The State Administration of Traditional Chinese Medicine pushed forward spreading traditional Chinese medical culture to the world and held the high-level international conference on the development of traditional Chinese medical culture with the theme of "promoting the natural, harmonious and healthy development of human beings".

VII. The construction of the legislation, standardization and informatization of the traditional Chinese medical science and medicines was promoted

The State Administration of Traditional Chinese Medicine accelerated the promotion of the standardized work, held the first working conference on the standardization of the traditional Chinese medical science and medicines since the founding of new China, clarified the fundamental, strategic and overall position and the leading role in the development of the undertaking of the traditional Chinese medical science and medicines, put forward the general train of thought and objective tasks in the new era and established three standardization committees responsible for the management and coordination, the experts and techniques and the international advisory. Efforts were made to speed up the formulation and revision of the standards for the traditional Chinese medical science and medicines and organize the China Association of Chinese Medicine to draw up and issue 195 standards. The Construction of informatization was strengthened. The State Administration of Traditional Chinese Medicine further optimized the information statistics, supplemented the statistical indexes for the traditional Chinese medical science and medicines to the *National System for Survey on Health Resources and Medical Service,* intensified supervision and informed people of the characteristics and harms of false and illegal advertisements through media.

VIII. The foreign exchange and cooperation of the traditional Chinese medical science and medicines was pushed forward

In 2012, in cooperation with the Ministry of Commerce and other 13 ministries, the State Administration of Traditional Chinese Medicine issued the *Several Opinions on Promoting the Development of Traditional Chinese Medical Service Trade* and further expanded international developmental fields. Special activities for the traditional Chinese medical science and medicines were carried out successfully on the First China (Beijing) International Fair for Trade in Services (CIFTIS) which were attached attention and importance by the leaders of the Party Central Committee. Cooperation with the WHO and the ISO was furthered and positive progress was made in the international classification of disease and the formulation of international standards for the traditional Chinese medical science and medicines. The State Administration of Traditional Chinese consolidated and developed bilateral cooperation, further promoted practical cooperation with foreign governments and signed the agreements, the memorandums and the summaries of talks on cooperation in the traditional Chinese medical science and medicines with 6 countries and regions. Connection with four districts of Cross-Straits was deepened, with cooperative mechanisms further perfected and cooperative level continuously improved. Satisfactory results were gained in cooperation with Hong Kong in smoking control with TCM acupuncture and moxibustion.

(Zhao Yinghong)

2. Work of the Integration of Traditional Chinese Medicine and Western Medicine

In 2012, the State Administration of Traditional Chinese Medicine printed and issued the *Standards for the Evaluation on Grade-3 Hospitals of Traditional Chinese Medicine and Western Medicine (2012 Edition)*, the *Detailed Rules for the Evaluation on Grade-3 Hospitals of Traditional Chinese Medicine and Western Medicine (2012 Edition)*, the *Scoring Criteria and Core Indicators for the Evaluation on Grade-3 Hospitals of Traditional Chinese Medicine and Western Medicine (2012 Edition)*, the *Manual for the Experts in the Evaluation of Grade-3 Hospitals of Traditional Chinese Medicine and Western Medicine (2012 Edition)* and a series of documents concerning the evaluation and basically fulfilled the work of the evaluation. After evaluation, 18 hospitals were designated as the third batch of key construction units of the State Administration of Traditional Chinese Medicine and construction work was launched.

(Zhao Yinghong)

3. Compilation of the *Collection of Chinese Medicine* was Initiated Formally

The *Collection of Chinese Medicine* was another important project on the collation of ancient books and the protection of culture after our country organized the compilation of the *Collection of Chinese Taoism, the Collection of Chinese Buddhism,* and the *Collection of Chinese Confucianism,* which was an integrated work combining the collation, research and protection of ancient books on the traditional Chinese medical science and medicines together. In recent two years, standards for collecting books, forms of publication, organizational structure and working mechanisms were discussed systematically and more than 2300 kinds of books were basically selected for the *Collection.* At the suggestions of experts concerned, selected books were further discussed and the implementation plan on comprehensively promoting the compilation was worked out. In August 2012, the work of compilation was formally launched. At present, the State Administration of Traditional Chinese Medicine and the Ministry of Culture were actively coordinating and jointly made the implementation plan more specific, strived to secure grants and the project was expected to be launched comprehensively at the end of the year.

(Zhao Yinghong)

4. 11 Projects on the Traditional Chinese Medical Science and Medicines Won 2012 National Science and Technology Awards

Of all the National Science and Technology Award in 2012, 2 projects on the traditional Chinese medical science and medicines respectively won the second prize of the National Award for Natural Sciences and the National Award for Technological Invention. Of all the National Science and Technology Progress Award in 2012, projects in medical and health fields won 30 prizes (including 1 prize for innovative team), of which 1 project on the traditional Chinese medical science and medicines won the first prize and other 8 won the second prize. The National Science and Technology Award went to 330 projects and 7 experts in science and technology in 2012. 2 persons won the National Highest Science and Technology Award; 41 projects won the second prize of the National Award for Natural Sciences; 3 projects won the first prize of the National Award for Technological Invention and other 74 projects won the second prize. 3 projects, 22 projects and 187 projects respectively won the grand prize, the first prize and second prize of the National Science and Technology

Progress Award.

(**Zhao Yinghong**)

5. The Symposium on Foreign Exchange and Cooperation in the Traditional Chinese Medical Science and Medicines was Held in Guangzhou

The Symposium on Foreign Exchange and Cooperation in the Traditional Chinese Medical Science and Medicines was held in Guangzhou on December 18, 2012, at which progress in foreign exchange and cooperation in recent years was reviewed and summarized and key work in the 12th Five-Year-Plan period such as how to promote TCM international standardization, service trade and construction of bases was discussed. Wang Xiaopin, head of the Department of International Cooperation of the State Administration of Traditional Chinese Medicine, Wu Dong, deputy head of the Department of Planning and Finance of the State Administration of Traditional Chinese Medicine, Tu Zhitao deputy director of Beijing Administration of Traditional Chinese Medicine and Cao Lizhong, Deputy Director of Guangdong Provincial Administration of Traditional Chinese Medicine respectively delivered speeches on the progress in foreign exchange and cooperation, the thinking of budgeting for TCM international cooperation and the progress in it, the TCM cultural travel and the cooperation with Hong Kong, Macao and Taiwan in the traditional Chinese medical science and medicines. Representatives from Guangzhou University of Chinese Medicine, Shanghai University of Traditional Chinese Medicine, Guangdong Provincial Hospital of Traditional Chinese Medicine, the Secretariat of the Technical Committee of Traditional Chinese medicine of the ISO, Hong Kong Baptist University, Shanxi Zhendong Pharmaceutical Co. Ltd and other units respectively made reports on recent years' implementation of the *Outlines* and the development in such key work as TCM international standardization, the construction of bases and the service trade and they also exchanged experience. With focus on the main tasks and major issues of TCM foreign exchange and cooperation, the representatives analyzed the current situations thoroughly, fully discussed the focal and difficult work and made clear of the major work for future. Activities of investigation and survey were arranged during the conference; Yu Wenming, vice-commissioner of the State Administration of Traditional Chinese Medicine, led the representatives to visit Guangdong Provincial Hospital of Traditional Chinese Medicine, the Science Park of Guangzhou University of Chinese Medicine, Guangdong Zisun Group and Guangzhou Jinxiu Xiangjiang Hot-spring Center and listened to the reports made by relevant units on the intensification of international cooperation in TCM science and technology, the cooperation with Comorin in anti-malarial treatment, the development of medicated food and the services of TCM health preservation and travel.

(Zhao Yinghong)

6. The Seminar on Sino-Luxembourg TCM Cooperation and 7th Framework Oncology Program of EU was Held in Beijing

On October 29, 2012, the State Administration of Traditional Chinese Medicine and the Luxembourg national health research center jointly held the Seminar on Sino-Luxembourg TCM Cooperation and 7th Framework Oncology Program of EU, at which Carlo Krieger, Luxembourg's Ambassador to China, attended the seminar and delivered a speech and the current China-Luxemburg cooperative projects and the way forward were discussed mainly. The cooperative partners undertaking the 7th Framework Oncology Program of EU, Liu Xinmin, professor of the Institute of Medicinal Plant Development (IMPLAD) of the Chinese Academy of Medical Sciences and the director of the Department of Plant Molecular Biology of the Luxembourg Public Research Centre for Health respectively introduced the research progress in the project made by two sides and offered proposals on such issues as future cooperative areas and joint publication of articles.

(Zhao Yinghong)

7. Diao Xin Xue Kang Capsule (a Traditional Herbal Medicinal Product) was Registered Successfully in the Netherlands

On March 22, 2012, Diao Xin Xue Kang Capsule, developed and manufactured by Diao Chengdu Pharmaceuticals with China's completely independent intellectual property, passed the registration of the Dutch Medicines Evaluation Board (MEB) as a therapeutic drug (Registration Number: RVG102142) and gained the marketing authorization in the Netherlands. Diao Xin Xue Kang capsule made a breakthrough from zero on the therapeutic drug with China's independent intellectual property entering the mainstream market in developed countries and was also the first herbal medicinal product that gained marketing authorization from outside European Union countries.

(Zhao Yinghong)

8. The World Health Organization (WHO) Designated the Chinese Medicine Division (CMD) of the Department of Health (DH) of the Government of the Hong Kong Special Administrative Region as the Collaborating Centre for Traditional Medicine (CCTM) in Hong Kong

For the significant contribution made by the Department of Health to the popularization and development of traditional medicine, the World Health Organization (WHO) designated the Chinese Medicine Division (CMD) of the Department of Health (DH) as the 15th Collaborating Centre for Traditional Medicine in Western Pacific Region. The inauguration ceremony on May 9, 2012 was attended by about 200 international experts from Australia, Brazil, Canada, India, the United States and the Mainland as well as local experts. The Collaborating Centre for Traditional Medicine was the first of its kind in the world as the Centre that would focus on assisting the WHO to formulate policies and strategies as well as setting regulatory standards for traditional medicine, assisting the strategies in the regions of traditional medicine to be carried out, developing and perfecting global strategies for traditional medicine, establishing and training professional teams and offering professional advice and support to traditional medical fields. The establishment of the Collaborating Centre for Traditional Medicine was beneficial to further play of the characteristics and superiorities of Hong Kong and Hong Kong could function as a bridge connecting different countries so as to promote the cooperation and international development in traditional medicine.

(Zhao Yinghong)

9. The Anniversary Networking Meeting on WHO's Project of the International Classification of Diseases of Traditional Medicine was Held in Hong Kong

On May 2, 2012, sponsored by the World Health Organization, hosted by the Department of Health of the Government of the Hong Kong Special Administrative Region, the Anniversary Networking Meeting on WHO's Project of the International Classification of Diseases of Traditional Medicine was held in Hong Kong, which was attended by about 40 experts from 6 countries, including China, Australia, Japan, South Korea, Holland and the United States. The experts discussed and exchanged opinions on the Project of the International Classification of Diseases of Traditional Medicine. The Project of the International Classification of Diseases of Traditional Medicine was aimed to formulate the coordinated and unified international standardized terms and classification and promote traditional medicine to integrate with international classification system of the World Health Organization, which would not only develop a set of standardized terms and classification contributing to information communication inside and outside the field of traditional medicine, but also lay foundation for future medical information systems.

(Zhao Yinghong)

10. The Top Ten News Events of Traditional Chinese Medicine in 2012 Were Released

The Information Office of the State Administration of Traditional Chinese Medicine and the China News of Traditional Chinese Medicine jointly organized the selection of the top ten news events of traditional Chinese medicine and the results were as follows:

I. The *12th Five-Year Plan for the Development of the Undertaking of the Traditional Chinese Medical Science and Medicines (hereinafter referred to as Plan)* was issued and implemented and key projects were pushed forward effectively. In May 2012, the *Plan* was issued and implemented. The *Plan* defined the leading thought, basic principles and goals for development, attached importance to the connection of the development of TCM undertaking and deepening the medical and health care reform and adhered to overall and coordinated development of a combination of six parts, including TCM treatment, health care, scientific research, education, industry and culture. It pointed out that management system as well as operation mechanism that adapted to the development TCM undertaking would have been formed by 2015, so that TCM would make more contribution to China's economic and social development. In addition, major projects involved in the plan were to be pushed forward step by step.

II. Traditional Chinese medicine played an active role in the medical and health care reform and national project for improvement of TCM services capacity at the grassroots level was carried out. In September 2012, as a main part in "improving the service capacity of grassroots medical and health care institutions", the State Administration of Traditional Chinese Medicine, the Ministry of Health, the Ministry of Human Resources and Social Security, the State Food and Drug Administration and the Health Bureau of the PLA Logistic Department jointly carried out the project of improvement of TCM services capacity in grassroots medical and health care institutions and required that by 2015, over 95% of community health service centers, 90% of township health care centers, 70% community health service stations and 65% of village clinics would be able to provide traditional Chinese medical services and basically set up the service networks of traditional Chinese medical science and medicines so as to satisfy urban and rural residents' needs for medical treatment and health protection with the traditional Chinese medical science and medicines. Governments of all the localities also successively issued measures and launched such projects.

III. Service trade of the traditional Chinese medical science and medicines was incorporated into the national strategy for trade development. In April 2012, 14 ministries and commissions including the Ministry of Commerce, the Ministry of Foreign Affairs, the State Administration of Traditional Chinese Medicine and some others jointly issued and implemented the *Several Opinions on Promoting Development of TCM Trade in Services*, which defined the guidelines, basic principles and goals for TCM trade in services and required that, based on the demands of international market, systems for promoting TCM service trade and international marketing be initially set up in five years, indicating that national trade development strategy would include TCM trade in services. In May 2012, special activity of traditional Chinese medicals science and medicines was successfully organized at the First China (Beijing) International Fair for Trade in Services (CIFTIS) and Wen Jiabao, Li Keqiang and other top leaders of the Central Government visited the exhibition booths of the traditional Chinese medical science and medicines.

IV. The *Encyclopedia of Tibetan Medicine and the Chinese Military Materia Medica* were published. The *Encyclopedia of Tibetan Medicine* was the largest project on the compilation of Tibetan medical literatures in our country's history, which consisted of 60 volumes totaling 60 million words, including 638 ancient classic books as well as modern representative books on Tibetan medicine during the period of more than 2900 years and comprehensively and systematically reviewed the theory, practice and historical achievements of Tibetan Medicine. It took more than 20 years to accomplish the *Encyclopedia* and nearly 1,000 experts and scholars successively worked for the book. The *Chinese Military Materia Medica* was the first monograph of our county on materia medica in the military field, which collected 530 species of medicinal plants, more than 800 simple recipes and 2000 photos, covering all kinds of war injuries and illnesses in military medical science and giving a clear account of the classification and distribution of Chinese medicinal herbs for military throughout the country and the officinal animals and plants and the ecological and geographical environment concerned in military sensitive areas or military management areas. The book was an important initiative in the field of traditional medicine in the world for it integrated our country's traditional Chinese medicine with modern military pharmacy closely.

V. The *Outlines for the Medium- and Long-Term Development Program on the Standardization of Traditional Chinese Medicine* was issued and implemented. In September 2012, the State Administration of Traditional Chinese Medicine held the

National Forum on the Standardization of Traditional Chinese Medicine for the first time since the founding of new China and the TCM Standard Management and Coordination Committees, Expert Technical Committee and International Consultation Committee were established. The *Medium- and Long-Term Development Program on the Standardization of Traditional Chinese Medicine* (2011-2020) issued at the meeting defined the basic, strategic and overall status and role of the standardization of traditional Chinese medicine in the development of the undertaking, which was of significant importance in leading and supporting the development.

VI. The first batch of workrooms for the inheritance of 64 academic schools of traditional Chinese medical science and medicines were selected. In December 2012, the State Administration of Traditional Chinese Medicine released the units that constructed the first batch of workrooms for the inheritance of 64 academic schools of the traditional Chinese medical science and medicines. The aim was, on the basis of the exploration and arrangement of the experience, to cultivate an inheritance contingent that had outstanding characteristic superiorities, profound academic impact, remarkable clinical effects, complete inheritance echelon, powerful radiation function and horizontal integrated resources, which was of significant importance to promote the inheritance and innovation of the traditional Chinese medical science and medicines.

VII. Chinese medicine gained access to the European market for the first time. Diao Xin Xue Kang Capsule, developed and manufactured by Diao Chengdu Pharmaceuticals, was allowed to register in the EU market with the Netherlands as the first registered country. Diao Xin Xue Kang capsule made a breakthrough from zero on the therapeutic drug with China's independent intellectual property entering the mainstream market in developed countries and was also the first herbal medicinal product that gained marketing authorization from outside European Union countries, which signified that internationalization of Chinese medicine took another important step.

VIII. The two topics on the traditional Chinese medical science and medicines, "bears farmed for their bile" and "dredging Ren and Du meridians", attracted public concern. At the beginning of 2012, a topic concerning seeking listing by the FJ (fujian) into Allah Pharmaceutical Co., a bearing farming enterprise, initiated an argument on "extraction of gallbladder from a live bear" and protection of wild animals, from which a problem was reflected on how to deal with the relation between the protection of rare and endangered animal and plant resources and the use of Chinese medicinal raw materials. In May 2012, the news on the website of the Health Department of Gansu Province that "medical workers in Gansu Province cultivated intrinsic energy (genuine Qi) and over 40 persons connected Ren and Du meridians" attracted public concern and argument. The argument indicated some people's knowledge on Qigong came from martial arts novels and they knew little about Qigong in traditional Chinese medicine, therefore, popularization of the traditional Chinese medical science and medicines should be strengthened further.

IX. The first batch of 15 kinds of popular science books on traditional Chinese medical culture were recommended to the public. To solve the problem in recent years that good and bad books were intermingled in the market, the General Administration of Press and Publication and the State Administration of Traditional Chinese Medicine jointly launched the first national activity for recommendation of excellent popular science books on traditional Chinese medical culture. The first batch of 15 kinds of books were finally selected and recommended to the public, including *A series of Books on Sinology and Regimen and the Pictorial Handbook on Acupuncture and Moxibustion*. The activity was to ensure people to have popular knowledge on the traditional Chinese medical science and medicines and of significance to guide the sound development of book market, safeguard people's rights and interests and glorify traditional Chinese medical culture.

X. Emergency medical response systems with the traditional Chinese medical science and medicines were initially formed and the capacity for response to emergencies improved. In November 2012, the State Administration of Traditional Chinese Medicine held the National Working Conference on TCM Emergency Response the first time since the founding of new China, at which the leading group of TCM emergency response and the Committee of Experts on TCM emergency response were established and the objectives and tasks were defined. The traditional Chinese medical science and medicines played an active role in fighting against SARS and mitigating the impact of the massive Wenchuan earthquake, the strong Yushu earthquake, the huge Zhouqu mudslide and other natural disasters. With the rapid development in construction in recent years, the emergency medical response systems with the traditional Chinese medical science and medicines were initially formed and the capacity for response to emergencies improved substantially.

(Zhao Yinghong)

Chapter XIII   Management of Pharmaceutical Industry

Analysis on the General Operation Conditions of Pharmaceutical Industry in 2012

In 2012, the pharmaceutical industry grew steadily; the production and sales increased as compared with the same period in the previous year and tail-raising phenomenon appeared in the increment speed of grass profits. The deficit scale and deficit value both dropped to a certain degree. The overall economy of pharmaceutical industry exhibited a good tendency.

I. Production grew steadily

(1) The amplitude of the gross output value of the industry picked up steadily.

In 2012, the accumulated gross output value of the pharmaceutical industry reached 1,814.79 billion yuan, a year-on-year increase of 21.7%, and the increment speed increased by 1.5% as compared with the previous three quarters.

The increment speeds of the sub-industries, namely Chinese traditional medical herbal pieces processing industry, health materials and medicinal supplies manufacturing industry, chemical medicine preparation manufacturing industry and Chinese patent medicine manufacturing industry, were higher than the average of the pharmaceutical industry. Compared with the previous three quarters, except that the increment speeds of Chinese traditional medical herbal pieces processing industry and chemical medicine preparation manufacturing industry dropped slightly (0.7 % and 0.2% respectively), all the other sub-industries experienced various levels of increment speeds, among which biological & biochemical product manufacturing industry and chemical material medicine manufacturing industry took the lead, increasing by 3.7% and 3.6% respectively.

In 2012, the added value of pharmaceutical industry experienced a year-on-year increase of 14.5%, higher than the average of the national industry (10.0%), flat from the previous three quarters.

Analyzed from the monthly increase in the gross output value of the pharmaceutical industry since 2011, the increase in every month in 2011 was balanced, the increment speed remained between 25% and 28% with little fluctuation; while in 2012 there was a large amplitude, though it decreased by 5% after March, there was a steady recovery after the second quarter and the increase remained at more than 20% every month in the second half of the year.

Table 1   Total accumulated gross output value of the pharmaceutical industry in 2012

Sub-industry	Accumulated gross output value (100 million yuan)	Year-on-year increase (%)
chemical material medicine manufacturing industry	3,304.6	16.6
chemical medicine preparation manufacturing industry	5,088.7	24.7
Chinese medical herbal pieces processing industry	1,019.8	26.4
Chinese patent medicine manufacturing industry	4,136.5	21.3
b biological product manufacturing industry	1,852.7	20.5
health materials and medical supplies manufacturing industry	1,172.2	24.9
medical equipment, device & machine manufacturing industry	1573.4	20.6
pharmaceutical industry	18,147.9	21.7

(2) The increment speeds of sales value increased slightly.

In 2012, the accumulated sales value of the pharmaceutical industry reached 1,735.52 billion yuan, a year-on-year increase of 21%, the increment speed increasing by 1% as compared with the previous three quarters.

Of the total sales value, except for chemical material medicine manufacturing industry, biological and biochemical product manufacturing industry and Chinese patent medicine manufacturing industry, the increment speeds of the other four sub-industries were higher than the average of the pharmaceutical industry, particularly, the rise of Chinese medical herbal pieces processing industry was 6.5% higher than the average. Compared with the previous three quarters, except for chemical material medicine manufacturing industry and Chinese patent medicine manufacturing industry, which experienced decrease in increment speed (decreasing by 1.2% and 1.3% respectively), all the other sub-industries experienced various levels of rebound in the increment speed, with health materials and medical supplies manufacturing industry, biological and biochemical product manufacturing industry and chemical material medicine manufacturing industry taking the lead, rebounding by 4.1%, 3.8% and 2.4% respectively. The sales value resembled the gross output value.

Since 2012, the monthly increase of sales value of the pharmaceutical industry resembled that of the gross output value of the industry, the increment showed steady tendency of first drop and then increase after March, the there was a rebound in the third quarter to 20%, and increased steadily in the fourth quarter with the amplification increasing every month.

Table 2   Total finished sales value of the pharmaceutical industry in 2012

Sub-industry	Accumulated gross sales value (100million yuan)	Year-on-year increase (%)
chemical material medicine manufacturing industry	3,136.4	16.5
chemical medicine preparation manufacturing industry	4,846.0	22.8
Chinese medical herbal pieces processing industry	999.4	27.5
Chinese patent medicine manufacturing industry	3,914.8	20.8
biological product manufacturing industry	1,778.8	19.4
health materials and medical supplies manufacturing industry	1,143.1	24.8
medical equipment, device & machine manufacturing industry	1,536.8	21.1
pharmaceutical industry	17,335.2	21.0

(3) Production and sales ratio dropped naturally.

The production and sales ratio of the whole industry rebounded in 2012, (95.6%), dropping by 0.5% compared with the previous three quarters, lower than that at the end of 2011. The drop of production and sales ratio indicated that the enterprises increased production since the third quarter, and the amplitude of the gross output value exceeded that of the sales value, thus the production and sales ratio dropped naturally, but the production and sales of the industry were in a state of gradual coordination.

Analyzed from the production and sales ratios of all the sub-industries in 2012, the production and sales ratios of Chinese patent medicine manufacturing industry, chemical material medicine manufacturing industry, chemical medicine preparation manufacturing industry and biological and biochemical product manufacturing industry were lower than the average of the pharmaceutical industry, while the production and sales ratio of Chinese medical herbal pieces processing industry took the lead with 98.0%, higher than the whole industry by 2.4%.

Compared with the same period in 2011, except for Chinese medical herbal pieces processing industry and medical equipment, device & machine manufacturing industry, all the other sub-industries experienced various levels of drop in the production and sales ratio, with Chinese patent medicine manufacturing industry experiencing the biggest drop, dropping by 1.4%.

Compared with the first three quarters in 2012, the production and sales ratios of chemical material medicine manufacturing industry, chemical medicine preparation manufacturing industry and Chinese medical herbal pieces processing industry dropped to certain degrees, which led to the drop of production and sales ratio of the whole industry. Of all the sub-industries, Chinese medical herbal pieces processing industry and Chinese medical herbal pieces processing industry dropped the most, both by 0.9%.

Table 3   Production and sales ratio of the pharmaceutical industry in 2012

Sub-industry	Production and sales ratio (%)	Year-on-year increase (%)
chemical material medicine manufacturing industry	94.9	−0.1
chemical medicine preparation manufacturing industry	95.2	1.4
Chinese medical herbal pieces processing industry	98.0	0.8
Chinese patent medicine manufacturing industry	94.6	0.4
biological product manufacturing industry	96.0	−0.8
health materials and medical supplies manufacturing industry	97.5	−0.1
medical equipment, device & machine manufacturing industry	97.7	0.4
pharmaceutical industry	95.6	−0.5

II. The increase in foreign trade slowed down

(1) The increment speed of export delivery value dropped slightly.

In 2012, the accumulated export delivery value reached 147.84 billion yuan, a year-on-year increase of 7.3%. Compared with that of the first three quarters, the amplitude increased by 1.2%.

Viewed from the accumulated export delivery value of all the sub-industries in 2012, the percentage of chemical material medicine manufacturing industry, which used to accounted for the largest percentage of export value, dropped by 0.9%, while that of medical equipment, device & machine manufacturing industry, which used to accounted for the second largest percentage of export value, increased by 0.3%. Compared with that in the same period in 2011, the export delivery value of Chinese medical herbal pieces processing industry, chemical medicine preparation manufacturing industry, health materials and medical supplies manufacturing industry and Chinese patent medicine manufacturing industry, all of which accounted for less than 10%, increased by more than 15%, but the increment speed of biological and biochemical product manufacturing industry was much lower then that in the same period last year (decreasing by 5%). Compare with the first three quarters, except for biological and biochemical product manufacturing industry and Chinese patent medicine manufacturing industry, the increment speeds of the expert delivery values for all the other sub-industries increased slightly.

Table 4   Finished export delivery value of the pharmaceutical industry in 2012

Sub-industry	Export delivery value (100 million yuan)	Year-on-year increase (%)
chemical material medicine manufacturing industry	550.2	6.8
chemical medicine preparation manufacturing industry	146.3	23.5
Chinese medical herbal pieces processing industry	27.9	24.4
Chinese patent medicine manufacturing industry	45.5	15.6
biological product manufacturing industry	184.25	−5.0
health materials and medical supplies manufacturing industry	144.85	17
medical equipment, device & machine manufacturing industry	379.55	4.2
pharmaceutical industry	178.4	7.3

(2) The increment of import and export at the customs slowed down at the bottoming process.

Customs data showed that the total accumulated import-export amount of pharmaceuticals reached $80.95 billion, a year-on-year increase of 10.5%, and the year-on-year amplitude decreased by 0.9% as compared with the first three quarters, which meant a huge gap as compared with the year-on-year increase of 39.7% in 2011.

The export value was $47.60 billion, a year-on-year increase of 6.9%, down by 1% compared with the first three quarters, much lower than the 34.9% at the end of 2011, while the import value was $33.35 billion, a year-on-year increase of 15.9%, down by 1.1% compared with the first three quarters, down by over 30% compared with the 46.1% at the end of 2011; the increase of import value outnumbered that of the export value, the export was subdued, and the trade surplus was $14.25 billion, down by 9.5%, the decrease enlarged compared with the 8.4% in the first three quarters, but the gap between the increase of 18.3% in 2011 was large and trade surplus decreased.

Viewed from the three major categories, medical equipment and devices ranked first in the year-on-year increase of the total import-export amount and traditional Chinese medicines came next. Of all the western medicines, the western medicines already prepared by a pharmacy had the biggest increase of export value, bio-chemical products came next, while the year-on-year increase of that of the raw materials for western medicines was only 3.2%. Viewed respectively, the western medicines already prepared by a pharmacy had the biggest year-on-year increase of export value, and medical equipment and devices came next; while the bio-chemical products had the biggest year-on-year increase of import value and the western medicines already prepared by a pharmacy came next.

Table 5 Import and export of pharmaceuticals in 2012

	Amount of export (100 million dollar)	Year-on-year increase (%)	Percentage (%)	Amount of import (100 million dollar)	Year-on-year increase (%)	Percentage (%)
Chinese medicines(including health care products, plant extracts,Chinese patent medicines、 Chinese herbal medicines and Chinese medical herbal pieces)	25.0	7.2	5.3	8.7	22.0	2.6
Western medicines(including raw materials, preparations and bio-chemical products)	275.2	3.9	57.8	200.1	16.6	60.0
medical equipment and devices (including dressing, disposable medical supplies, products of hospital diagnosis and treatment, health protection and rehabilitation, dental equipment and materials)	175.9	12.0	36.9	124.7	14.6	37.4
total	476.0	6.9	100	333.5	15.9	100

Analyzed from the increasing tendency of monthly accumulated import values from 2011 to 2012, the increment speeds of bio-chemical products, western medicines and traditional Chinese medicines were obviously higher than the average of the pharmaceutical import, while analyzed from the increasing tendency of accumulated export values, the increment speeds of western medicines and medical equipment and devices were higher than the average of pharmaceutical export.

As for export, the increment speed of western medicines was remarkable in 2012; even though the increment speeds tended to decline, the growth was far higher than that of other medicines while bio-chemical products showed negative growth. The export increases of the whole industry were all far lower than those in the same period in 2011, which led to the sharp drop in the export increase of the whole industry.

As for import, the import growths of bio-chemical products, western medicines and traditional Chinese medicines were higher than the import growth of the whole industry. Meanwhile, the import growths of all the products were lower than that in the same period in 2011, which drove down the import growth of the whole industry. The import growth of the traditional Chinese medicine in the first three quarters showed an upward tendency but there was a downturn in October. The growth decreased after the rebound in October with bio-chemical products and western medicines taking the lead.

III. Growth in economic profits rebounded steadily.

(1) Main business income increased steadily.

The accumulated main business income reached 1,784.53 billion yuan in 2012, a year-on-year increase of 20.1%, increasing by 0.5% compared with the previous three quarters.

Analyzed from the increase of quarterly main business income from 2008 to 2012, the main business income rebounded in the third quarter after the drop of increase for two successive quarters in 2012. Compared with the growth of 28.9% at the end of 2011, the gap of 9.8% accumulated in the first half year narrowed in the second half year and reached 20% at the end of the year.

Analyzed from the finished main business income, compared with the previous three quarters, there were year-on-year increases in biological product manufacturing industry, medical equipment, device & machine manufacturing industry and health materials and medicinal products and preparation manufacturing industry, the increment speed of Chinese patent medicine manufacturing industry remained the same and there were slight decline in the year-on-year in chemical medicine preparation manufacturing industry and Chinese medical herbal pieces processing industry, with Chinese medical herbal pieces processing industry suffering the largest decline, down by 2.9%. Biological product manufacturing industry experienced the largest increase, up by 2.7%.

Table 6   Finished main business income of the pharmaceutical industry in 2012

Sub-industry	Main business income (100 million yuan)	Year-on-year increase (%)
chemical material medicine manufacturing industry	3,289.7	14.0
chemical medicine preparation manufacturing industry	5,023.7	22.5
Chinese medical herbal pieces processing industry	990.3	24.2
Chinese patent medicine manufacturing industry	4,079.2	21.4
biological product manufacturing industry	1,775.4	18.8
health materials and medical supplies manufacturing industry	1,122.4	19.9
medical equipment, device & machine manufacturing industry	1,564.5	21.4
pharmaceutical industry	17,845.3	20.1

Compared with that in 2011, the growth of monthly main business income of pharmaceutical industry in 2012 decreased by nearly 8%. The price reduction at the end of March led to the successive decline in the growth for three months and the effects of price reduction began to show. In the second half year the main business income gradually increased.

(2) Growth of the total profits rebounded slightly.

The accumulated total profits finished fin 2012 amounted to 182.05 billion yuan, a year-on-year increase of 20.4%, the increment speed increased by 2.5% compared with that in the previous three quarters and dropped by 2.8% compared with that at the end of 2011.

The increase in the quarterly total profits of the pharmaceutical industry from 2008 to 2012 showed that the first quarter of 2012 had the least increase since 2008, record low in four years time. In the second quarter, the increase in the quarterly total profits of the pharmaceutical industry began to rebound and it remained steady in the second half year. Chemical material medicine manufacturing industry had the positive growth in the total profits in the second half year and the growth amplitude gradually enlarged (15.9%), which reversed the negative growth in the first half year and also led the total profits of the whole industry to rebound in the end.

Compared with the growth of total profits in the first three quarters, health material and medical supplies manufacturing industry and medical equipment, device & machine manufacturing industry had a decline of 2.4% and 1.6% respectively, while chemical material medicine manufacturing industry had an increase of 11.5%, showing a sharp increase. Chinese medical herbal pieces processing industry had an increase of 3.6% and other sub-industries had slight increases. The sales in the second half year gradually returned normal.

Table 7   Total finished profits of the pharmaceutical industry in 2012

Sub-industry	Total profits (100 million yuan)	Year-on-year increase (%)
chemical material medicine manufacturing industry	243.0	15.9
chemical medicine preparation manufacturing industry	556.0	25.3
Chinese medical herbal pieces processing industry	71.0	27.5
Chinese patent medicine manufacturing industry	436.0	16.5
biological product manufacturing industry	230.1	14.3
health materials and medical supplies manufacturing industry	114.8	26.2
medical equipment, device & machine manufacturing industry	169.1	24.4
pharmaceutical industry	1,820.5	20.4

Since 2012, the monthly growth of total profits of pharmaceutical industry firstly dropped sharply at the beginning of the year and then rebounded month by month. The first round of price reduction at the beginning of April put off the delayed effects of returned funds till June, the new round of price reduction in September caused slight decline in the year-on-year increase of accumulated total profits in September and October, and the profitability of the whole industry fluctuated slightly, but the benefit-oriented goals would promote the restructuring of the industry and enterprises. The sharp increase of the chemical material medicine manufacturing industry raised the profit growth of the whole industry.

(3) Sales profit ratio declined

In 2012, the sales profit ratio of the pharmaceutical industry reached 9.8%, down by 0.2% compared with the first half year, flat with the first three quarters and down by 0.2% compared with the same period in 2011. The drop in the sales profits indicated that the profitability of the pharmaceutical industry declined. Compared with the same period in 2011, the sales profit ratios of Chinese patent medicine manufacturing industry and biological product manufacturing industry declined, down by 0.4% and 0.5% respectively. While the sales profit ratios of health materials and medical supplies manufacturing industry and medical equipment, device & machine manufacturing industry increased by 0.5% and 0.3% respectively compared with the same period in 2011.

IV. Asset grew steadily.

(1) Total assets

In 2012, the total assets of the pharmaceutical industry amounted to 1,628.31 billion yuan, a year-on-year increase of 18.4%, up by 2% compared with those in the first three quarters.

Table 8   Total assets of the pharmaceutical industry in 2012

Sub-industry	Total assets (100 million yuan)	Year-on-year increase (%)
chemical material medicine manufacturing industry	3,101.6	16.6
chemical medicine preparation manufacturing industry	4,981.6	20.9
Chinese medical herbal pieces processing industry	646.1	29.9
Chinese patent medicine manufacturing industry	3,706.9	16.6
biological product manufacturing industry	1,848.1	14.9
health materials and medical supplies manufacturing industry	707.7	20.2
medical equipment, device & machine manufacturing industry	1,291.1	17.2
pharmaceutical industry	16,283.1	18.4

Compared with that in the first three quarters, only medical equipment, device & machine manufacturing industry experienced a slight decline in the year-on-year increase of total assets (down by 0.2%), while Chinese medical herbal pieces processing industry and chemical material medicine manufacturing industry ranked first and second in the total assets of all the sub-industries, up by 3.8% and 3.7% respectively. Other sub-industries all experienced slight rise in the increment speeds.

(2) Investment in the fixed assets

In 2012, the total accumulated fixed asset investment of the pharmaceutical industry reached 356.47 billion yuan, a year-on-year increase of 34.6%, and the growth decreased by 2.4% compared with that in the first three quarters. Compared with the year-on-year increment speed (45.5%) at the end of 2011, it decreased by nearly 10%. Since the beginning of the second half year, the growth of investment in the fixed assets is decreasing gradually.

V. Deficit

In 2012, there were 642 enterprises in deficit, a year-on-year drop of 4.9%. Deficit enterprises accounted for 9.8%, down by 3.1% compared with those in the first three quarters. The accumulated losses reached 6.18 billion yuan, a year-on-year increase of 17.7%, down by 13% compared with those in the first three quarters.

Of all the sub-industries, Chinese medical herbal pieces processing industry had the biggest deficit, more than doubled; next to it was chemical medicine preparation manufacturing industry, which had a year-on-year increase of 42.0%, up by nearly 31% compared with that in the first three quarters. Chemical material medicine manufacturing industry had a year-on-year increase of 10.6% in deficit, decreased sharply compared with the 110% in the first three quarters. Except in biological product manufacturing industry and health materials and medical supplies manufacturing industry, the numbers of enterprises in deficit in other sub-industries all decreased compared with the same period last year. Negative growth in deficit values appeared in health materials and medical supplies manufacturing industry (down by 24%), Chinese patent medicine manufacturing industry and medical equipment, device & machine manufacturing industry, and the numbers of enterprises in deficit in the later two sub-industries showed a declining trend.

Table 9 Deficit of the pharmaceutical industry in 2012

Sub-industry	Deficit enterprise (company)	Amount of losses (100 million yuan)	Year-on-year increase (%)
chemical material medicine manufacturing industry	150	20.9	10.6
chemical medicine preparation manufacturing industry	140	18.2	42
Chinese medical herbal pieces processing industry	23	0.8	102.5
Chinese patent medicine manufacturing industry	137	6.4	−0.6
biological product manufacturing industry	56	8.5	27.5
health materials and medical supplies manufacturing industry	41	1	−24
medical equipment, device & machine manufacturing industry	95	6	−0.5
pharmaceutical industry	642	61.8	17.7

VI. Summary

In 2012, the year-on-year increase of industry output value and sales value of the pharmaceutical industry experienced sharp fall in the first half year and rebounded to the increment speed of over 20% in the second half, showing a trend of falling first and rebounding then, but the trend for later development remained unclear. The year-on-year production and sales ration decreased, showing an abnormal falling trend, but the ratio remained comparatively high and production and sales linked up well. In the aspect of export, the increment speed of finished export delivery value rebounded. Chemical material medicine manufacturing industry still took lead in the finished export delivery value; however, its year-on-year increase was lower than the average of the pharmaceutical industry and the percentage it accounted for decreased, while the percentage of medical equipment, device & machine manufacturing industry, which ranked second in export delivery value, increased considerably. Of all the sub-industries, the export delivery value experienced negative growth. Compared with the first three quarters, except for biological product manufacturing industry and Chinese patent medicine manufacturing industry, all the other sub-industries had slight increase in export delivery values, indicating the severe situation for the sub-industries. Viewed from the overall customs data, the growth of both import and export fell and stabilized and the growth in trade surplus decreased. The export of western medicine increased remarkably while its import increased steadily. The export of bio-chemical products experienced negative growth and the growth in its import also decreased.

In 2012, the main business income and the total finished profit of the pharmaceutical industry both had year-on-year increase, but both of them showed trends of slight rise after stabilizing and the increment of total finished profit rebounded in the end after the fall. Chinese medical herbal pieces processing industry had the biggest fall in growth and among the three types of medicine products, only bio-chemical product manufacturing industry had a rebound in growth. In the aspect of profit growth, chemical material medicine manufacturing industry reversed the negative growth in the first half year and to the positive growth in the second half year with fast rebound. The year-on-year sales profits of the whole industry dropped, with Chinese patent medicine manufacturing industry and biological product manufacturing industry dropping the most.

The total assets grew steadily, the growth in fixed asset investment was larger than the growth of total assets, but growth amplitude of fixed asset investment of the pharmaceutical industry was gradually minishing. The deficit of pharmaceutical industry was turning for the better, the number of enterprises in deficit, and scale of deficit and the value of deficit all dropped compared with the same period last year; however, the values of deficit of Chinese medical herbal pieces processing industry and chemical medicine preparation manufacturing industry ranked first and second, with year-on-year increase of 102.5% and 42.0% respectively, which was related to the depressed international market, the domestic price reduction and the launching and carrying out of the new round of pharmaceuticals purchase by public bidding. The deficit of chemical material medicine manufacturing industry turned for the better, with only a 10.6% year-on-year increase, a sharp decrease compared with the 110% in the first three quarters.

(Zhao Xuemei)

Chapter XIV The Basic Medical Security System

Work of Medical Insurance in 2012

In 2012, human resources and social security departments at all levels focused on the overall situation of steady growth, livelihood improvement and stability maintenance, and stuck to the keynote of "making progress while maintaining stability". They also gave full play to the fundamental role of universal health care with the focus on "improving the quality of universal health care". As a result, everything went smoothly.

I. Continue to Extending the Coverage of Medical Insurance

Emphasis was laid on the management for the insured, including rural migrant workers, employees from non-public economic organizations, flexible employees, students, pre-school children and new-born babies. The work for the insured disadvantaged groups was promoted continually, including the retirees of closed bankrupt enterprises and the workers of enterprises in difficulties. By the end of 2012, there had been 536,410,000 people nationwide that participated in the basic medical insurance, 62,980,000 people more than the end of last year; 264,860,000 workers, 271,560,000 residents and 49,960,000 rural migrant workers participated in the medical insurance.

II. The Medical Insurance Treatment was Improved Steadily

In 2012, budgets at all levels raised the subsidy standard of urban-rural residents' medical insurance to no less than 240 yuan per capita. Meanwhile the individual (household) payment was adjusted appropriately. The payment for medical expenses of hospitalization within the range of medical insurance policy for workers universally reached 75%. The payment for medical expenses of hospitalization within the range of medical insurance of health care agencies at level II and below for urban residents' medical insurance reached 70% or so. The maximum payment limit of the overall fund for workers' medical insurance and urban residents' medical insurance were raised to 6 times of the average salary of local workers and per capita disposal income of local residents respectively, and no less than 60,000 yuan. In some cities in Jiangsu, Zhejiang and Shandong, the limit line for workers' large medical subsidy was cancelled. The residents' medical insurance treatment for outpatient service as a whole was steadily improved. The exploration of overall mechanism of outpatient service was promoted, and the management and service for outpatient service as a whole were strengthened. Its supporting role in the reform of primary health care agencies was given full play to.

III. The Reform of Payment Method was Promoted

The first was to implement the requirements of the Twelfth Five-Year Plan for medical reform, issue *Opinions on Total Payment Control of Basic Medical Insurance ([2012] No.70 issued by the Ministry of Human Resources and Social Security)*, and define the objective, principle, procedure and requirement of total payment control, which laid the foundation for strengthening the management of fund budget for medical insurance and deepening the payment method reform. In September of 2012, a forum on special topic was held in Changchun to conduct a comprehensive deployment, and business training and experience exchanges were carried out. The second was to sum up local experience, sort out the main points of handling and management under different payment methods, issue *Living Examples of Handling Cities for Payment Method of Medical Insurance*, compile *Handling Procedures for Total Payment Control of Medical Insurance*, and guide local authorities in the handling of payment method reform. The third was to strengthen the guidance over the key contact cities for payment method reform, and promote the multiple payment methods including payment according to disease type and capitation.

IV. The Management Service of Medical Insurance was Strengthened

The first was to strengthen the supervisory control and management for medical services. On the basis of sufficient investigation, business requirements for the supervisory control of medical services, basic indexes for the supervisory control, database standards and regulations for the supervisory control were made. Research and development were conducted for applied software of the supervisory control for medical services. Eighteen regions (Ningxia and Jilin as provinces) were chosen for the pilot construction of supervisory control of medical services, and initial results were achieved. The second was to extend the supervisory control for medical services from health care agencies to medical workers. Local authorities were guided in the exploration of establishing the system of "doctors for medical insurance". With explorations made in most of the regions nationwide, there was integral advancement in eight provinces including Shandong and Jilin. Refined management was conducted by the establishment of prescription right for medical insurance, credit management for medical insurance doctors and registered doctors' bank for medical insurance. The third was to consolidate the results of direct billing, and accelerate the promotion of issuance of "social security card", and there had been 341,000,000 card holders by the end of 2012. Long-distance medical treatment and settlement were promoted. As a result, direct settlement can be made for medical insurance within Chongqing, Fujian, Hainan and Yunnan, with the exception of Beijing, Tianjin and Shanghai. In sixteen provinces including Zhejiang, Hunan and Guangdong, the platforms for long-distance medical treatment and settlement got started. In some other regions, long-distance medical treatment and settlement for some people could be made by long-distance designated networking settlement and the establishment of long-distance offices. In Shanghai, Hainan and Guangzhou, explorations were being made for trans-provincial long-distance medical treatment and settlement with the focus on long-distance settlement of retirees.

V. The Establishment of Urban-Rural Residents' Critical Illness Insurance was Promoted

In August of 2012, the National Development and Reform Commission (NDRC), the Ministry of Health, the Ministry of Finance, the Ministry of Human Resources and Social Security, the Ministry of Civil Affairs and China Insurance Regulatory Commission jointly issued *Guiding Opinions on Carrying Out the Work of Urban-Rural Residents' Critical Illness Insurance ([2012] No.2605)*. In September of 2012, the Ministry of Human Resources and Social Security held a forum on special topic in Changchun to make deployment and arrangements. A liaison system for critical illness insurance was set up to strengthen the contact and communication with local authorities, and steadily promote the pilot work.

VI. The Operating Quality of Medical Benefits Fund was Improved

In 2012, the revenue of workers' medical benefits fund amounted to 606.2 billion yuan, and fund expenditure reached 486.8 billion yuan. The revenue of urban residents' medical benefits fund amounted to 87.7 billion yuan, and fund expenditure reached 67.5 billion yuan. With municipal medical insurance further consolidated, investigations were conducted to know the real situation of municipal medical insurance in various regions. Stress was laid on the inspection for the provinces where little progress was made, and categorized guidance was strengthened. Provincial medical insurance was achieved in Beijing, Tianjin, Shanghai, Chongqing, Tibet and Hainan.

VII. The Urban-Rural Medical Insurance was Promoted

Policy reserve for urban-rural medical insurance was made positively. A research group for urban-rural medical insurance was set up to conduct specific research and give guidance to local authorities in their work. In 2012, there were 6 provincial-level regions (Tianjin, Chongqing, Ningxia, Guangdong and Xinjiang Production and Construction Corps), 32 prefectures (cities) and 153 counties (cities, districts) which started urban-rural medical insurance with 160,000,000 insured people.

(Shan Yongxiang)

Chapter XV The Management of Planning and Finance

The 2012 Management of Health Planning and Finance

In 2012, based on the train of thought for work defined at the beginning of the year, the Ministry of Health earnestly fulfilled the responsibilities of planning, security, regulation and resource allocation. As a result, remarkable achievements were made in health planning and finance.

I. The medical and health system reform was pushed forward

The year 2012 witnessed an input of 176.8 billion yuan of the central treasury for health services, thereinto the budget fund of the central departments at the corresponding level reached 11.8 billion yuan, and 165 billion yuan went to the central subsidies for local special funds of health. We got involved in the Twelfth Five-Year Plan for medical reform, and the formulation of *Circular of the General Office of the State Council on Main Work Arrangements for 2012 Five Key Reforms of the Medical and Health System.* We organized the prospective study of four major policies, including the research on the relationship between the development of medical and health services and the rapid transformation of economic development way. We also gave guidance to the hospitals under the ministerial budget management in getting involved in local reform. The subsidies of financial authorities at all levels for the New Rural Cooperative Medical System (NCMS) were increased to 240 yuan, and the reimbursement rate for hospitalization expenses within the policy range was raised to 75% or so. The pilot work of critical illness security was comprehensively promoted, and the reform of payment way was accelerated. *An Internal Control System of Fund for the New Rural Cooperative Medical System* was revised and improved to guarantee the safe operation of fund. We continued to strengthen the system construction of medical and health services, and launched the construction projects of medical service system of pediatrics, general hospitals at the municipal level, and prevention and control agencies for major diseases and endemic diseases. The compilation of special planning was promoted simultaneously. The post-assessment of the construction projects for primary medical and health service system was started up, and the preliminary work for the planning formulation of the construction of the national center for medical sciences and medical services was carried out.

II. The Overall Plan was Made for the Development Plan of Health Services

The Twelfth Five-Year Plan for Health Services Development was made, which defined the development goal, guiding principles, key tasks, major projects and safeguard policies for health services in the period of the Twelfth Five-Year Plan. Circular of the Ministry of Health on Regional Health Planning and Installation Planning for Medical Agencies, and Promoting the Development of Non-public Medical Agencies was studied and issued. Measures were brought forward for the arrangements of non-public medical agencies, and work requests were made to all local authorities. The strategy research report on Health in China in 2020, and was released by Health Minister Chen Zhu at 2012 China Health Forum. We got involved in the research and formulation of national special planning, including The Twelfth Five-Year Plan for National Basic Public Service System.

III. The Health Economic Management was Improved

The project library for major special projects of medical reform in the period of the Twelfth Five-Year Plan was established, and the management system of project library was perfected. The database of central finance subsidies for major special projects of medical reform was set up. The information monitoring network for total expenditure on health was structured. The direct reporting system of monitoring network for governmental health input was perfected. The tracking system of monitoring progress for governmental health input was researched and developed. The declaration and verification of assets inspection for the hospitals under the budget management of the Ministry of Health were carried out. The hospitals under the budget management of the Ministry of Health were urged to have accountants-general. The comprehensive budget management was promoted and conducted. The columns and contents of information exchange platform for health planning and finance, instant messaging was developed, and a regular check-up system for the use of platform was established. The management information system for budget enforcement of the Ministry of Health was improved to promote the fulfillment of target tasks of budget enforcement schedule. The personalized control system of the Ministry of Health for financial accounting and budget management was developed to improve the accuracy of budget control. The 335 project for the construction of financial talent team of health planning was carried out. The trainings for financial and accounting rules of hospital were organized.

IV. The Departmental Budget Management was Intensified

The system was adhered to that major events and major decisions of the departmental budget management must go through group decision-making of departmental meeting, budget committee and ministerial meeting. Besides the resident supervision bureau of the Ministry of Supervision in the Ministry of Health and the auditing bureau of the auditing administration for health and drugs were invited to get involved in the supervision. Professional appraisal and on-site verification were conducted for the project of related major incremental expenditure to ensure the quality of project application. *Interim Measures of the Ministry of Health for Enforcement and Management of Departmental Budget* was revised, and regulations for the link-up between the budgeting and budget enforcement schedule were reinforced to promote the budget enforcement. The departmental budget, final settlement of account and the budget for three public consumption areas were made public. *Interim Measures of the Ministry of Health for Budget Performance Management of Budget Management Organizations* was worked out. Pilot projects were extended to 20 for 2013 performance evaluation of departmental budget.

V. The Economic Liability Audit, Fund Supervision and Specific Inspection were Under Way as Usual

We cooperated on the completion of Health Minister Chen Zhu's economic liability audit. *Provisions on the Economic Liability Audit of Main Leading Cadres of Organizations Directly under the Ministry of Health* was studied and mapped out. *Service Regulations for the Joint Session of the Ministry of Health on Economic Liability Audit* was printed and issued. The economic liability audit was conducted for nine leading cadres. We also coordinated with the Auditing Administration to complete the 2011 central budget implementation, other financial revenue and expenditure, annual audit for final accounts (draft) of the Ministry of Health, and audit investigation for the two major special science and technology projects in which the Ministry of Health took the lead. *Interim Measures of the Ministry of Health for Funds Management of Local Health Projects with Central Government Subsidies and Interim Measures of the Ministry of Health for the Regulation of Project Funds* were studied and mapped out. The evaluation and acceptance of special governance for "private savings" were organized. Spot checks for 13 departments and bureaus, 26 projects and 11 commissioned institutions were completed; so was the financial acceptance of the project topics of 513 major science and technology projects. The target responsibility assessment was conducted for the chief auditors of Beijing Hospital, Peking Union Medical College Hospital and China-

Japan Friendship Hospital, and the work report on chief auditor appointment was submitted. Supervision and inspection for 2012 project of central subsidies for local public health and construction projects of health infrastructure were conducted. Priority was given to the supervision and rectification for related provinces and cities in the audit investigation of the system construction for rural medical and health services. The check for radiological protection of township health care centers nationwide was organized.

VI. The Allocation of Large Medical Equipments and Basic Construction Management were Strengthened

The evaluation of clinical trial results, including TOMO, of Zhongshan Hospital affiliated to Fudan University was organized and completed. The review for the allocation of class A large medical equipments in 83 medical agencies was conducted. 1.417 billion yuan of investment in capital construction within 2012 central budget were used to support the budget management units of the Ministry of Health in the improvement of infrastructures. The exposure draft of *An Atlas of Standard Construction for Community Health Service Centers*, The *Construction Standard for Psychiatric Hospitals (Manuscript) and The Code of Building Design for Psychiatric Hospitals (for Approval)* were completed. The compilation of *The Construction Standard for Children's Hospitals* got started. The statistical work for energy consumption investigation got started. *A Circular on Further Strengthening the Energy Conservation and Emission Reduction* was printed and issued. The statistical work for energy and resources consumption of budget management units was fully carried out.

VII. The Price Control for Medical Services was Reformed

The Project Specifications for National Prices of Medical Service (2012 Edition) was printed and issued. *A Circular on Promoting the Reform of Medical Prices of Public Hospitals at the County Level* was printed and issued. The monitoring work of medical service cost of medical agencies was carried out. The names of 100 disease types were studied and screened, and experts were organized to study and set quality control criteria. The experiences and practices of various localities in payment reform including capitation and global budget were studied and summarized. Four administrative fee-charging items including the fee for hygienic quality inspection were retained by the Ministry of Finance. The circular on adjusting the fee-charging standard for the examination of practicing doctors' qualifications was printed and issued.

VIII. The Centralized Procurement of Drugs and High-value Consumables was Promoted

Jointly with the State Council Office for Rectifying, we held the national work meeting on the centralized procurement of drugs. The development of database for consumable prices was completed, while the information database for the centralized procurement of high-value consumables was set up and improved. *The Work Specifications for the Centralized Procurement of High-value Consumables (Trial Edition)* was studied and mapped out to define the procurement scope and ways of organizing the procurement of high-value consumables. A Circular on Specific Rectification for the Use of Invoices of Production and Business Units of Drugs and Medical Devices and Medical Agencies was printed and issued. The supervision and inspection for the specific rectification of the use of invoices in medical agencies were conducted.

IX. Poverty Alleviation & Development and Partner Assistance were Carried out

According to the new situation, new task and new requirement facing poverty alleviation and development and partner assistance, the leading group of the Ministry of Health for poverty alleviation and partner assistance was set up. Two plenary sessions of the leading group were held to study and formulate relevant documents for promoting the work. The system of inter-ministerial contact meeting for regional development and poverty alleviation in the area of Luliang Mountain was established, and the first session of inter-ministerial contact meeting was held. Researches for poverty alleviation in the area of Luliang Mountain were conducted successively for four times, covering all 20 counties in the area, and the status quo of economic and social development in the area was understood. We coordinated the implementation of 2012 project for children's nutrition improvement in the poverty-stricken area. We also coordinated People's Hospital of Peking University and China-Japan Friendship Hospital in giving their partner assistance to some medical agencies in the area of Luliang Mountain. We worked with China National School of Administration to organize the training class for deepening the reform of medical and health system in the area of Luliang Mountain. We coordinated China Telecom Corporation Ltd. and Life Care Networks (Beijing) in donating the long-distance heart monitoring system to the area of Luliang Mountain. We also got involved in the compilation of *A Planning for Regional Development and Poverty Alleviation in the Area of Luliang Mountain (2011-2020)*. The support for Huishui County and Zamtang County of Aba Autonomous Prefecture and of Sichuan and Zadoi County of Yushu Prefecture of

Qinghai was reinforced. Based on relevant requirements of the State Council Leading Group Office of Poverty Alleviation and Development, we coordinated the adjustment work of the designated counties of poverty alleviation by the Ministry of Health. The summary meeting of poverty alleviation of the Ministry of Health and a new round of meeting for poverty alleviation were organized and held to study and make arrangements for a new round of poverty alleviation.

The partner assistance was promoted. The 2012 forum on partner assistance of national health circles to Tibet and the 2012 forum on partner assistance of national health circles to Xinjiang were organized and held. We donated the long-distance heart monitoring system to Tibet Autonomous Region, and bought some medical kits and portable medical equipments for general practice. The pilot work plan for 17 provinces and cities giving partner assistance to the physical examination of Tibetan urban-rural residents was studied and suggested. The thinking and measures of work of the Ministry of Health in support of health service development of the Corps were studied and suggested. Nineteen and seventeen provinces and cities offering counterpart assistance were promoted to work out specific plans respectively for health assistance to Xinjiang and Tibet. The budget management units of the Ministry of Health which undertook the tasks of giving assistance to Xinjiang and Tibet were promoted to sign counterpart support agreements with the recipient organizations.

The work of post-disaster reconstruction was well done. The post-disaster reconstruction of medical and health system in Zhouqu was fully completed, and all the health reconstruction projects were completed and went into service. In Yushu, 78 projects have been under construction, and 52 projects have been completed and put to use (accounting for 66% of total projects).

(Shan Yongxiang)

Section 1   The Work Progress of the Center for Project Supervision and Management of the Ministry of Health

1. The World Bank-funded China Emerging Infectious Disease Preparedness and Control Project was officially Launched

The China Emerging Infectious Disease Preparedness and Control Project, funded by a grant from the Avian and Human Influenza Facility (AHIF) of the World Bank, officially came into effect and was launched on July 15, 2012. The Project was an international cooperation project of grant from the Avian and Human Influenza Facility (AHIF) applied for by Chinese government for the third time after the successful cooperation on the first and second phases of avian/human influenza prevention and control between Chinese government and the World Bank. The total grant amounted to US$2,566,400, and the project was scheduled to complete at the end of 2013. The Project was implemented jointly by the Ministry of Health and Ministry of Agriculture to sustainably enhance China's capacity to prevent and respond to emerging infectious diseases (EID). The project involved seven counties of Xinjiang Uygur Autonomous Region and Inner Mongolia Autonomous Region (thereinto, health group included only four counties of Inner Mongolia). The Project aimed to improve the country and Project areas' universal capacity to prevent and control emerging infectious diseases (EID), such as the capacity of impacting assessment, epidemiological survey, risk communication and emergency decision. It also aimed to strengthen the capacity to prevent and control brucellosis in the Project areas as well as the collaboration between China and its neighboring countries for joint prevention and control of emerging and re-emerging diseases.

(Shan Yongxiang)

2. The Promotion and Workshop for Experience of Payment Reform of New Rural Cooperative Medical System of WB/DFID China Rural Health Project was Successfully Held

To promote and exchange the innovations of WB/DFID China Rural Health Project in the payment reform, the Center for Project Supervision and Management of the Ministry of Health and the Department of Rural Health Management of the Ministry of Health jointly held the promotion and workshop for experience of payment reform of WB/DFID China Rural Health Project in Xi'an of Shaanxi on April 26-27, 2012. At the workshop, *Guiding Opinions on Promoting Payment Reform of the New Rural Cooperative Medical System* jointly issued by the Ministry of Health, National Development and Reform Commission and the Ministry of Finance on April 24 was read and interpreted. In addition, the pilot practices of some of the Project areas in the payment reform of inpatient service and outpatient service were presented, and comments were made on the innovations of the Project areas. The innovative significance of the payment reform carried out by the Project lied in going ahead and being a pioneer, with characteristics of diversity exploration, continuous improvement in explorations and simultaneous promotion of payment reform and other reforms.

(Shan Yongxiang)

3. The Experience Exchange Meeting for Comprehensive Reform of County Hospitals of WB/DFID China Rural Health Project was Held in Beijing

On October 18, 2012, the Center for Project Supervision and Management of the Ministry of Health and the Medical Reform Office of the Ministry of Health jointly held the Experience Exchange Meeting for Comprehensive Reform of County Hospitals of WB/DFID China Rural Health Project in Beijing. The Meeting aimed to promote the experience and practice of the Project in the comprehensive reform of county hospitals, and provide reference for the reform of public hospitals. The pilot Project for the comprehensive reform of county hospitals was carried out first in Henan, Chongqing and Shaanxi. After three years of explorations, a patient-oriented pilot mode has taken shape step by step, with clinical pathway as the standard service, integrated payment system as a means of expenses control, the improvement of regulatory system as the guarantee, the incentive mechanism as the impetus, and the supporting platform of informatization as the basis.

(Shan Yongxiang)

Chapter XVI International Cooperation and Foreign Exchange

International Cooperation and Exchange in 2012

I. Participating in global health issues to facilitate the nation's diplomatic activities.

The friendly relationship with the developing and developed countries was pushed forward by the international health cooperation of the Ministry of Health in 2012. With the efforts of Ministry of Health(MOH), *Protocol on the Dispatch of Medical Teams to South Sudan between the Republic of China and the Republic of South Sudan, Memorandum of Understanding Between China and ASEAN on Cooperation in Health Issues,* and *The Joint Declaration on Public Health and Disaster Response between Health Ministry of China and German Federal Ministry of Health* were signed. In addition, the ophthalmic medical team was sent to DPRK to carry out free cataract operations for the local people. The efforts put in the formulation and implementation of medical aid measures for *the Beijing Action Plan* (2013-2015), an outcome of the Fifth Ministerial Meeting of the Forum on China–Africa Cooperation (FOCAC), played an active role in facilitating the nation's diplomatic activities.

II. Participating in international cooperation to facilitate and give publicity to the health care reform in China.

The visiting ministerial delegations to other countries were well chosen to boost the healthcare reform. They went to other countries to learn the development in their health industry and their experience and practice in their reform of the medical and pharmaceutical systems. During the multilateral or bilateral international events, they introduced and publicized the experience and measures of China's health care reform to the international society. In February, Chen Zhu, Minister of Health, informed the international organizations and the embassies in China of the situation in China's health care reform and the 12th Five-Year Plan for the reform. On the 65th World Health Assembly (WHA) held in May, Chen Zhu, Minister of Health, introduced the process of the full coverage of China's health care and the reform and development of health care in China's rural areas. The officials and experts in the health field in countries like the UK, USA and Ecuador were invited to visit China to learn the situation in China's reform of the health care system and the mechanism of health care service. Centering on the themes of the general practitioner system and the appraisal of medical techniques, forums and health policy dialogs were organized. Active actions were taken to apply for new international cooperative projects. 1 million euros was granted by the Foundation Merieux to the cooperative project and over 2 million dollars was granted to the China-US collaborative program on emerging and re-emerging infectious diseases. In addition, *the Western Area Health Initiative* was signed with the support of the World Health Organization and the five-year China-UK Global Health Support Program (GHSP) was launched with a fund of a total 12 million pounds. All these projects lent great support to the local areas to form the policies in disease control and prevention, public health and health care. Meanwhile, the projects also facilitated the training of international health talents and the study of international health strategy.

III. Carrying out comprehensive and in-depth collaboration in global health issues to push forward the multilateral health cooperation.

Active participation was conducted in the board meetings and the activities of the international organizations like the World Health Organization (WHO), the Joint United Nations Program on HIV/AIDS(UNAIDS) and the Global Fund to Fight AIDS, Tuberculosis and Malaria (the Global Fund). With China's promotion, Margaret Chan Fung Fu-chun, was successfully re-elected as the Director-General of WHO. The exchange with WHO was enhanced in the fields like health policy, control of major infectious diseases, response to public health emergence, maternal and child health care, community health and food safety. The exchange promoted the declaration of polio-free status of China, the confirmation of the eradication of tetanus among pregnant women and newborns and the pre-authentication of the medicines and vaccines made in China. Encouragement and support were given to the health technical institutions like the WHO collaborating centres in China to help the health care reform and development in China. Close communication with the international organizations like UNICEF, UNFPA and APEC was maintained and the applications and plans for the UN Millennium Development Goals like women's and children's health and food safety were successfully carried out. In response to the emergencies like emerging infectious diseases of new coronary virus and food safety, China collaborated closely with the international organizations and institutions, which gained understanding and support from the international society.

IV. Expanding the bilateral and regional health exchange and cooperation

The bilateral contact with high-level health officials of the developed countries was maintained and enhanced and the cooperation and exchange with these countries were carried out in the fields like the health care system, the health insurance system, the reform of public hospitals, the general practitioner system, the reform of payment system and the purchase of medicines. The cooperation with the neighboring countries like Japan, South Korea and North Korea in the aspects like public health, staff training, food safety, supervision of large medical equipment and health care reform was actively conducted. The joint programs on the prevention and control over AIDS, malaria and dengue fever along the borders of China with Vietnam, Laos and Myanmar were earnestly continued.

V. Making new progress in foreign medical aiding teams

The negotiation and subscription of the agreements on dispatch of medical aiding teams to other countries were continued and more medical teams were sent. In 2012, another 432 medical workers were sent abroad and by the end of the year, 1,029 medical workers were working in 49 foreign countries. 26 agreements on dispatch of medical aiding teams were signed and 17 were under negotiation. The measures and directions for the cooperation between China and African countries under the new circumstances were explored. In order to celebrate the 50th anniversary of the dispatch of medical aiding teams to other countries in 2013, detailed action plans were formed and carried out. Two training courses for the team leaders, translators and accounts in the medical aiding teams were conducted. The training of French translators was carried out and the Portuguese textbooks were compiled and put to use. The information management software for the medical teams was also officially in use.

VI. Deepening the cooperation with Hongkong, Macao and Taiwan in the medical and pharmaceutical fields.

The Hongkong experts were invited to the west regions in China to give lectures on the new concepts of community health and general practitioners. In addition, many mainland presidents of the first class hospitals of Grade 3 were organized to be trained in Hongkong within the framework of the agreements signed with Hongkong Hospital Authority. The cooperative programs with Health Express and Huaxia Foundation were carried out to give more training to the specialized talents and community health workers in the poverty-stricken areas. CEPA9 was signed, which would allow more service providers from Hongkong and Macao to set up medical institutions in mainland in terms of joint venture, cooperation and sole proprietorship.

Meanwhile, CEPA9 prescribed that part of the review and approval should be done by the related provincial health department. The reporting system of infectious diseases with Hongkong and Macao was maintained and a total of 351 reports were conducted among each other. 11,031 cataract operations were done by Health Express in the mainland China. 125 medical students and young doctors from Taiwan were invited to the mainland China. The medical media like "Health News" were introduced to Taiwan.

VII. Strengthening the administration of traveling abroad for official business

The joint meeting of the Health Ministry continued the systematic and normalized administration over the traveling abroad for official business of the staff of the Health Ministry and the departments directly under the Health Ministry. The routine examinations and reviews were strengthened, meetings were held regularly to discuss the major events related to traveling abroad for official business, and inspection and supervision of the administration of foreign affairs over the departments directly under the Health Ministry were conducted. *The Administrative Provisions of the Ministry of Health on Further Standardizing the International Cooperation with Foreign Enterprises* [No. 39 of 2012 of the general office of the Ministry of Health] was formulated and issued. Support was given to the departments directly under the Health Ministry to apply for the international technological cooperation programs from the Ministry of Science and Technology and for the programs on the introduction of foreign talents from the State Administration of Foreign Experts Affairs. Guidance was given to the foreign NGOs in China to organize their health cooperation activities. Attention was given to the analysis of the international situation to track the dynamics of the global health issues and studies were done on the themes like measures for aging in different countries and the establishment of medical institutions by foreign capital. The training courses for division chiefs of foreign health affairs were organized and the fourth recruitment examination for the international staff reserve was conducted to discover and cultivate talents for foreign health affairs.

(Qu Yang)

Section 1   Important Visits to Foreign Countries

1. Zhang Mao, Party Group Secretary and Vice Minister of Ministry of Health, Attended the 130th Session of WHO Executive Board

The WHO Executive Board's 130th session took place in Geneva from January

16–23, 2012. Zhang Mao, Party Group Secretary Ministry of Health, attended the session. The meeting was respectively chaired by Rahhal El Makkaoui, Secretary General, Ministry of Health Rabat, Morocco and 3 Assistant Director-Generals from Norway, Japan and Mozambique. Approximately 800 people were present at the session and they were from the 34 board members, 71 non-members, observers, specialized institutions of UN, the African Union (AU), the European Union (EU) and 46 NGOs. The Executive Board nominated Dr Margaret Chan for a second term as Director-General of WHO and reviewed her report and 32 issues, including the reform of WHO, mental health, social determinants of health, prevention and control of non-communicable diseases, global eradication initiative of poliomyelitis, global immunization plans. The Executive Board also listened to the report of the program, budget and administration committee of the Executive Board, the report from the related experts committee and the report over the progress in relevant fields. 20 decisions and resolutions, including prevention and control of noncommunicable diseases, global burden of mental disorders and elimination of schistosomiasis were made by the board.

(Qu Yang)

2. Vice Health Minister Yin Li Visited the Bahamas and the USA

On invitation of the Health Ministry of the Bahamas and the Bill & Melinda Gates Foundation (BMGF) of the USA, Vice Health Minister Yin Li, with the delegation headed by him, visited the Bahamas and USA from March 10–16, 2012. During his stay in the Bahamas, Yin Li met with Hubert Minnis, Health Minister of the Bahamas, and Camille Johnson, Permanent Secretary of Health Minister of the Bahamas. He also investigated the local medical institutions. During his stay in the USA, Yin Li met with Bill and Melinda Gates, chairs of BMGF and visited BMGF and the related institutions.

(Qu Yang)

3. Minister of Health Chen Zhu Visited France and was Awarded the Legion of Honor

On invitation of speaker of the French National Assembly, Minister of Health Chen Zhu, with the delegation headed by him, visited France from April 11-15, 2012. On 12 April, Chen Zhu was bestowed the Legion of Honor medal by Bernard Accoyer, speaker of the French National Assembly, on behalf of French President Nicolas Sarkozy in Hôtel de Lassay to honor his contribution to the China-France cooperation. During his visit, Chen Zhu attended the signing ceremony of the agreement on the cooperation between Chinese Academy of Medical Sciences and Paris Public Hospitals Group (AP-HP) and invested the French medical institutions.

(Qu Yang)

4. Vice Minister of Health Liu Qian Paid a Visit to the Kingdom of Lesotho and Went to the South Africa to Attend the Global Forum for Health Research

From April 18-27, 2012, Vice Minister of Health Liu Qian, with the delegation headed by him, visited the Kingdom of Lesotho and the South Africa. He extended solicitude to the Chinese medical team in Lesotho and attended the Global Forum for Health Research in the South Africa. During his stay in the Kingdom of Lesotho, Liu had a talk with Health and Social Welfare Minister of Lesotho Mphu Ramatlapeng. The two sides spoke highly of the achievements in the bilateral health cooperation and exchanged opinions over further strengthening the cooperation. Liu also visited the hospital where the Chinese medical team worked, witnessed the signing ceremony on China's donating medical equipment to the hospital and went to dorms of the Chinese medical workers to chat with them. From April 23-26, Liu attended the 2012 session of the Global Forum for Health Research. The theme of this session was "Beyond Aid—Research and Innovation as Key Drivers for Health, Equity and Development." During the session, Liu made a keynote speech—*Rely on the Advance of Science and Technology, Enhance the Capacity of Self-development and Improve the People's Health*. He also introduced China's management over scientific research and development and the contribution of scientific research and development to the prevention and control of H1N1.

(Qu Yang)

5. Chen Zhu, Minister of Ministry of Health, Paid a Visit to Mongolia

Minister of Health Chen Zhu, with the delegation headed by him, visited Mongolia on invitation of the Mongolian Ministry of Health. He investigated the health care system in Mongolia, especially the aspect of disease control and prevention from May 2-4, 2012. Mongolian Prime Minister Sukhbaataryn Batbold met with Chen Zhu in Mongolia's State Palace. Batbold spoke highly of the bilateral comprehensive strategic cooperative partnership and he hoped that the bilateral health departments would deepen their cooperation and the good-neighborly relationship would be strengthened. Earlier, Chen met Health Minister N. Khurelbaatar to discuss bilateral health cooperation. The two sides agreed to strengthen their cooperation in health system construction, hospital management and the establishment of border-region infectious disease control mechanism. After the meeting, the two ministers signed the Health Cooperation Plan from 2012 to 2016 between the two ministries. Chen was accompanied by Chinese Ambassador to Mongolia Wang Xiaolong and other related people. In addition, during his visit, Chen also went to investigate the Mongolian National Center for Communicable Diseases and made a speech in Mongolia Medical University.

(Qu Yang)

6. Vice Minister of Health Huang Jiefu Attended the First China-Ukraine Health Sub-committee Meeting and Paid a Visit to Greece

From May 10-19, 2012, Vice Minister of Health Huang Jiefu visited Ukraine and Greece on invitation the two countries' ministries of health. During his stay in Ukraine, Huang together with Vice Ukraine Minister of Healthcare presided over the First Health Sub-committee Meeting of the China-Ukraine Inter-government Cooperation Committee and signed the Regulations of the Health Sub-committee of China-Ukraine Inter-government Cooperation Committee. During Huang's stay in Greece, he met Vice Greek Minister of Health and President of IASGO Markus Bolaris and visited the Athens Medical Center.

(Qu Yang)

7. Minister of Health Chen Zhu, with the Delegation Headed by Him, Attended the 65th World Health Assembly

From May 21-26, 2012, the 65th World Health Assembly was held in Geneva, Switzerland. The Chinese delegation, headed by Minister of Health Chen Zhu, attended the annual meeting. Nearly 3, 000 delegates from 194 member states of the World Health Organization, related international organizations and NGOs were present. Margaret Chan was reappointed as WHO Director-General. The assembly discussed 32 technical and administrative issues, including reform of WHO, health research and fund-raising, prevention and control of noncommunicable diseases, monitoring of the United Nations millennium development goals and so on. 24 resolutions and decisions were passed by the assembly. Head of the Chinese delegation Chen Zhu made remarks at the general discussion on "universal health coverage." During the assembly, Chen Zhu also met the health ministers from different countries like Ivory Coast, USA, UK, Italy, Switzerland, Sweden, Pakistan, Australia and Israel and the directors of different international organizations like WHO, UNAIDS, the Global Fund, Secretariat of FCTC. Margaret Chan expressed her gratitude for China's support to herself and WHO and hoped that China would play a more active role in global health issues like the reform of WHO. At the seminar sponsored by the Secretariat of WHO on "Sharing the Achievements in Preliminary Health Care Reform in Brazil, China and India", Chen Zhu introduced the situation in China's health care reform in the rural areas. He also attended the breakfast meeting over the global premature infant initiative and shared China's experience in this field. The Chinese delegates actively participated in the assembly meetings, the committee meetings, the draft panel meetings and the technique introductions and fully participated in the discussion over the issues on the agenda. In addition, the Assembly awarded the United Arab Emirates Health Foundation Prize to Chen Bowen nominated by the Ministry of Health of China to honor his contribution to community health. Chen Bowen is Vice President and Secretariat of Community Health Association of China and Deputy Director and research associate of the Capital Institute of Pediatrics.

(Qu Yang)

8. Health Minister Chen Zhu Went to Canada to Investigate the General Practitioners System

Health Minister Chen Zhu, with the delegation headed by him, paid a visit to Canada from May 24-28, 2012. During his visit, Chen Zhu focused on the investigation of the general practitioners system in Canada. He had exchange with the staff of Canadian Association of General Practitioners and the University of Toronto Faculty of Medicine and visited the local training center for general practitioners. He also accepted the honorary doctorate degree from University of Montreal. In addition, Chen Zhu met the Director-General of the health department of Quebec and the directors of CSTAR and ICAV and he also visited the Clinical Research Institute of Montreal.

(Qu Yang)

9. Li Xi, the Discipline Inspection Team Leader to Ministry of Health, Paid a Visit to Sweden and Italy

On invitation of the Swedish Ministry of Health and Social Affairs and the Italian Ministry of Health, Li Xi, the Discipline Inspection Team Leader to Ministry of Health, with the delegation he headed, visited Sweden and Italy from June 12-21, 2012. During his stay in Sweden, Li Xi met Karin Johansson, State Secretary of Ministry of Health and Social Affairs. The two sides agreed to set up a bilateral cooperative team and worked out the plan for the team. The delegation also visited the Swedish Medical Products Agency and the local community health center and attended the seminar on hospital management. During his stay in Italy, Li Xi met Italian Minister of Health Renato Balduzzi and Lazio President Renata Polverini and visited the Italian Medicines Agency and medical institutions.

(Qu Yang)

10. Vice Health Minister Wang Guoqiang Paid a Visit to Serbia,Macedonia and Germany

On invitation of the Serbian Ministry of Health, the Macedonian Ministry of Health and the German Bavarian State Ministry of the Environment, Public Health and Consumer Protection, Wang Guoqiang paid a visit respectively to the three countries. During his stay in Serbia, Wang Guoqiang met Zoran Stankovic, Health Minister of Serbia and he expressed that his visit was the first ever visit paid by ministerial officials between the two countries' ministries of health. China would actively implement the cooperative memorandum and send experts of traditional Chinese medicine to give support in terms of the design of the outline of traditional Chinese medicine textbooks, the training of teachers of acupuncturists and the registration of acupuncturists. Wang also visited Serbian Medical Society, Academy of Military Medical Sciences of Serbia and other medical institutions. During his stay in Macedonia, Wang had talks with Macedonian Health Minister Nikola Todorov and other health officials and visited the local hospitals. During his stay in Germany, Wang had a talk with the Bavarian State Minister for Environment and Health, Dr. Marcel Huber and signed *The Understanding Memo over the Cooperation on Traditional Medicine between the State Administration of Traditional Chinese Medicine of China and the Free State of Bavaria*. The two sides agreed to enhance the cooperation in the clinical practice, research and development, teaching and training courses of traditional medicine. Wang visited the first traditional Chinese medicine hospital in Bavaria and the Chinese experts of traditional Chinese medicine who were working there. The delegation also visited the German Proton Therapy Center and the Medical School of Technical University of Munich.

(Qu Yang)

11. Vice Minister of Health Ma Xiaowei Visited Switzerland and France

From June 28- July 5, 2012, on invitation of the Swiss Interior Ministry and the French Ministry of Social Affairs and Health, a Chinese delegation headed by Vice

Minister of Health Ma Xiaowei, paid a visit respectively to these two countries. During his stay in Switzerland, Ma Xiaowei met Swiss Interior Minister Pascal Struopler and visited the hospital affiliated to University of Basel and the hospital affiliated to University of Geneva. These two hospitals were the cooperative partners of the public hospitals in China. During his stay in France, Ma Xiaowei had a talk with French Minister of Social Affairs and Health Marisol Touraine and Director of Division of Medical Service Francois Xavier Selleret. They looked back the cooperation among the two countries' 17 cooperative hospitals and reached a preliminary agreement to hold the China-France Forum on Hospitals in France in 2013. In addition, the delegation also visited the hospital of University Of Montpellier I and had talks with the chiefs from the Foundation Mérieux, the French Federation of Public Hospitals and Paris Public Hospitals Group (AP-HP).

(Qu Yang)

12. Vice Minister of Health Huang Jiefu Visited Thailand and Indonesia

From July 4-12, 2012, a Chinese delegation of 7 people, headed by Vice Minister of Health Huang Jiefu, attended the Fifth Health Ministers' Meeting of the ASEAN Plus China, Japan and South Korea (10+3) and the Fourth Health Ministers' Meeting of ASEAN Plus China (10+1) held in Thailand and visited Indonesia. During his stay in Indonesia, Huang Jiefu met the newly-appointed Indonesian Minister of Health Nafsiah Mboi and they had a talk over the bilateral health cooperation and the signing of the understanding memorandum between the two countries. Huang Jiefu also visited the Indonesian medical institutions. The delegation exchanged experience with delegates from the ASEAN countries, Japan and South Korea over the issues like the universal coverage of health and tobacco control and signed *The Memorandum of Understanding between the Member States of ASEAN and the Government of the People's Republic of China on Health Cooperation.*

(Qu Yang)

13. Zhang Mao, Party Group Secretary and Vice Minister of Ministry of Health, Visited the Republic of Belarus and the Republic of Latvia

From July 25-August 3, 2012, a Chinese delegation headed by Zhang Mao, Party Group Secretary and Vice Minister of Ministry of Health, visited the Republic of Belarus and the Republic of Latvia. During his stay in Belarus, Zhao Mao met the Deputy Health Minister Dmitry Pinevich and visited the related medical institutions. During his stay in Latvia, Zhang Mao had a talk with Ingrda Circene and they inked

The Implementation Plan for Health Cooperation between the Ministry of Health of P.R.C. and the Ministry of Health of Latvia(2012-2015). Zhang Mao also visited the medical institutions like the National Health Service of Latvia.

(Qu Yang)

14. Vice Minister of Health Chen Xiaohong Paid a Visit to Japan and South Korea

From September 3-12, 2012, the Chinese delegation, headed by Vice Minister of Health Chen Xiaohong, visited Japan and South Korean on invitation. The delegation attended the Exchange on China-Japan Health Policies held in Japan and investigated the supervision of food safety and health planning in South Korea. During his stay in Japan, Chen Xiaohong attended the Exchange on China-Japan Health Policies and met the Senior Vice Minister of Health, Labor and Welfare. During his stay in South Korea, Chen Xiaohong had a talk with Vice South Korea's Vice Minister of Health and Welfare Sohn Gunnyikk and met the Chief of Korea Food & Drug Administration Lee Huiseong. He also visited the South Korea's Institution of Food Safety Evaluation, the Samsung Medison and the Gil Hospital of Gachon University.

(Qu Yang)

15. Minister of Health Chen Zhu Paid a Visit to USA

From October 4-6, 2012, Minister of Health Chen Zhu with the delegation headed by him visited USA. During his stay in USA, Chen Zhu attended the ceremony of the 50th founding anniversary of St. Jude Children's Research Hospital, the Roundtable on Future of Bio-treatment of Leukemia and the Roundtable on the Challenges in the Health Care Reform in Minnesota and USA. Chen Zhu received an honorary doctorate degree from University of Minnesota. Chen Zhu also attended the signing ceremony of the cooperation agreement between the He'nan Provincial People's Government of China and Hormel Institute of USA, had an informal discussion with Chinese-American young scholars and met the representatives from some USA companies. In addition, Chen Zhu was interviewed by the press and he introduced the development in China's reform of the medical and pharmaceutical systems and the progress in organ transplantation.

(Qu Yang)

16. Vice Minister of Health Huang Jiefu Attended the 13th Meeting of the Health Sub-committee of the China-Russia Committee on Humanities Cooperation and Paid a Visit to Poland

From December 3-12, 2012, Vice Minister of Health Huang Jiefu, with the delegation headed by him, visited Russia and Poland on invitation of the two countries' ministries of health. Huang Jiefu and Russian Deputy Minister of Health and Social Development co-hosted the 13th Meeting of the Health Sub-committee of the China-Russia Committee on Humanities Cooperation. The two sides had in-depth discussions over the issues like infectious disease control alone the border, response to disasters, cooperation in supervision of medical products and collaboration in traditional medicine. A minute was signed after the meeting. During his stay in Poland, Huang Jiefu had a talk with Poland Undersecretary of State for Health Krzysztof Chlebus and they exchanged ideas mainly over Poland's health care system reform, health funding, organ transplantation and so on. The delegation also visited the Central Clinical Hospital of the Ministry of Interior in Warsaw.

(Qu Yang)

17. Wang Guoqiang, Vice Minister of the Ministry of Health, Visited Vietnam

On invitation of Vietnamese Ministry of Health, Vice Minister of the Ministry of Health and Commissioner of the State Administration of Traditional Chinese Medicine (TCM) Wang Guoqiang, paid a visit to Vietnam from December 3-8, 2012 to discuss the bilateral cooperation in the administration of practitioners of TCM, the recourses of traditional Chinese medicinal materials and the development of new drugs. The two sides signed *the Minute of the Ministerial Meeting on China-Vietnam Cooperation in Traditional Chinese Medicine.*

(Qu Yang)

Section 2   Important Visits from Other Countries

1. Vice Minister of Health Liu Qian Met UNICEF's Regional Director Dan Toole

On February 28, 2012, Vice Minister of Health Liu Qian Met UNICEF Regional Director for East Asia and the Pacific Dan Toole. The two sides exchanged opinions over the issues like improving children's nutrition and enhancing women and children's health. Liu Qian expressed gratitude to UNICEF for the long-term support to China's health industry especially in the field of women and children's health. He also introduced the situation of the major public health programs on women and children's health in China's health care reform and hoped that UNICEF would enlarge cooperation over the issues like children's nutrition and birth defects through the exchange of techniques and management. Toole wished to strengthen the cooperation in health education and project supervision. The two sides agreed to share the successful experience between China and other countries and push forward the South-South cooperation within the framework of UNICEF and other organizations. The relevant officials from the International Cooperation Department and the Department of Maternal and Child Health Care and Community Health of Ministry of Health attended the meeting.

(Qu Yang)

2. Minister of Health Chen Zhu Met Secretary-general of the OECD Angel Gurria

On March 20, 2012, Minister of Health Chen Zhu had a meeting with Secretary-general of the OECD Angel Gurria. Chen Zhu thanked OECD for its concern over China's health industry and wished to carry out dialogue and exchange with OECD and explore the cooperation in evaluation of health care reform, control of chronic diseases and telemedicine. Gurria expressed willingness to share the relevant data and experience of the OECD countries with China and conduct comparative study. The two sides agreed to strengthen the communication and organize activities in specialized fields to push forward the bilateral cooperation. The relevant officials from the International Cooperation Department and the Department of Health Policy and Regulation of Ministry of Health attended the meeting.

(Qu Yang)

3. Mr. Roy Quek, Deputy Secretary of the Singapore Ministry of Health, Paid a Visit to China

From March 20-22, 2012, a Singapore delegation of 20 people, headed by Secretary of the Ministry of Health Mr. Roy Quek, visited China to investigate the health care system. Chinese Minister of Health Chen Zhu had a meeting with the delegation. The delegation had a briefing on Singapore's health care system and the reform of it in the Ministry of Health. Over 100 people from the departments and the subordinate institutions of the Ministry of Health attended the briefing. The delegation also visited the China's CDC.

(Qu Yang)

4. Minister of Health Chen Zhu Met the Head of the Russian Presidential Property Management Department Vladimir Igorevich Kozhin

On March 21, 2012, Minister of Health Chen Zhu met the Head of the Russian Presidential Property Management Department Vladimir Igorevich Kozhin. Chen Zhu spoke highly of the bilateral health cooperation and thanked Kozhin for the importance he attached to the bilateral health exchange and cooperation. He hoped that the two sides would strengthen the cooperative mechanism between the two countries' health departments, explore new health cooperative platforms, carry out in-depth cooperation in the fields of common interests like traditional Chinese medicine, push forward the direct connection between the two countries' medical and health institutions, enhance the exchange of medical personnel and share information. Kozhin praised the progress in the bilateral cooperation and was willing to explore new cooperative channels. The two sides also exchanged ideas over the issues like the health care system and rehabilitation. Kozhin was invited over to China by the National Government Offices Administration. During their stay in China, the delegation also visited the Peking Union Medical College Hospital, the China National Pharmaceutical Group Cooperation and other organizations.

(Qu Yang)

5. Minister of Health Chen Zhu Met the Singapore Minister of Health Gan Kim Yong

On April 27, 2012, Minister of Health Chen Zhu Met the Singapore Minister of Health Gan Kim Yong and the Singapore's new ambassador to China. They had discussions over the working mechanism on the exchange of management personnel between the two countries' health ministries, the bilateral cooperation in chronic disease control and the coping strategies of the aging of population.

(Qu Yang)

6. Vice Minister of Public Health of Vietnam Nguyen Thanh Long Paid a Visit to China

From May 7-11, 2012, a Vietnamese delegation of 14 people, headed by Vice Minister of Public Health Nguyen Thanh Long, visited China. On 8 May, Vice Minister of Health Huang Jiefu met the delegation. The delegation visited the China's CDC and the CDC of Beijing. In addition, the delegation visited Yunnan Province.

(Qu Yang)

7. Minister of Health Chen Zhu Met Iran's Minister of Health and Medical Education Marzieh Vahid-Dastjerdi

On May 14, 2012, Minister of Health Chen Zhu met Iran's Minister of Health and Medical Education Marzieh Vahid-Dastjerdi and his entourages. The two sides had a friendly talk over the strengthening of the bilateral health cooperation. Chen Zhu introduced China's health care system and progress in the reform of it. He expressed willingness to explore cooperative fields and strengthen the bilateral health collaboration. Dastjerdi introduced Iran's health system and he wished to carry out active cooperation with China in medical equipment, medicine, chronic disease prevention and treatment and so on to push forward the. concrete cooperation in the health field.

(Qu Yang)

8. Cyprus's Health Minister Stavros Malas Paid a Visit to China

On invitation of Chinese Ministry of Health, Cyprus's Health Minister Stavros Malas visited China from May 13-17, 2012. Chinese Minister of Health Chen Zhu met Malas and the delegation headed by him. The two sides agreed to further strengthen the cooperation and exchange over the fields like prevention and treatment of thalassemia and traditional medicine within the framework of the action plan signed by the two countries' ministries of health and encourage the medical institutions of the two countries to carry out collaboration. During their stay in Beijing, the delegation also visited the Traditional Chinese Ophthalmology (TCO), the Guang'anmen Hospital, the Institute of Materia Medica of Chinese Academy of Medical Sciences, the China National Pharmaceutical Group Corporation and other organizations.

(Qu Yang)

9. Deputy Minister of Yemen Ministry of Public Health and Population Dr. Jamal Thabet Nasher Paid a Visit to China

From May 20-25, 2012, Deputy Minister of Yemen Ministry of Public Health and Population Dr. Jamal Thabet Nasher and his entourage visited China. They had discussions with the Chinese side to strengthen the bilateral cooperation and exchange in the health field and signed the agreement on sending the new medical aid team to Yemen. They also visited Liaoning Province which had sent medical aid team.

(Qu Yang)

10. Minister of Health Chen Zhu Met the Executive Director of UNAIDS Michel Sidibé

On June 25, 2012, Minister of Health Chen Zhu met the Under-Secretary-General of the United Nations and the Executive Director of UNAIDS Michel Sidibé. The two sides exchanged opinions over the prevention and control of AIDS. Chen Zhu thanked UNAIDS for its long-term support to China's control of AIDS and introduced the recent achievement of the Chinese government in the prevention of mother-to-child transimission and the involvement of NGOs in the prevention of AIDS. Sidibé praised China for the achievements in AIDS prevention and control, especially in terms of the political commitment, the promotion of effective prevention measures and the mobilization of the whole society. The two sides also had exchanges over the issues like helping developing countries, carrying out South-South cooperation and the prevention and control of AIDS. The relevant officials from the International Cooperation Department and the Disease Control and Prevention Bureau of Ministry of Health attended the meeting.

(Qu Yang)

11. Margaret Chan, Director-General of the World Health Organization (WHO), Paid a Visit to China

From July 16-21, 2012, Margaret Chan, Director-General of the World Health Organization(WHO) visited China on invitation and attended the opening ceremony of the Fifth Ministerial Conference of the Forum on China-Africa Cooperation. Vice President Xi Jinping, Vice Premier Li Keqiang, and Foreign Minister Yang Jiechi met respectively with Margaret Chan. Margaret Chan also had a formal talk respectively with Health Minister Chen Zhu, Party Group Secretary and Vice Minister of Ministry of Health Zhang Mao, Vice Health Minister Wang Guoqiang and Vice Health Minister Chen Xiaohong, Vice Health Minister Yin Li and Minister of General Administration of Quality Supervision, Inspection and Quarantine Zhi Shuping. Margaret Chan thanked China for its support to WHO and her work. She said that she would live up to the expectations during her second term, give full play to her leadership and expertise, and push forward the development of global health cause. Margaret Chan spoke highly of China's tremendous achievements in the medical and health fields. She pointed out that, in past 10 years, China had increased the capital and human input in the health field. The effective measures against H1N1, the response to Wenchuan earthquake and the block of polio had proved that the capability of China's health system had been enhanced and that the health input would contribute greatly to the economic development and social stability. During her stay in Beijing, Margaret Chan and Chen Zhu inked the agreement on donation to WHO by Chinese Ministry of Health. Together with Vice Health Minister Ma Xiaowei, she also attended the Chinese version launch ceremony of *Patient Safety Curriculum Guide* and visited the China National Center for Food Safety Risk Assessment. In addition, Margaret Chan met with Peng Liyuan, the image ambassador of Chinese Ministry of Health for control and prevention of HIV/AIDS and tuberculosis and WHO's goodwill ambassador for Tuberculosis and HIV/AIDS and thanked her for her contribution to tobacco control and the prevention and control of HIV/AIDS and tuberculosis.

(Qu Yang)

12. The Irish Minister of Health James Reilly Pain a Visit to China

On invitation of Chinese Ministry of Health, Irish Minister of Health James Reilly visited China from August 13-19, 2012. On August 16, Minister of Health Chen Zhu met the delegation headed by Reilly. The two sides agreed to give priority to the cooperation in training of general practitioners and specialized doctors, construction of the information system and preliminary health care. After the meeting, they signed *The Memorandum of Understanding on Health Cooperation between Chinese Ministry of Health of P.R. China and Ministry of Health of Ireland* (2012-2017). During his stay in China, Reilly attended the 3rd China Health Forum and visited some medical facilities like Peking Union Medical College Hospital and Beijing Children's Hospital.

(Qu Yang)

13. Permanent Secretary at the Irish Department of Health of UK Una O'Brien Paid a Visit to China

On invitation of Chinese Ministry of Health, Permanent Secretary at the Irish Department of Health of UK Una O'Brien visited China from August 14-20, 2012. During her stay in China, Una O'Brien attended the 3rd China Health Forum and introduced at the forum the development and experience in the reform of medical and pharmaceutical systems in UK. In addition, she visited the community Health Service Center of Changying Village, Chaoyang District, Beijing.

(Qu Yang)

14. Ecuador's Minister for Public Health Carina Isabel Vance Mafla Paid a Visit to China

On August 14, 2012, Ecuador's Minister for Public Health Carina Isabel Vance Mafla, on invitation of Chinese Ministry of Health, visited China and attended the 3rd China Health Forum. Minister of Health Chen Zhu met the delegation headed by Mafla. The two sides had a talk over carrying out further cooperation in fields like training of medical workers, construction of medical facilities and traditional medicine. During their stay in Beijing, the delegation visited Health Science Center of Peking University, Jishuitan Hospital, China's CDC, China National Pharmaceutical Group Corporation and other organizations.

(Qu Yang)

15. The Iranian Delegation, Headed by Deputy Health Ministers Hossein and Ahmad, Attended the 3rd China Health Forum

From August 15-19, 2012, the Iranian deputy ministers of the Ministry of Health and Medical Education Mohammad Hossein Nicknam and Ahmad Sheibani, with the delegation headed by them, attended the 3rd China Health Forum held in Beijing. On August 16, Chinese Vice Minister of Health Huang Jiefu met with the delegation. On August 17, Nicknam made a speech—*The Achievements in the Past 30 Years in Iran's Health Undertaking since the Islamic Revolution* at the forum.

(Qu Yang)

16. Donville Inniss, the Health Minister of Barbados, Paid a Visit to China

On invitation of Chinese Ministry of Health, the Health Minister of Barbados Donville Inniss with the delegation headed by him paid a visit to China on August 17, 2012. Chinese Health Minister Chen Zhu met with the delegation. Chen Zhu pointed out that the two countries were faced with many common challenges in the health field. Therefore, the two sides should strengthen the cooperation in chronic disease control and expand the range of collaboration. Inniss described the development plans in the health industry of Barbados and the needs in public hospital construction and training of clinical and research personnel. The two sides agreed to fix the prioritized fields of health cooperation and start negotiation on health cooperation. During his stay in Beijing, Inniss also visited Peking Union Medical College Hospital.

(Qu Yang)

17. Vice Minister of Health Chen Xiaohong Met the Federal Secretary of the German Federal Ministry for Food, Agriculture and Consumer Protection Müller

On August 29, 2012, Vice Minister of Health Chen Xiaohong met the visiting German delegation headed by the Federal Secretary of the Federal Ministry for Food, Agriculture and Consumer Protection Müller. The two sides exchanged opinions over strengthening the cooperation in food safety and attended the signing ceremony of *The Memorandum of Understanding on Cooperation between China National Center for Food Safety Risk Assessment and German Federal Institute for Risk Assessment.*

(Qu Yang)

18. Zhang Mao, Party Group Secretary and Vice Minister of Ministry of Health, Attended China-Germany Government Consultation and Met German Health Minister Daniel Bahr

On August 30, 2012, Zhang Mao, Party Group Secretary and Vice Minister of Ministry of Health attended the 2nd China-Germany Government Consultation and had a consultation meeting with his counterpart, German Health Minister Daniel Bahr. The two sides spoke highly of developments in the bilateral health cooperation since the first round of the China-Germany Government Consultation and agreed to deepen the exchange and cooperation in public hospital management, public health emergency response, disaster medicine and prevention of infectious diseases by means of high-level policy forums, academic exchanges and so on. After the meeting, witnessed by the two countries' premiers, the two sides signed *The Joint Declaration on Public Health and Disaster Response between Health Ministry of China and German Federal Ministry of Health.*

(Qu Yang)

19. Vice Minister of Health Huang Jiefu Met Health Minister of UK Simon Burns

On August 30, 2012, Chinese Vice Minister of Health Huang Jiefu met with Health Minister of UK Simon Burns at Ministry of Health of China and they exchanged opinions over deepening the bilateral health cooperation. Huang Jiefu introduced the progress and achievements made in the past 3 years in China's reform of the medical and pharmaceutical systems. He also pointed out that there would be more challenges in the health care reform and wished to study the mature experience and measures from UK and other countries. China was willing to strengthen the exchange and cooperate with UK over the issues like the training system of medical majors, certification of doctors and global health. Burns said that the health care in UK was also faced with the challenges like the increasing medical expenses, the growing health demand of people and the shortage of government investment. He wished to strengthen the bilateral cooperation and the exchange of experience.

(Qu Yang)

20. Vice Minister of Health Chen Xiaohong Met Deputy Minister of Commerce for Ministry of Agriculture, Food and Rural Affairs (South Korea) Kim Jong jin

On August 31, 2012, Vice Minister of Health Chen Xiaohong met with the visiting Deputy Minister of Commerce for Ministry of Agriculture, Food and Rural Affairs (South Korea) Kim Jong jin and they had a talk over the issues like food safety standards. Chen Xiaohong pointed out that when formulating food safety standards the government should take the influence of people's health into consideration, refer to the existing international standards and solicit the views of all walks of life in the society. After the standards were promulgated, the interpretation of them should be done properly so the public would understand them. China was willing to have exchange with South Korea and other countries in food safety standards and absorb the useful experience and measures from the international society. During the talk, the Chinese side explained the progress in formulating the food safety standards on fermented wine and other foods and the procedures of the formulation on request. The relevant officials from the Health Supervision Bureau and the International Cooperation Department of Ministry of Health attended the talk.

(Qu Yang)

21. Vice Minister of Health Chen Xiaohong Met Jean Besson, Chairman of the French Parliament's France-China Friendship Group

On August 31, 2012, Vice Minister of Health Chen Xiaohong met with Chairman of the French Parliament's France-China Friendship Group Jean Besson and the delegation headed by him. The two sides had in-depth discussions over the issues like reform of public hospitals, community health service, training of medical workers and the health insurance system.

(Qu Yang)

22. Minister of Health Chen Zhu Met Jean-Pierre Raffarin, Former French Prime Minister and Currently Vice President of the Senate

On September 17, 2012, Minister of Health Chen Zhu met with the visiting Former French Prime Minister and currently Vice President of the Senate Jean-Pierre Raffarin and they exchanged opinions over strengthening the bilateral health cooperation. Chen Zhu spoke highly of the long-term Sino-French cooperation and thanked Raffarin for his efforts for the cooperation. On Raffarin's request, Chen Zhu gave an introduction to the recent progress in China's reform of the medical and pharmaceutical systems, the 12th Five-Year Plan for the health industry and the prevention and treatment of beast cancer and cervical cancer. Raffarin expressed his admiration for the achievements in China's health undertaking. He said he was willing to push forward the cooperation between the relevant institutions and enterprises in the two countries on.

(Qu Yang)

23. Bartosz Arłukowicz, Minister of Health of Poland Paid a Visit to China

From September 19-21, 2012, Minister of Health of Poland Bartosz Arłukowicz visited China on invitation of Chinese Ministry of Health. On September 20, Minister of Health Chen Zhu met with Arłukowicz and the delegation headed by him. The two sides had exchanges over the issues like the development and reform of the health care system, the drug policies and the basic drug system in both countries. They agreed to give priority to the cooperation in the fields like the research and development of drugs, the supervision of medicine, the training of general practitioners and medical sciences and techniques. During their stay in Beijing, the delegation also visited the State Food and Drug Administration and Beijing Children's Hospital.

(Qu Yang)

24. Joe Cassar, Minister for Health, the Elderly and Community Care of Malta Paid a Visit to China

From September 22-28, 2012, Minister for Health, the Elderly and Community Care of Malta Joe Cassar with the delegation headed by him visited China on invitation of Chinese Ministry of Health. On September 25, Minister of Health Chen Zhu met with the delegation. The two sides had exchanges over the bilateral health cooperation and signed the protocol on the bilateral cooperation in traditional Chinese medicine. Cassar hoped that the two countries' ministries of health would carry out collaboration in the fields like treating tumors and mental disorders with traditional Chinese medicine and that the Traditional Chinese Medicine Center of the Mediterranean region would be expanded. Cassar also visited the relevant medical institutions.

(Qu Yang)

25. Minister of Health, Welfare and Sport in the Netherlands Edith Schippers Paid a Visit to China

On September 24, 2012, Minister of Health, Welfare and Sport in the Netherlands Edith Schippers with the delegation headed by him visited China. Minister of Health Chen Zhu met with the delegation. The two sides had a talk over strengthening the bilateral health cooperation in fields like control of infectious diseases, rational use of antibiotics, E - medicine, life science, aging of population and control of chronic diseases. Schippers also introduced the reform of the health care system in the Netherlands, the challenges they were faced with like the aging of population, supply of health service and control of medical expenses and the measures they took to address the challenges. After the talk, the two side sign *The Action Plan for Health Cooperation between Ministry of Health of P.R. China and Ministry of Health, Welfare and Sport of the Netherlands(2013-2015)*.

(Qu Yang)

26. Chairman of Cambodia National AIDS Authority Nuth Sokhom Paid a Visit to China

From November 4-9, 2012, Chairman of Cambodia National AIDS Authority Nuth Sokhom visited China on invitation of Chinese Ministry of Health. Minister of Health Chen Zhu met with Nuth Sokhom and the delegation headed by him. Chen Zhu said that the China-Cambodia health cooperation covered a wide range and Chinese Ministry of Health was willing to strengthen the cooperation with Cambodia in the various fields like prevention and control of HIV/AIDS. Nuth Sokhom praised China for the development of the health industry and the achievements in HIV/AIDS prevention and control in recent years. The two sides introduced to each other the situation of the AIDS epidemic and the measures against it. They exchanged opinions over the contents and forms of further cooperation and agreed to put emphasis on closer connection and communication. In the future, the exchange of experience and training of personnel concerning the relevant policies and techniques would be carried out. In addition, the delegation also went to visit Yunnan Province.

(Qu Yang)

27. Managing Director of the Global Fund to Fight AIDS, Tuberculosis and Malaria (the Global Fund) Gabriel Jaramillo Paid a Visit to China

From November 29 – December 5, 2012, the delegation, headed by Managing Director of the Global Fund to Fight AIDS, Tuberculosis and Malaria (the Global Fund) Gabriel Jaramillo, visited China. They went to Beijing and Shanghai and attended the relevant activities of World AIDS Day. On November 30, Jaramillo was invited over to the discussion presided over by Premier Wen Jiabao in Zhongnanhai of Beijing. The participants of the discussion were AIDS patients, orphans, petitioners, medical workers, researchers and volunteers, and the representatives from the relevant international organizations. Jaramillo spoke highly of China's achievements in the fight against AIDS and was proud of the cooperation of the Global Fund with China. He praised the Chinese leaders for their outstanding leadership in the fight and thought that China had assumed more and more important role in the global health and that China's experience could be shared with the international society. During his stay in Beijing, Jaramillo attended the charity activity of World AIDS Day and the release of a short film—*Forever Together on HIV/AIDS* as well as the evening party held by China Red Ribbon Foundation. He had discussions with the relevant representatives from the multilateral or bilateral international organizations and the NGOs. He also visited the methadone clinics under China's CDC and Shijingshan Hospital. During his stay in Shanghai, Jaramillo visited National Institute of Parasitic Diseases of China's CDC and the health service center in Litian Community of Xuhui District. He also met with the representatives from Chinese or jointed enterprises and called on them to participate in the actions of the Global Fund.

(Qu Yang)

28. Shin Young-soo, WHO's Regional Director for the Western Pacific, Paid a Visit to China

From December 10-14, 2012, WHO's Regional Director for the Western Pacific Shin Young-soo visited China. During his stay in China, Shin Young-soo paid a visit to Shaanxi and Chongqing to inspect the project of Health Campaign in Western China and investigated the local health care reform. During his stay in Shaanxi, Shin Young-soo had a talk with vice governor Zhen Xiaoming and visited the local community health facilities in Zhen'an County and Weiyang District. He praised Shaanxi for the achievements in health care reform and affirmed the outstanding progress of Zhen'an County in its development of the local health with relatively scarce resources. He said that WHO would strengthen the cooperation with Shaanxi on the platform of Health

Campaign in Western China over the issues like evaluation of health care reform, chronic disease control and healthy cities. During his stay in Chongqing, Shin Young-soo had a talk with deputy mayor Tong Xiaoping and investigated the local health facilities in Wulong County and Shapingba District. He said Chongqing had made many innovations in the health industry that benefited more people. He also said that the WHO project–Health Campaign in Western China aimed to boost the health industry in China's west regions and improve the health of people in those regions. He expressed willingness to cooperate with Chongqing.

(Qu Yang)

29. Minister of Health Chen Zhu Met Health Minister of Zambia Joseph Kasonde

On November 1, 2012, Minister of Health Chen Zhu met Health Minister of Zambia Joseph Kasonde and they exchanged opinions over the health care reform in both countries and discussed the direction for future bilateral cooperation. Chen Zhu said that China and Zambia were actively pushing forward the reform in the medical and pharmaceutical systems and the exchange and cooperation of the two sides would boost the development of the health industry in both countries. In addition, China wished to carry out collaboration with Zambia in fields like health policies, continuing medical education and training of medical talents. Kasonde praised China for the achievements in the health care reform and thanked China for sending the medical aiding teams. He also said that the two countries were faced with common challenges in the health industry and Zambia was willing to cooperate and exchange with China in dealing with the challenges. The relevant officials from the Department of International Cooperation of Ministry of Health of China attended the meeting.

(Qu Yang)

30. Vice Minister of Health Chen Xiaohong Met Minister of Plantation Industries and Commodities of Malaysia Tan Sri Bernard Giluk Dompok

On November 28, 2012, Vice Minister of Health Chen Xiaohong met the visiting Minister of Plantation Industries and Commodities of Malaysia Tan Sri Bernard Giluk Dompok. The two sides exchanged opinions over strengthening the bilateral cooperation on the formulation of the standards for palm oil. Chen Xiaohong said that China was one the major countries that imported palm oil from Malaysia and China attached great importance to the cooking standards of palm oil and was willing to solicit the opinions from the relevant countries when formulating the new national food safety standards. He suggested that the cooperative mechanism of the research of the palm oil cooking standards be set up and the fixed liaisons be chosen to actively push forward the cooperation and information sharing in the field of food safety standards of palm oil. Giluk Dompok agreed to Chen's suggestion and he hoped that the cooperation with China on food technology and information sharing would be enhanced. He said that the cooking standards of palm oil would be bettered to ensure the quality of palm oil. The relevant officials from Bureau of Food Safety and Health Supervision, and the International Cooperation Department of Ministry of Health attended the meeting.

(Qu Yang)

31. Vice Minister of Health Chen Xiaohong Met Canadian Associate Deputy Minister of Health Paul Glover

On December 12, 2012, Vice Minister of Health Chen Xiaohong met the visiting Canadian Associate Deputy Minister of Health Paul Glover and they exchanged opinions over the bilateral cooperation in food safety. Chen Xiaohong made an introduction to the overall situation of China's food safety and the existing supervisory system. And he hoped that China and Canada would continue to strengthen the exchanges and carry out cooperation in food safety supervision, risk assessment and response to food safety emergencies. Glover praised China for the efforts to improve food safety and expressed willingness to strengthen the cooperation in the field.

(Qu Yang)

Section 3　Important International Conferences

1. Delegates from Chinese Ministry of Health Attended the 2012 APEC Health Working Group (HWG) Meeting

From February 7-9, 2012, the 2012 APEC Health Working Group (HWG) Meeting was held in Moscow, Russia. The issues like trade and investment liberation and human safety topped the agenda of APEC 2012.The Health Working Group (HWG) Meeting called on the economies of APEC to strengthen the cooperation on prevention and treatment of noncommunicable diseases, maternal and child health and so on. Delegates from Chinese Ministry of Health attended the meeting and reported to the meeting the implementation of the following projects: the Early Warning Platform against Health Effects of Climate Change, the Program on Health Emergency Response Capacity and the Seminar on How to Attract, Retain and Manage Rural

Health Manpower. From June 24-27, the Second 2012 APEC Health Working Group (HWG) Meeting was held in St. Petersburg, Russia. The meeting had 3 sessions: a routine meeting of HWG, a high level dialogue on health and economy and a high level forum. During the meeting, the delegates from Chinese Ministry of Health explained the project- Strengthening the Nursing Capacity and Regional Cooperation to Meet an Ageing Society and reported to the meeting the implementation of the following projects: the Program on Health Emergency Response Capacity and the Seminar on How to Attract, Retain and Manage Rural Health Manpower. The dialogue on health policies was held on June 26 with the theme of application of information technology in health system. On June 27, the high level forum was hosted by APEC Life Science Innovation Forum and APEC Health Working Group with the theme— investments along the life course.

(Qu Yang)

2. The 2012 Directors' Meeting of WHO Collaborating Centers in China Was Held in Beijing

From February 9-10, 2012, the 2012 Directors' Meeting of WHO Collaborating Centers in China was held in Beijing. The meeting made an introduction to the issues like the global role of WHO collaborating centers, the status quo of them and the policies concerning their appointment and succession. The meeting also discussed the development of WHO collaborating centers in China, the challenges they were faced with and their future directions. The report on the external evaluation on the collaborating centers was made and two WHO collaborating centers in China shared their experience at the meeting. Over 260 participants from Beijing Health Bureau, Shanghai Health Bureau, China's CDC, Chinese Academy of Medical Sciences, WHO's representative office in China, WHO collaborating centers in China and other relevant organizations attended the meeting.

(Qu Yang)

3. Delegates from Chinese Ministry of Health Attended the Conference on Reform of World Health Organization

From February 26-28, 2012, the Conference on Reform of World Health Organization was held in Geneva, Switzerland. A Chinese delegation consisting of delegates from Chinese Ministry of Health and the relevant officials from Chinese mission in Geneva attended the conference. The meeting was initiated by WHO member countries, aiming to discuss the issues like the priorities, standards, categories, measures and schedule of the reform of World Health Organization. After the discussion, the participants suggested that the responsibilities of WHO fall into the following five categories: infectious diseases, non-communicable diseases, health alone the life course, health care system and health emergency response.

(Qu Yang)

4. Vice Minister of Health Chen Xiaohong Attended the 44th Session of the Codex Committee on Food Additives (CCFA)

From March 12-16, 2012, the 44th Session of the Codex Committee on Food Additives (CCFA) was held in Hangzhou, China. Vice Minister of Health Chen Xiaohong attended the session and addressed the opening ceremony. Chen Xiaohong made an introduction to the development in China's food safety in terms of the amendment of food safety regulations and laws, the comprehensive management of food safety, the acceleration of the establishment of national food safety standards, the enhancement of the evaluation and monitoring of food safety risks and so on. It was the 6th session since China's election as the presiding country. The session was attended by over 200 delegates from 51 member countries, 1 member organization and 31 international organizations. They focused on the studies over the relevant issues like GSFA and JECFA priorities.

(Qu Yang)

5. China-Canada Seminar for General Practice Was Held in Beijing

On March 15, 2012, China-Canada Seminar for General Practice was held in Beijing. Ren Minghui, director of the International Cooperation Department of Chinese Ministry of Health and Sarah-Taylor, deputy head of mission of Canadian Embassy in Beijing attended and addressed the seminar. At the seminar, the experts from the two sides explored the issues concerning general practice like the perfection of China's existing system, the curriculum design, the determination of the training bases and the examination and evaluation. They also discussed the possible cooperative intentions by way of forming partnership and the specific fields of cooperation. The seminar was sponsored by the General Practitioners Training Center of the Ministry of Health, the Health Human Resources Development Center (HHRDC) of the Ministry of Health, Canadian embassy to China and the University of British Columbia. Approximately 250 participants from Chinese Ministry of Health, National Development and Reform Commission, 27 provinces/autonomous regions/municipalities of China, the Canadian Association of General Practitioners and some medical colleges attended the seminar.

(Qu Yang)

6. Delegates from Chinese Ministry of Health Attended the Second Senior Officials' Meetings on Health Development of ASEAN plus China, Japan and South Korea (10+3) and ASEAN plus China (10+1)

From March 29-30, 2012, a Chinese delegation, headed by deputy director of the International Cooperation Department of Chinese Ministry of Health Wang Liji, attended the Second Senior Officials' Meetings on Health Development of ASEAN plus China, Japan and South Korea (10+3) and ASEAN plus China (10+1) in Cebu City of Malaysia. The meetings required that priority be given to health cooperation within the framework of ASEAN plus China, Japan and South Korea (10+3) and ASEAN plus China (10+1). China pledged to actively participate in the health cooperation and carry out the relevant programs.

(Qu Yang)

7. Minister of Health Chen Zhu Attended the Bo'ao Forum for Asia (BFA)

On March 31, 2012, the 2012 Bo'ao Forum for Asia was held in Bo'ao of Hainan, China. Minister of Health Chen Zhu attended the opening ceremony, made a speech-International Cooperation on Chronic Diseases at the breakfast meeting and attended the roundtable on international medical tourism.

(Qu Yang)

8. Vice Minister of Health Yin Li Attended the World Health Day 2012 Activities and the Seminar "Aging and Health in China"

On April 7, 2012, the theme activities of 2012 World Health Day were held in Beijing with the theme of Aging and Health in China. A seminar on aging and health was sponsored by Chinese Ministry of Health, China National Committee on Aging, World Health Organization and UNFPA. Participants of seminar included Vice Health Minister and Director of the State Food and Drug Administration Yin Li, WHO Representative in China Dr. Michael O'Leary and the UNFPA Representative to China Arie Hoekman. Yin Li indicated that Chinese Ministry of Health attached great importance to the health of senior citizens and had given priority to their health issues. The senior citizens were the key group that would benefit first from the basic public health service and the relevant policies were being formulated. Yin Li noted that China was still faced with many difficulties and challenge in addressing the aging problems though certain achievements had been made. China had a large population of senior citizens, many of them lived with chronic diseases, the medical expenses were high and the policies and measures were not sound. In addition, the specialized medical service for the seniors was not available and the medical facilities at different levels lacked the capacity for serving the senior citizens. Yin Li also said that more actions would be taken during the 12th Five-Year Plan to improve the health of the senior citizens. The actions included the perfection of the policies and measures concerning medical insurance for the seniors, the elevation of the service ability for the seniors and more support to the industries concerning the health of the seniors.

(Qu Yang)

9. Delegates from Chinese Ministry of Health Attended the Board Meetings of the Global Fund

In 2012, the Global Fund to Fight AIDS, Tuberculosis and Malaria held 3 board meetings in Geneva, Switzerland. Chinese Ministry of Health attended the meeting as the board member representing the West Pacific Region. The Twenty-Sixth Board Meeting was held in Geneva, Switzerland, from May 10-11, 2012. Aiming to finish the selection of the Executive Director, the Board approved *The Executive Director Selection Process* and decided to set up a nomination committee consisting of 6 board members and 3 independent members. The Board considered a new financial forecast that $1.6 billion was available for funding for the 2012-14 period, and voted to implement available funds in effective programs that save lives. The 27th Board Meeting was held from September 12 - 14, 2012. The delegation of West Pacific Region, consisting of delegates from Chinese Ministry of Health, China's CDC, Lao People's Democratic Republic and the Solomon Islands, attended the meeting. The meeting approved the new funding model. The Global Fund would adopt the strategic investment, which would divide the recipient countries into different levels according to their national disease burden and payment ability, combine the funding with the prevention strategies of the recipient countries and enhance the involvement of all the stakeholders, especially the civil societies and target groups. The application would be simpler and more predictable and utilization of the funds would be more flexible. The representatives at the meeting hoped that the grant of funds would be more transparent, the interaction between recipient countries would be intensified, the share of information would be timely, the fund application procedures would be simpler and the technical support would be provided to the recipient countries. The Twenty-Eighth Board Meeting was held from November 13-15. The delegation of West Pacific Region, consisting of representatives from China, Laos and Cambodia, attended the meeting. The Board appointed Mark Dybul as the new Executive Director and approved the new funding model. The Global Fund adopted the strategic investment, which would divide the recipient countries into different levels according to their national disease burden and payment ability, combine the funding with the prevention strategies of the recipient countries and enhance the involvement of all the stakeholders, especially the civil societies and target groups. The application would be simpler and more predictable and the utilization of the funds would be more flexible. The Board agreed that the Secretariat would maintain the Affordable Medicines Facility – malaria (AMFm) in the next 12 months to integrate the resources and pass the transitional period. The Board approved the detailed evaluation and discussion on the performance of Inspector General John Parsons and determined to terminate his employment.

(Qu Yang)

10. Minister of Health Chen Zhu Attended the Health Conference of BRICS

The BRICS countries represented by the Ministers of Health of China, Brazil and South Africa, Permanent Representative of the Russian Federation and the Secretary of Health and Family Welfare, Government of India met on May 22, 2012 on the sideline of the 65th session of the World Health Assembly in Geneva and signed *The Joint Communiqué of the BRICS Member States on Health*. The meeting emphasized the importance and the need of technology transfer as a means to empower developing countries and the important role of generic medicines in the realization of the accessibility to health. The meeting also required the member states to give priorities in research and development and cooperate with one another especially in fields like the treatment of tuberculosis, malaria, neglected diseases, non-communicable diseases and the availability of new drugs. The Chinese delegates, including Health Minister Chen Zhu and the Permanent Mission Ambassador in Geneva Liu Zhenmin, attended the meeting.

(Qu Yang)

11. Delegates from Chinese Ministry of Health Attended the 131st Session of the Executive Board of WHO

The 131st Session of the Executive Board of WHO was held in Geneva, Switzerland, from May 28-29, 2012. Over 250 participants from 34 member states, 53 non-member states, the relevant international organizations and the relevant NGOs attended the meeting. The Chinese delegation headed by Ren Minghui, Director of the International Cooperation Department of Chinese Ministry of Health and the Vice Chairman of the Board, attended the meeting. Dr Joy St. John, the Chief Medical

Officer of Barbados, was Chairman of the WHO Executive Board during this session. The meeting briefed the outcomes of the 65th World Health Assembly and discussed the issues like WHO reform, WHO evaluation policy and the ratio of donation of the partners within the framework of Pandemic Influenza Preparedness Framework. The session aslo decided the constitution of the committees under the Board and the meeting schedules of the Administration Committee of the Executive Board.

(Qu Yang)

12. The Third International Roundtable on China-Africa Health Collaboration was Held in Beijing

The Third International Roundtable on China-Africa Health Collaboration was held in Beijing from June 12-13, 2012. Over 100 participants attended the meeting, including Han Qide, Vice Governor of the Standing Committee of NPC, Bience Gawanas, Commissioner of Social Affairs on the African Commission, and Richard Sezibera, Secretary General of the East African Community.

Chinese Minister of Health Chen Zhu attended and addressed the meeting. He said that health collaboration was a microcosm of China-Africa friendship and had made innumerable great achievements. By the end of 2011, 65 Chinese medical aiding teams with a total of 20,000 medical workers had been sent to the Africa. At present, there were 42 Chinese medical teams working in 41 African countries and nearly 1000 Chinese medical workers stationed there annually. The Chinese government gave support to African countries for the development of their health systems and medical abilities by way of conducting training courses and helping construct medical facilities. Chen Zhu emphasized that 2012 was an important year for the realization of UN's Millennium Development Goals. There was still a long way to go to realize of the millennium development goals for health. China was willing to exchange experience with African countries, give support to their health industry and continue to deepen the China-Africa health cooperation. Within the China-Africa cooperation framework, China would earnestly implement the action plans formulated by Chinese national leaders and make the health cooperation the key and outstanding point in China-Africa cooperation. The health projects that would benefit the common people should be carried out continuously. The dispatch of medical aiding teams to Africa would be continued and new health cooperation programs would be explored. The two sides should collaborate closely in the global health affairs and cooperate with the multinational organizations like WHO to push forward the fairness and availability of global health. The roundtable meeting was sponsored by Institute for Global Health of Peking University and supported by Chinese Ministry of Health, Department for

International Development of UK, WHO and UNAIDS. The key issues of the meeting included: developing potential resources to enlarge the South-South Cooperation; increasing the medicine supply and the technology transfer; and strengthening the cooperation evaluating measures to give guidance to policy formulation.

(Qu Yang)

13. Symposium on the China-World Health Organization Country Cooperation Strategy was Held in Beijing

Symposium on the China-World Health Organization Country Cooperation Strategy was held in Beijing on June 21, 2012. It discussed the goals and priorities of the China-World Health Organization Country Cooperation Strategy 2013-15. The strategy outlines a medium-term framework for cooperation between the Chinese government and WHO to improve the health and well-being of Chinese people. The meeting pointed out that the priority should be given to China's reform of health care system and other key health issues in China. China would make full use of WHO's support in formulation of policies and standards, development of technology and cooperation with multilateral partners. The relevant officials and experts from the departments of Ministry of Health, the State Food and Drug Administration, State Administration of Traditional Chinese Medicine, Beijing Health Bureau and the World Health Organization office in China attended the symposium.

(Qu Yang)

14. Delegates from Chinese Ministry of Health Attended the 63rd Session of the World Health Organization (WHO) Regional Committee for the Western Pacific Region

The 63rd Session of WHO Regional Committee for the Western Pacific Region was held in HaNoi, Vietnam, from September 24-28, 2012. The Chinese delegation with delegates from the four departments of Chinese Ministry of Health attended the meeting. Approximately 350 participants from 31 countries and regions, 3 UN organizations, 7 observers and 24 NGOs were present. Nguyen Thi Kim Tien, Health Minister of Vietnam, was elected chairman. Nguyen Thi Doan, Vietnamese Vice President, attended the opening ceremony and delivered a welcome speech. Shin Young-soo, Regional Director of the WHO West Pacific, indicated in his report that the overall development was achieved in the work of measles, *International Health Regulations*, nutrition and food safety. The meeting also reviewed the end-cycle report on the execution of the annual budget of the West Pacific Region 2010-2011 and passed

10 resolutions. The 10 resolutions included the draft of the annual budget 2014-2015, nutrition, prevention of violence and injuries, elimination of measles, implementation of *International Health Regulations*, the appointment of the regional director and so on. The Chinese delegation also attended sideline meetings sponsored by the Vietnamese government and WHO with the themes of the universal coverage of medical insurance, concise packaging of tobacco, funding for health development and research and so on.

(Qu Yang)

15. Minister of Health Chen Zhu Attended the Second Sino-French Symposium on Transdisciplinary Infectious Diseases

The Second Sino-French Symposium on Transdisciplinary Infectious Diseases was held in Wuhan, China on October 29, 2012. Minister of Health Chen Zhu attended the opening ceremony and delivered a speech. Chen Zhu looked back on the long history of Sino-French health cooperation and affirmed the remarkable achievements in the cooperation. He pointed out that in the past 3 decades, the influence of emerging and re-emerging infectious diseases had expanded and posed a treat to people's health and the development of the society. Effective prevention and control of emerging infectious diseases was a challenge faced by the whole international society. China attached great importance to it and had set up the prevention and control system. In recent years, large-scaled programs against the major infectious diseases had been carried out with remarkable periodical outcomes. Chen Zhu suggested that the experts in the two countries set up cooperative platforms, strengthen exchanges, share experience, expand collaboration and enhance the scientific cooperation to create a win-win situation in order to meet the challenge of the emerging infectious diseases. The symposium was sponsored by Chinese Academy of Engineering and French National Academy of Medicine, organized by Wuhan Institute of Virology of Chinese Academy Of Sciences and supported by Chinese Ministry of Health and Chinese Ministry of Science and Technology. Over 100 scientists from China and France had discussions and exchanges over etiology and epidemiology, anti-infection immunity and infectious disease control, biosafety, bioethics and other issues.

(Qu Yang)

16. Minister of Health Chen Zhu Attended the Second Global Symposium on Health Systems Research

The Second Global Symposium on Health Systems Research was held in Beijing, from November 1-4, 2012. Minister of Health Chen Zhu attended the meeting and delivered a keynote speech-*Universal Health Coverage, Development and Achievements in China's Health Care Reform*. Chen Zhu introduced to the meeting the efforts China had made in deepening the health care reform and realizing the universal health coverage. He said that the Chinese government attached great importance to the health of people and had given priority to the universal health coverage. The concept of universal coverage was actively practiced, thus, the policies of health care reform could benefit the mass people, encourage the medical workers and make the supervision easy to handle. Chen Zhu indicated that over years' practice in the reform of health care system, China had realized the universal coverage of the basic medical insurance and national basic drugs. The grassroots health service network had covered the urban and rural areas, the basic public health care was available to all Chinese citizens and the pilot reform of public hospitals had been steadily pushed forward. All these practices laid the foundation for China's realization of universal health coverage. Chen Zhu also pointed out the priorities of the health care reform during the 12th Five-Year Plan, including accelerating the perfection of the national health insurance system and pushing forward the pilot reform of the public hospitals. Chen Zhu thanked the international society for their concern over China's health care reform and hoped that China and the international society would strive together for the realization of universal health coverage globally. Thus, more people would enjoy the benefit. The Symposium was sponsored by WHO, organized by Peking University Health Science Center and supported by Chinese Ministry of Health. Approximately 1,800 scholars from over 110 different countries participated in this symposium. The issues like the latest research findings and major strategies on universal health coverage were discussed at the symposium. In addition, World Health Organization's strategy on health systems research and the *Beijing Statement* were launched.

(Qu Yang)

Section 4   Other Important Foreign Affairs

1. Minister of Health Chen Zhu Met Director of Paris Public Hospitals Group (AP-HP) Mireille Faugere

Minister of Health Chen Zhu met Director of Paris Public Hospitals Group (AP-HP) Mireille Faugere and the delegation headed by her on January 4, 2012. The two sides exchanged opinions over strengthening the bilateral cooperation of the public hospitals. Chen Zhu spoke highly of the cooperation that had been in progress between the two countries' public hospitals. He gave a brief introduction to China's deepening of the health care reform and the further plan for the pilot reform of public hospitals. Faugere shared the measures and experience of Paris Public Hospitals Group (AP-HP) in emergency treatment, medical quality control, certification of medical institutions and clinic paths. The two sides agreed to further strengthen the cooperation on public hospitals.

(Qu Yang)

2. Center for Health Statistics and Information of Ministry of Health Become the Collaborating Information Center of WHO

Center for Health Statistics and Information of Ministry of Health was appointed as the Collaborating Information Center of WHO for the next 4 years on February 8, 2012. As the collaborating center of WHO, it would enhance its cooperation with WHO and the relevant organizations home and abroad to boost construction of China's health information system and lend support to the development the global health statistics.

(Qu Yang)

3. Minister of Health Chen Zhu Briefed the Progress in China's Health Care Reform to the Diplomatic Missions in China

A briefing on the progress in China's health care reform was held in Beijing, on February 14, 2012, which was cosponsored by Chinese Ministry of Health and WHO office in China. Minister of Health Chen Zhu briefed the progress and achievements in China's health care reform and the priorities of the reform during the 12th Five-Year Plan to the diplomatic missions in China. Over 130 participants were present, including representatives from the UN agencies, relevant international organizations, embassies of relevant foreign nations, certain international NGOs and the press. Dr. Michael O'Leary, WHO Representative in China, presided over the briefing. Chen Zhu thanked the multilateral and bilateral international organizations for their support to China's health work. He hoped that the international society would give more support to China in the evaluation of the progress and achievements in health care reform so that China could set up an evaluation system that was suitable for China.

(Qu Yang)

4. Minister of Health Chen Zhu Met French Ambassador for Science, Technology and Innovation Catherine Bréchignac

On February 21, 2012, Minister of Health Chen Zhu met French Ambassador for Science, Technology and Innovation Catherine Bréchignac and French Chair of China-France Cooperation Committee on Traditional Chinese Medicine. The two sides exchanged opinions over the cooperation on traditional Chinese medicine. Chen Zhu thanked the French experts for their suggestions on pushing forward the bilateral cooperation on traditional Chinese medicine and congratulated the cooperation committee for the progress made over the year. He said that Ministry of Health would spare no efforts to support the cooperation in various fields within the framework of the cooperation committee. He encouraged the French side to strengthen the research of clinical techniques of the traditional Chinese medicine with the cooperation partners in China.

(Qu Yang)

5. Chinese Scientists Wang Zhenyi and Chen Zhu Awarded 7th Annual Szent-Gyorgyi Prize for Progress in Cancer Research

Minister of Health Chen Zhu went to New York, USA to attend the awarding ceremony of the 7th annual Szent-Gyorgyi Prize for Progress in Cancer Research held by the National Foundation for Cancer Research of USA from March 5-7, 2012. Health Minister Chen Zhu and Academician of the Chinese Academy of Engineering Wang Zhengyi had been awarded the 7th annual Szent-Gyorgyi Prize for Progress in Cancer Research for their innovative research that led to the successful development of a new therapeutic approach to acute promyelocytic leukemia (APL). By combining traditional Chinese medicine with Western medicine, Drs. Wang and Chen had provided dramatic improvement in the five-year disease-free survival rate of APL patients - from approximately 25 percent to 95 percent - making this therapy a standard of care for APL treatment throughout the world, and turning one of the most fatal diseases into a highly curable one. During his stay in USA, Chen Zhu had a seminar with over 20 young Chinese-American scholars, visited Columbia University and was interviewed by the press media like Xinhua News Agency, CCTV, the Wall Street Journal and Nature.

(Qu Yang)

6. Minister of Health Chen Zhu Attended the Singing Ceremony of Memorandum of Understanding on the Cooperation on Multi-drug Resistant Tuberculosis Prevention and Treatment

Minister of Health Chen Zhu Attended the Singing Ceremony of China's CDC-Lilly Foundation Memorandum of Understanding on the Cooperation on MDR TB Prevention and Treatment on March 20, 2012. Chen Zhu said that Ministry of Health welcomed all sectors of the society to participate in the TB prevention and treatment and he hoped that the program with Lilly Foundation would an excellent model for the cooperation between Chinese government and enterprises.

(Qu Yang)

7. Vice Minister of Health Yin Li Met WHO Representative in China Dr. Michael O'Leary in Xinjiang Uygur Autonomous Region

Vice Minister of Health Yin Li met with WHO Representative in China Dr. Michael O'Leary and the experts of WHO and UNICEF in Xinjiang Uygur Autonomous Region on April 15, 2012. Dr. O'Leary and the experts were participating in the fifth vaccination campaign against polio in Xinjiang. Yin Li welcomed the experts to witness the vaccination campaigns against polio. He said that Chinese authorities and the Xinjiang government responded aggressively immediately after the outbreak of the wild polio virus (WPV). The relevant measures were taken, including the publicity through multiple channels, the involvement of various departments and the mobilization of the whole society. He thanked WHO and UNICEF for their support in the first four vaccination campaigns. In addition, he pointed out that WHO had removed China from polio-active list, which showed that the international society had affirmed China's control of the polio epidemic. It was the result of the cooperation between China and the international society and China was willing to share the experience. Dr. O'Leary praised China for the aggressive and effective measures against the outbreak of polio epidemic. He said that China's experience in handling the outbreak should be shared with other countries and he suggested that China continue the monitoring on AFP. The officials of UNICEF praised China for the multi-channel mobilization of the society and suggested that the routine vaccinations be done with the methods. WHO and UNICEF both promised to continue the support to China's eradication of polio. The relevant officials from the Disease Control and Prevention Bureau of Ministry of Health, the International Cooperation Department of Ministry of Health, China's CDC and the Health Department of Xinjiang attended the meeting.

(Qu Yang)

8. Chinese Health Minister Dr. Zhu Chen Met Mr. Trevor Mundel, President of Global Health at Bill and Melinda Gates Foundation

Chinese Health Minister Dr. Zhu Chen met Mr. Trevor Mundel, President of Global Health at Bill and Melinda Gates Foundation on April 18, 2012 and they exchanged opinions over the further bilateral health collaboration. The two sides agreed to strengthen the collaboration in the fields like translational medicine, eradication of polio and elevation of the availability of medicine.

(Qu Yang)

9. Vice Health Minister Huang Jiefu Met Arie Hoekman, the UNFPA Representative to China

Vice Health Minister Huang Jiefu Met Arie Hoekman, the UNFPA Representative to China in Chinese Ministry of Health on April 23, 2012. They exchanged opinions over strengthening cooperation. Huang Jiefu thanked UNFPA for its long-term support to China's health development. He suggested that the two sides sum up the cooperative experience, combine the priorities of UNFPA with China's 12th Five-Year Plan and the reform of the medical and pharmaceutical systems and perfect the cooperative mechanism by way of annual consultation. The two sides agreed to intensify the cooperation in fields like reproductive health and aging. The relevant officials from the International Cooperation Department and the Department of Maternal and Child Health Care and Community of Ministry of Health attended the meeting.

(Qu Yang)

10. Chinese Ministry of Health Sent Experts to Cambodia

An undiagnosed illness had killed more that 60 children in Cambodia since April 2012. On request of Cambodian Ministry of Health, an expert team was sent to Cambodia by Chinese Ministry of Health on 11 July. The team quickly identified the virus-Enterovirus 71 (EV-71), which caused a lethal strain of hand, foot and mouth disease. During their stay in Cambodia, the experts also helped with the clinical treatment and the training of Cambodian medical workers. They also shared their experience in prevention and treatment of severe hand, foot and mouth disease.

(Qu Yang)

11. Minister of Health Chen Zhu Published the Article – *China's Health Diplomacy: sharing experience and expertise* **in the Special Issue of** *Global Health* **2012**

On request of Graduate Institute of International Studies of Geneva, Chinese Minister of Health Chen Zhu published the article – *China's Health Diplomacy: sharing experience and expertise in the special issue of Global Health 2012* while attending the 65th World Health Assembly in May of 2012. In his article, Chen Zhu explained the policies of China's health diplomacy and China's standpoint and expectation over the global health issues. He pointed out in his article that in the 21st century, globalization had achieved unprecedented depth and breadth, exerting a profound influence on health. Health existed at every moment and everywhere. Its strategic relevance was increasingly highlighted in the global arena. Health had entered into the global development agenda and lay at the core of the Millennium Development Goals (MDGs). As a component of a country's diplomatic policies, health reflected that country's soft power. Today, a health minister should not only protect national health from a biomedical perspective but must also view public health from a broader and global perspective. That person shouldered dual responsibilities: to ensure the health of his or her people and to contribute to the improvement of global health. He noted in the article that the following 3 convictions must be abided by in health diplomacy. First, global health diplomacy should respect the norms of international laws and fully consider specific conditions. Second, global health diplomacy should strengthen coordination. When formulating relevant policies and rules, countries and international organizations need to review the mutual impacts of the related factors and of public health in a general context. Third, global health diplomacy should focus on real effects. Developed countries should honor their international commitments as soon as possible and provide more support and assistance to developing countries in areas such as technology transfer and the promotion of drug accessibility and affordability. Developing countries should enhance their health systems, increase fiscal inputs, coordinate resources and strengthen South-South cooperation.

(Qu Yang)

12. Minister of Health Chen Zhu Attended the China-Harvard Medical School Translational Medicine Consortium MOU Signing Ceremony

Minister of Health Chen Zhu attended the opening ceremony of 14th Shanghai International Forum on Biotechnology and Pharmaceutical Industry and the China-Harvard Medical School Translational Medicine Consortium MOU Signing Ceremony on May 10, 2012. Chen Zhu indicated that translational medicine was one of the fastest developing disciplines of the medical sciences. The four cooperative institutions- Chinese Academy of Medical Sciences (CAMS), Peking Union Medical College, SJTU School of Medicine , Fudan University Shanghai Medical College and Harvard Medical School would form a win-win partnership in the study of it. China-Harvard Medical School Translational Medicine Consortium would establish a new cooperation mechanism to launch cooperative researches on the diagnosis, treatment, prevention and pathogenesis of type 2 diabetes, immunological disease and malignant cancer (cancer of lung and liver, and leukemia). It would also boost cooperation and exchanges in the cultivation of talents in translational medicine and the joint master degree programs.

(Qu Yang)

13. Minister of Health Chen Zhu Met Andrew Hamilton, President of Oxford University

Minister of Health Chen Zhu met Andrew Hamilton, President of Oxford University, on May 14, 2012.

Chen Zhu thanked Oxford University for its fruitful cooperation with China in fields like chronic diseases, women depression and response to disasters. Through the cooperation the latest achievements in medical research, as well as the new ideas in health policies, were introduced into China. Chen Zhu praised Mr. Hamilton for his efforts in pushing forward the bilateral cooperation in the medical research. Chen Zhu hoped that the cooperation between Oxford University and Chinese medical research institutes would be strengthened and that the cooperation between the two countries in medical education and translational medicine would be expanded as well.

(Qu Yang)

14. Margaret Chan Fung Fu-chun, Was Successfully Re-elected as the Director-General of WHO

On May 23, 2012, the nomination of Chinese candidate Margaret Chan was approved by the member states of the Executive Board of WHO at the 65th World Health Assembly. Margaret Chan was successfully re-elected as the Director-General of WHO and her new term ran from July 1, 2012 to June 30, 2017. Margaret Chan had previously served as Director of Health in the Hong Kong Government (1994–2003), representative of the WHO Director-General for Pandemic Influenza and WHO Assistant Director-General for Communicable Diseases (2003–2006). Margaret Chan was first elected by the Executive Board of WHO on November 8, 2006.

(Qu Yang)

15. Vice Minister of Health Xu Ke Met World Health Organization Polio Officials

Vice Minister of Health Xu Ke met the delegation headed by World Health Organization Polio Official Roland Sutter on June 12, 2012. Xu Ke briefly introduced the measures against the outbreak of the polio epidemic taken by the Chinese governments at all levels since the imported wild polio virus case in Xinjiang in June of 2011. She indicated that in order to consolidate the achievements in the previous campaigns, eliminate the blind points in vaccination and regain the polio-free status Chinese Ministry of Health would guide the vaccination in Xinjiang back from the emergency state to the regular state. The monitoring and sensitivity to AFP would be continued to ensure the indexes of monitoring and quality control would reach the standards of WHO. Favorable policies would be formulated and training courses carried out to elevate the grassroots vaccination ability in Xinjiang. Ministry of Health would cooperate closely with WHO and the neighboring countries to improve the cross-border prevention and control mechanism, strengthen the capacity of the vaccination planning and service, intensity the development and cooperation in manpower, enhance the research and application of vaccines and do well the eradication of polio. The World Health Organization polio officials fully affirmed the China's achievements in polio prevention and control and reckoned that China's national monitoring systems worked well. They also thought that the existing monitoring system in Xinjiang was sensitive enough to identify the polio cases promptly. According to statistics from the monitoring system, the WHO polio officials believed that the wild polio virus epidemic and the wild polio virus cases had been eradicated in Xinjiang. The relevant officials from Chinese Ministry of Health and Xinjiang Health Department attended the meeting.

(Qu Yang)

16. Minister of Health Chen Zhu Met Chairman of Cancer Research UK Michael Pragnell

Minister of Health Chen Zhu met Chairman of Cancer Research UK Michael Pragnell and the delegation headed by him on June 12, 2012. Chen Zhu thanked Cancer Research UK for its down-to-earth suggestions on China-UK cooperation on cancer research. He encouraged the UK side to intensify the exchange with its Chinese partners and Chinese Academy of Medical sciences. The cooperation in the translational medicine and clinic research on cancer should be deepened and the cooperative programs should be explored by starting from the commonly interested research of lung cancer and esophagus cancer.

(Qu Yang)

17. Minister of Health Chen Zhu Was Awarded the Director-General's Special Recognition Certificate for World No Tobacco Day

On July 18, 2012, Chinese Minister of Health Chen Zhu was awarded the Director-General's Special Recognition Certificate for World No Tobacco Day in Beijing by WHO Director-General Margaret Chan for his and Chinese Health Ministry's accomplishments in the area of tobacco control. Chen Zhu said that since China was the largest tobacco producer and consumer in the world, there were a lot of challenges in tobacco control and health promotion. The health system in China would take the lead in tobacco control and mobilize the whole society to implement *the Framework Convention on Tobacco Control*. And more efforts would be made to fully ban smoking in public places to realize the tobacco control goals of the 12th Five-Year Plan.

(Qu Yang)

18. The 2012 Global Health Diplomacy Executive Education Training Course Was Held in Shanghai

The 2012 Global Health Diplomacy Executive Education Training Course was held in Shanghai from July 23-27, 2012. 37 trainees from the relevant Chinese ministries, the relevant Chinese medical institutions and colleges, Australia, Cambodia, Indonesia and other 9 countries of the Asian-Pacific region participated in the training. Ren Minghui, Director of the International Cooperation Department of Ministry of Health attended the ceremony and delivered a speech on behalf of Chen Zhu, Minister of Ministry of Health. The main purpose of the week-long course was to provide the trainees with updated knowledge and perspectives on global health diplomacy and promote China's involvement in the collective actions on global health issues. The course covered the topics of concepts of global health and global health diplomacy, relation between health and diplomacy, governance of global health, global health strategies and so on. The trainees had discussions over the issues like China's global health strategy and policy of medical aid to other countries. The Global Health Diplomacy Executive Education Training Course was sponsored by Center for Global Health of Peking University and the Graduate Institute, Geneva.

(Qu Yang)

19. Vice Minister of Health Liu Qian Attended the Signing Ceremony of Partnership Agreement between China's National Center for Cardiovascular Diseases(Fuwai Hospital) and Merck Research Laboratories

Vice Minister of Health Liu Qian attended the signing ceremony of Partnership Agreement between China's National Center for Cardiovascular Diseases(Fuwai Hospital) and Merck Research Laboratories on August 1, 2012. In his speech, Liu Qian placed great expectation on the cooperation and he hoped that the two sides would figure out more rational strategies on the prevention and control of cardiovascular diseases.

(Qu Yang)

20. Minister of Health Chen Zhu Met Former Secretary of Health and Human Services of USA Mike Leavitt

Minister of Health Chen Zhu Met the visiting former US Secretary of Health and Human Services and currently board director of Medtronic, Inc. Mike Leavitt in Ministry of Health on August 6, 2012. Chen Zhu hoped that the cooperation between Medtronic, Inc. and its Chinese partners would be strengthened and the multidisciplinary study on the health path management for chronic diseases would be carried out. The Chinese institutions participating in the cooperation included National Center for Cardiovascular Diseases, National Health Development Research Center and Ruijin Hospital of Medical College of Shanghai Jiaotong University.

(Qu Yang)

21. Minister of Health Chen Zhu Met the Delegation from the Cancer Research Institute of USA

Minister of Health Chen Zhu met Director of the Cancer Research Institute of USA Frank McCormick and the delegation headed by him on August 16, 2012. They had in-depth exchange over intensifying the bilateral cooperation. Chen Zhu said that he would actively support the practical cooperation carried out by the institute in China, especially the collaboration and exchange in the fields like the translational medicine and the clinical research of cancer. Thus, more people would benefit from the cooperation.

(Qu Yang)

22. Minister of Health Chen Zhu Met GAVI's CEO Seth Berkley

Minister of Health Chen Zhu met Seth Berkley, CEO of the Global Alliance for Vaccines and Immunization (GAVI) on September 10, 2012. Chen Zhu spoke highly of the bilateral cooperative program on hepatitis B vaccine and gave a brief introduction to the development in China's vaccination planning. He hoped that the two sides would expand the cooperation in cancer vaccine, mother to child transmission of hepatitis B, hepatitis B vaccination strategy, and the development and research of vaccines against hepatitis and other diseases. In addition, he wished to push forward the pre-authentication of the medicines and vaccines made in China by WHO with the support of GAVI so that the Chinese vaccines could be exported. Berkley expressed his willingness to cooperate with China in new vaccine development and technology transformation and hoped that China would get more involved in GAVI's activities in terms of vaccine development and export. The two sides agreed to popularize China's experience and make efforts to push forward the vaccination planning in other developing countries by means of tripartite cooperation. Relevant officials from the International Cooperation Department of Ministry of Health, the Disease Control and Prevention Bureau of Ministry of Health and China's CDC attended the meeting.

(Qu Yang)

23. Minister of Health Chen Zhu Attended the 2012 Summer World Economic Forum (the Summer Davos) in Tianjin

The World Economic Forum's sixth Annual Meeting of the New Champions (also known as the Summer Davos) was held in Tianjin from September 11-13, 2012. Minister of Health Chen Zhu attended the opening ceremony and the discussion session- Sustainable Health Systems in the Future Economy. During the session, Chen Zhu gave a brief introduction to the concepts and development of China's health care reform and analyzed the relation between health and economy. He put forward 5 opinions. First, the Chinese health authorities welcomed the private sectors and foreign enterprises to invest in China's health industry. Second, better care at lower cost should be provided alone with high-end health service and the service models and contents should be diverse to meet the meet the needs of different people. Third, China's biomedicine industry was promising. Fourth, there was a huge market for commercial health insurance that could meet various needs. Fifth, the health care industry in China had great development potential. He called on the national capital to take the opportunity and become more engaged in the thriving health care industry. After the discussion, Chen Zhu met with Klaus Schwab, Executive Chairman of World

Economic Forum, had a meeting with the relevant officials from Tianjin Municipal Government, and observed the seminar of the Tianjin First Center Hospital on public hospital reform.

(Qu Yang)

24. Vice Minister of Health Liu Qian Attended the Ceremony for the 30th Anniversary of China's Cooperation with UNICEF and Was Conferred an Honorary Award

Vice Minister of Health Liu Qian attended the ceremony for the 30th anniversary of China's cooperation with UNICEF held in the UNICEF office in Beijing and accepted an honorary partnership award for China's cooperation in maternal and child health on September 19, 2012. Liu Qian thanked UNICEF for its support to China's work in the maternal and child health over the past 30 years. He hoped that the bilateral cooperation would be enhanced to improve the health of women and children in China. UNICEF Deputy Executive Director Yoka Brandt and UNICEF representative to China Gillian Mellsop thanked Chinese Ministry of Health for its cooperation and praised China for signing the Convention on the Rights of the Child. China pledged to carry out national activities and international cooperation to improve the rights of the child. The relevant officials from the International Cooperation Department and the Department of Maternal and Child Health Care and Community Health attended the ceremony.

(Qu Yang)

25. The Chinese Medical Team Went to DPRK to Perform Free Cataract Operations and Donate Medical Equipment and Medicine

On request of the Ministry of Public Health, DPRK, Chinese Ministry of Health and Sichuan Provincial People's Government sent a medical team of 16 people to DPRK. From September 19-28, 2012, the team performed free cataract operations and donated equipment and medicine worth more than 3 million yuan. During their stay in DPRK, they screened over 430 patients and performed 233 cataract surgeries. In addition, the team gave on-the-spot guidance and training to DPRK's medical workers. On behalf of Chinese Ministry of Health and Sichuan Provincial People's Government, Deputy Director of Sichuan Health Department Zhao Wanhua donated the relevant equipment and medicine to the Ministry of Public Health, DPRK. Chinese ambassador to DPRK Liu Hongcai and Deputy Minister of Public Health of DPRK Kang Ha kook attended the donation. Liu Hongcai fully affirmed the performance of the Chinese medical team and praised Chinese Ministry of Health and Sichuan Provincial People's Government for their efforts to improve the health of the people in both countries and their efforts to strengthen the bilateral friendship. Deputy Minister of Public Health of DPRK Kang Ha kook thanked the Chinese medical team for their hard work and indicated that the free surgeries and the donation of equipment and medicine would boost the development of DPRK's health industry. The medical team consisted of experts from Sichuan Provincial People s Hospital and West China Hospital of Sichuan University.

(Qu Yang)

26. Vice Minister of Health Huang Jiefu Met the Delegation from China Medical Board(CMB) in USA

On September 22, 2012, Vice Minister of Health Huang Jiefu met with CMB Chair Mary Bullock and President Lincoln Chen and they exchanged opinions over further strengthening the bilateral cooperation. Huang Jiefu thanked CMB for its long-term support and assistance to China's medical education and training of grassroots medical workers. He also appreciated CMB's efforts in promoting the study of global health policies and fostering global health medical talents. Huang Jiefu hoped that new cooperation would be explored to give support to the priorities in China's health care reform.

(Qu Yang)

27. 3 Foreign Experts Recommended by Ministry of Health were Awarded the Chinese Government Friendship Award

On September 28, 2012, the awarding ceremony of the 2012 "Friendship Award" of the Chinese government was held at the Great Hall of the People. 3 foreign experts recommended by Ministry of Health got the award. On the afternoon of September 29, Premier Wen Jiabao of the State Council met at the Great Hall of the People with the foreign experts winning the award and their families on behalf of the Chinese government and people. Premier Wen congratulated the award-winning foreign experts, thanked them for their outstanding contribution to China's economic development and social progress and extended his cordial greetings to all the foreign experts and international friends working in China and their families. The "Friendship Award" was set up by the Chinese government for the foreign experts who had made outstanding contributions to the economic and social development in China. The 50 winners of 2012 award came from 22 countries. Since 1991, a total of 1,249 foreign experts from 65 countries had received this award.

(Qu Yang)

28. Vice Minister of Health Chen Xiaohong Met AERAS CEO James Connolly

On October 18, 2012, Vice Minister of Health Chen Xiaohong met AERAS CEO James Connolly and they exchanged opinions over the prevention and treatment of tuberculosis and the development and manufacture of tuberculosis vaccine. Chen Xiaohong thanked AERAS for its concern and support to China's prevention and treatment of tuberculosis and hoped that the development and research of tuberculosis vaccine could be combined with the preventive policy to realize social value of the vaccine research. Connolly praised China for the achievements and contributions in the prevention and treatment of tuberculosis and he expressed his willingness to intensify the exchange and cooperation with China in the development and manufacture of tuberculosis vaccine. The relevant officials from the Disease Control and Prevention Bureau, the Science and Education Division and the International Cooperation Department of Ministry of Health attended the meeting.

(Qu Yang)

29. Minister of Health Chen Zhu Met the Outgoing United Nations Country Coordinator on AIDS in Beijing Mark Stirling

On October 18, 2012, Minister of Health Chen Zhu met the Outgoing United Nations Country Coordinator on AIDS in Beijing Mark Stirling. Chen Zhu praised UNAIDS and the international society for the long-term support to China's prevention and control of AIDS and thanked Mark Stirling for his efforts and contribution to China's AIDS control. He emphasized that China would like to cooperate with UNAIDS and the international society to promote the development in global health and AIDS control. Mark Stirling thanked China for the support to his work and spoke highly of the accomplishments and innovations China made in AIDS prevention and control.

(Qu Yang)

30. Vice Minister of Health Huang Jiefu Attended the China-Australia Symposium on the Improvement of Organ Donation System

On October 23, 2012, Vice Minister of Health Huang Jiefu attended the China-Australia Symposium on the Improvement of Organ Donation System and made a keynote speech on organ donation and social development of China. Huang Jiefu gave an overall introduction to the general situation of organ donation in China, the donation system and the pilot work of it. Later, the experts from the two sides had in-depth discussion and exchange over the issues like allocation of the organs, transplantation of kidney and liver in China, and ethics, laws and system of organ transplantation. As one of the key activities of the 100th anniversary of Peking University Health Science Center, the symposium was sponsored by Peking University Health Science Center and Sydney Medical School of the University of Sydney, co-sponsored by Peking University Organ Transplantation Center and attended by 150 experts and scholars from Chinese Ministry of Health, the University of Sydney, Peking University, Tsinghua University, the University of Hong Kong, Huazhong University of Science and Technology, Peking Union Medical College and the 309th Hospital of PLA.

(Qu Yang)

31. Minister of Health Chen Zhu Wrote a Letter to Condole the Passing of Cambodian King-father Norodom Sihanouk

On the morning of December 15, 2012, Cambodian King-father Norodom Sihanouk passed away in Beijing. Minister of Health Chen Zhu wrote a letter to the Cambodian embassy in China to express his deepest condolences. Chen Zhu spoke highly of King-father Norodom Sihanouk for his contribution to China-Cambodia relation and asked the Cambodian embassy to relay his condolences to the family. In addition, specially-assigned persons from Ministry of Health went to the Cambodian embassy to offer condolences.

(Qu Yang)

32. Ministry of Health Organized the Lecture on Health Care Delivery Science

On November 2, 2012, director of Dartmouth Center for Health Care Delivery Science and academician of the American National Academy of Sciences Albert Mulley was invited by Chinese Ministry of Health to give a lecture-*Take Opportunity of Health Care Reform and Enjoy the Benefits of Innovation*. Chinese Health Minister Chen Zhu, Vice Health Minister Huang Jiefu and the representatives from the departments and bureaus of Ministry of Health attended the lecture.

(Qu Yang)

33. Minister of Health Chen Zhu Met Joanna Rubinstein, Assistant Director of the Earth Institute for International Programs at Columbia University

On November 3, 2012, Minister of Health Chen Zhu met Joanna Rubinstein,

Assistant Director of the Earth Institute for International Programs at Columbia University, and they exchanged opinions over the development of global health, the cooperation with Africa and the sustainable development after 2015.

(Qu Yang)

34. World Health Organization Announced that China Regained the Polio-free Status

The 18th meeting of the Regional Commission for the Certification of Poliomyelitis Eradication was held in Beijing from November 26-29, 2012. After the review of the commission, the meeting announced that China had regained its polio-free status. After four cases of wild poliovirus infection were confirmed in Xinjiang Uygur Autonomous Region in August of 2011, the Chinese government promptly launched emergency response plans and a massive vaccination campaign which had effectively blocked the spread of the polio epidemic. Approximately 100 participants, including commissioners from the Regional Commission for the Certification of Poliomyelitis Eradication and the Commissions for the Certification of Poliomyelitis Eradication of 17 countries and regions, officials from WHO and Secretariat of WHO West Pacific Region and representatives from UN agencies, foundations and NGOs, attended the meeting.

(Qu Yang)

35. LOI of the China-HMS Collaboration in Transitional Medicine was Signed

On December 12, 2012, Vice Health Minister Liu Qian attended Signing Ceremony for LOI of the China-HMS Collaboration in Transitional Medicine and Forum and witnessed the signing of the LOI together with Deputy Mayor of Shanghai Shen Xiaoming. Chen Zhu, Minister of Health delivered a speech over the video. He congratulated the signing of the LOI and had great expectation on the high-end cooperation with HMS on translational medicine.

(Qu Yang)

36. Training Course for Division Chiefs of Health Diplomacy was Organized in Fujian

The national training course for division chiefs of health diplomacy was organized in Quanzhou City of Fujian Province from December 19-21, 2012. Approximately 70 trainees from the provincial or municipal health departments and the departments of Ministry of Health participated in the course. Director of the International Cooperation Department Ren Minghui attended the course and delivered a speech. He said that under the new circumstances, the nationwide health workers should study and implement the spirit of the Eighteenth Congress of Chinese Communist Party and spare no efforts to service the course of all-round construction of well-off society, the development of the health undertaking and the deepening of the health care reform. With the globalization of health issues, their position in the global development became increasingly prominent. China would get more engaged in the global health actions and practices. All the medical workers in China should think strategically and practice innovatively to push forward the formulation of China's global health strategies and the development of China's health undertaking. The scholars from Peking University and Renmin University of China gave lectures on the international situation, China's diplomatic strategies, global health, China's cooperation with WHO and dispatch of foreign medical aiding teams. Comprehensive quality-oriented training of the trainees was organized and the trainees also had filed trips to the foreign medical institutions in China.

(Qu Yang)

Section 5   International Cooperation Projects

1. Progress in China-US Cooperation—Global AIDS Program (GAP)

China-US Cooperation—Global AIDS Program (GAP) went well in 2012. The actions of the program were carried out within the framework of China's AIDS prevention and control plan and had positive influence on the formulation of AIDS policies. Meanwhile, the abilities of China's AIDS technicians and laboratories were elevated. The execution rate of the program reached 96.62%. The main accomplishments covered the following five aspects. First, surveillance of cases was strengthened. Great support was given to the surveillance, survey, consultation and testing. 2,059,000 people were screened and 2,480 were found HIV positive with 2,280 of them transferred to CDC. Second, the case management ability was elevated. Support of GAP was given to the development of *the National Handbook on Free Access to HIV/AIDS-related Treatment(Version 3)* and the analysis of the data of national programs on antiviral treatment of HIV/AIDS. Relevant activities were conducted within the national framework of the prevention of mother-to-child transmission. GAP participated in the formulation of the national handbook on diagnosis and treatment of TB/HIV and piloted in Sichuan and Hunan the programs on TB/HIV and HIV/HCV/HBV. And surveys on the factors that contributed to low rate of treatment among the IDU group were done. Third, the construction of laboratory system was enhanced. Assistance was given to the national reference laboratory for passing the certification as the laboratory of the highest international level. Meanwhile, the progress to get College of American Pathologists (CAP) Laboratory Accreditation was started. Fourth, the ability of AIDS medical technicians was elevated. Trainings on clinical treatment were conducted in regions with a high incidence. 185 doctors were trained and 66% of them became experts in clinical treatment in the local medical facilities. Fifth, the applied research was done. The evaluation program on methadone maintenance treatment (MMT) and the prevention of HIV/HBV infant infection among HIV/HBV affected pregnant women in mid-term and late stage of pregnancy by antiviral treatment were carried out.

(Qu Yang)

2. China-US Collaborative Program on Emerging and Re-emerging Infectious Diseases

China-US Collaborative Program on Emerging and Re-emerging Infectious Diseases went well in 2012. Reform was done in the management of the program and the execution of the fund was optimized with an execution rate of 98%. The program was conducted in close collaboration with the major national health issues like the control of major diseases and response to public health emergencies and it was fruitful. 149 symposiums, consultations or coordinating meetings were organized, 80 training courses held and 26 documents, including summaries, development plans, drafts, handbooks, proposals and translations, compiled. 173 times of surveys or evaluations were carried out, 21 people were trained overseas and 24 American experts came to China. 184 articles were published home and abroad, 4,035 persons/ times were trained in the training courses of the program and 46,438 samples were tested.

(Qu Yang)

3. China-Australia Health and HIV/AIDS Facility was Completed

In December of 2012, China-Australia Health and HIV/AIDS Facility was successfully completed and the yearly executive rate was 100%. On November 22, 2012, the completion ceremony of China-Australia Health and HIV/AIDS Facility was held in Beijing. The Facility carried out fruitful activities in collaboration with the main tasks of Chinese Ministry of Health. The activities were mainly conducted in perfecting the new rural cooperative medical system, strengthening the national basic drug system, pushing forward the fairness of the basic health service, intensifying the pilot reform of public hospitals and enhancing AIDS prevention and control. The 5-year program submitted 70 suggestions for policy formulation and had positive influence. 29 project institutions of the 52 sub-programs collaborated closely with 26 Australian institutions and formed sustainable cooperative partnership. The administrative ability of the health departments, the ability of the medical workers, the ability in health information collection and utilization, the ability of the relevant organizations in policy solicitation and development and the ability in participating in the global health issues were elevated. The Facility gave more opportunities for China to have practice in crass-border prevention and control of AIDS and other global health issues and accumulated experience for China's future involvement in global health issues.

(Qu Yang)

4. China-UK Global Health Support Program was Launched

In September 2012, China-UK Global Health Support Program was launched. It was a five-year initiative with a UK investment of £12 million. The programmed would build capacity for DFID and low income countries to learn lessons from China's unparalleled success in reducing infant, child and maternal mortality rates, disease prevention and control and so on. The program would also help to improve China's capacity to contribute to global health. The Ministry of Health's Centre for Project Supervision and Management would provide program management. The launching ceremony and the first meeting of the strategic committee were held. The plans for the first year and the expert panel of the program were decided. At present, the management regulation, the program budget and the purchase procedures were being drafted.

(Qu Yang)

5. China-US Partnership on Smoke-free Workplaces was Launched

On August 17, 2012, *the Joint Statement on Establishing the China-United States Partnership on Smoke-free Workplaces* was issued by Chinese Ministry of Health and United States Department of Health and Human Services and the China-US Partnership on Smoke-free Workplaces was launched. On September 7, the launching ceremony was held in Beijing. Huang Jiefu, China's vice health minister and Howard Koh, assistant secretary of the US HHS attended the ceremony. China's CDC would provide program management and set up an office to manage the popularization and implementation of the program. Smoking in workplaces was a serious health problem in China, as over 63 percent of employees were exposed to secondhand smoke in workplaces. The program would conduct aggressive publicity campaigns and mobilize the whole society, especially the companies. The logo and the publicity materials were designed to recruit participants from companies operating in China for the promotion of 100-percent smoke-free workplaces. The charity salon would be set up for the company participants to share their experience in creating smoke-free workplaces. By the end of 2012, 68 companies in China joined in the program and approximately 288,000 employees would benefit.

(Qu Yang)

6. Progress of the AIDS and Tuberculosis Prevention and Treatment Program of Chinese Ministry of Health-Bill & Melinda Gates Foundation (BMGF)

In 2012, the AIDS Prevention and Treatment Program of MOH with Bill & Melinda Gates Foundation mainly made preparations for the pilot of the comprehensive models. The preparations included the recruitment and determination of the piloting regions in Jiangsu, Hubei, Shaanxi and Ningxia, the completion of implementation plans for the comprehensive models of tuberculosis control and the Ningxia project, the establishment of the national laboratories and the infection control expert panel, and the commencement of evaluation of the program and baseline survey. The fund executed in the first phase was 11,920,000 yuan with an execution rate of 88.90%. For the selection of pilot regions, the plan for the second phase was delayed and the actual fund executed was 2,820,000 yuan. The main program activities included the pilot of HIV/AIDS screening and case management at the community health service centers, terminal assessment and summary of service models, and the review, exchange and share of program experience. Progress was made in the AIDS screening among MSMs, the screening rate of AIDS in the medical facilities and the case management. The total budget for 2012 was 37,431,600 yuan, the actual expenditure was 34,338,200 yuan and the executive rate was 91.7%.

(Qu Yang)

7. China-MSD HIV/AIDS Partnership

In 2012, the China-MSD HIV/AIDS Partnership (hereinafter referred to as C-MAP) focused mainly on the AIDS prevention and control in Liangshan prefecture and the review and popularization of experience. The transition of the program was done well. The assessment of the first stage of the program was done and the application for the second stage was under way. The number of patients receiving the antiviral treatment in Liangshan prefecture was 4,859. The number of people covered by the AIDS prevention publicity in Sichuan was 973,468 and the number of people covered among the migrating population was 288,552. The program expenditure of 2012 was 14,940,000 yuan.

(Qu Yang)

8. Progress of the Advanced International Courses of Health Development and Reform (Harvard Program)

From December 2-22, 2012, the seventh Advanced International Courses of Health Development and Reform (Harvard Program) were held. 25 trainees from Ministry of Health, Research Office of the State Council, Ministry of Finance and some provincial health departments took the courses in Tsinghua University for a week and went to Harvard University to continue the training. The courses covered the issues like policy formulation, implementation and evaluation and health development and reform. The trainees also visited some health institutions in USA. Centering on the priorities and difficulties in the health care reform, the trainees compiled their study reports on topics of the development of health industry, reform of payment system, enhancement of the quality control, and management of public hospitals. They presented the reports at the end of the training courses.

(Qu Yang)

9. Progress of Smile Train—the Cleft Lip and Palate Repair Program

Smile Train—the Cleft Lip and Palate Repair Program was an initiative jointly carried out by Chinese Ministry of Health, US Smile Train, China Charity Federation and Chinese Stomatological Association. In 2012, the program sponsored 26,954 repair operations with a total donation of approximately 120,000,000 yuan. In September 2012, the 8th academic conference of Smile Train was held and the number of trainees reached 1,500. In addition, two training courses on anesthesia were held with 116 anesthetists trained. Documentaries and charity publicity videos about the program were made as well. Other activities like rehabilitation training and aid were also conducted.

(Qu Yang)

10. Health Cooperation Program with Dartmouth College

The cooperation program with Dartmouth College was carried out by the

International Cooperation Department of Ministry of Health and Dartmouth College and it mainly covered the fields like health care service, training of specialists and academic exchanges. In April 2012, the Chinese delegation headed by director of the International Cooperation Department Ren Minghui visited Dartmouth College. The two sides held the first steering committee meeting and discussed the cooperative fields, priorities and the five-year plan for the program. In October and November of 2012, the program organized the lecture *"Take Opportunity of Health Care Reform and Enjoy the Benefits of Innovation"* in Shanghai and Beijing and shared the solutions to the improvement of doctor-patient relation and the rational allocation of medical resources with Chinese health officials and health policy researchers.

(Qu Yang)

11. The Progress of the Sino-French Program on Prevention against Emerging Infectious Diseases

In 2012 the construction of the building for the P4 laboratory for the Sino-French Program on Prevention against Emerging Infectious Diseases was basically completed. The seventh steering committee meeting and the eighth secretariat meeting of the program were held from October 29-30, 2012. During the meetings, the progress in the construction of the P4 laboratory, bio-safety laws and regulations, laboratory standards, personnel training and scientific research was reported. *The Operation Handbook of the Sino-French Program on Prevention against Emerging Infectious Diseases* was officially approved. The two sides reached a series of agreements and they expressed that they would soon reach the supplementary agreement, carry out evaluation and set up the on-the-spot working team as soon as possible. And they would push forward the establishment of the lab with a positive and constructive attitude.

(Qu Yang)

12. The International Cooperation Department of MOH-Foundation Mérieux Cooperation on Prevention against Tuberculosis and Nosocomial Infection

The second round of the International Cooperation Department of MOH-Foundation Mérieux Cooperation on Prevention against Tuberculosis was successfully launched on 23 March, 2012. The two sides signed the LOI (2012-2017) for the second round. Minister of Health Chen Zhu attended the signing ceremony and delivered a speech. On October 30, 2012, the first meeting of the administrative committee was held in Wuhan and approved the implementation plans. The first round of the

International Cooperation Department of MOH-Foundation Mérieux Cooperation on Prevention against Tuberculosis was completed. From October 21-28, 2012, the last activity of the first round was held in France. The presidents and testing technicians from the program hospitals attended the training on nosocomial infection. The trainees had in-depth and extensive exchanges and discussions with French experts.

(Qu Yang)

13. The Progress of the Belgian Damien Foundation Project on Tuberculosis/ Leprosy Prevention and Treatment in China

In 2012, the Belgian Damien Foundation Project on Tuberculosis/Leprosy Prevention and Treatment in China went well. The program carried out activities mainly in personnel capacity building, discovery and treatment MDR-TB patients, control of nosocomial infection and popularization of new TB diagnosis techniques. The expenditure in 2012 was 3,357,526 yuan. The regions covered were Inner Mongolia, Guizhou, Tibet, Qinghai and Ningxia province/autonomous region. In-service training and on-the-spot training of TB prevention personnel at provincial, municipal, county, township and village levels in the project provinces/autonomous regions were conducted. The trainings mainly covered laboratory techniques, quality control of the laboratories, collaboration of the treatment and prevention departments, statistics management, project management, MDR-TB infection control, prevention and treatment and so on. The treatment of the newly-discovered MDR-TB patients would be continuously sponsored. The program would provide for the expenses of the two-year treatment, the regular examinations, the initial hospitalization and the incentive-based patient management. Support was given by the program to organize the national training courses in Zhejiang, which was conducted by China's CDC and provided systematic training on the TB infection control for the backbone doctors in the designated provincial hospitals. The pilot of using the light-emitting diode fluorescence microscopy in TB testing was carried out in Tibet and the relevant training was done as well. By the piloting and the popularization of the new international techniques, the local TB diagnosis ability was greatly enhanced.

(Qu Yang)

14. Progress of "Go to the West"—County-level Hospital Doctors Training Program between Ministry of Health and the Bayer Company

"Go to the West"—County-level Hospital Doctors Training Program was a strategic initiative between Chinese Ministry of Health and the Bayer Company, aiming to cultivate a health talent contingent consisting of backbone medical technicians and management personnel in the county hospitals in the mid-west provinces/autonomous regions/municipalities. The activities of the program conducted in 2012 covered mainly two aspects. First, 9 training courses for doctors were organized with 456 doctors in the hospitals trained. And 21 training courses for management of the county public hospitals were organized with 4,235 people trained. Second, 3 sets of textbooks tailored to the doctors in the county and grassroots hospitals were compiled by Lanzhou University and published by People's Medical Publishing House in 2012.

(Qu Yang)

15. Community Health Program of the Novartis Foundation

The following activities of the program were carried out. First, the review of national demonstration community health centers was conducted. The reference indexes to the selection of the 2012 national demonstration community health centers were formulated. 161 communities were awarded the 2012 National Demonstration Community Health Center. Second, the national training bases for community health service were set up. By the end of August 2012, 17 training bases had qualified as the national training centers. Third, the specialized funds for community health service research were established and support given to the relevant studies. Fourth, the evaluation and survey on the national primary public health service regulations were performed. A survey panel of 35 relevant experts was established and two meetings of the panel were held. The range, methods and specific action plans of the survey was determined. At the end of 2012, the panel meeting was held and the annual summary of the work conducted. Fifth, the training for the administrative personnel of community health was performed. Two training courses were organized in Beijing and Changchun with nearly 100 trainees. Sixth, training courses on the construction of the community health service abilities were conducted. Over 300 trainees participated in the courses.

(Qu Yang)

16. Progress of Health Campaign in Western China

On July 18, 2012, Minister of Health Chen Zhu, Director-General of WHO Margaret Chan and WHO's Regional Director for the Western Pacific Shin Young-soo signed *the MOU on Improving People's Health in Western China* respectively with Vice Chairwoman of Guangxi Zhuang Autonomous Region Li Kang, Deputy Mayor of Chongqing Wu Gang and Vice Governor of Shaanxi Zheng Xiaoming. In November of 2012, the International Cooperation Department of MOH and WHO respectively went to Guangxi, Chongqing and Shaanxi to study and discuss the action plans and the management framework of the Health Campaign in Western China. From December 10-14, 2012, WHO's Regional Director for the Western Pacific Shin Young-soo went to Shaanxi and Chongqing to investigate the development of the health campaign and the local health care reform.

(Qu Yang)

17. Program on "Improving Nutrition, Food Safety and Food Security for China's Most Vulnerable Women and Children" of the UN-Spain Millennium Development Goals Achievement Fund (UN-Spain MDG-Fund)

Two meetings of the executive committee of Program on "Improving Nutrition, Food Safety and Food Security for China's Most Vulnerable Women and Children" of UN-Spain MDG-Fund were held in 2012. On May 2, the first executive committee meeting was held in Beijing. The developments of the program in 2011 were reviewed, the accomplishments and experience summed up, the 2012 plans of the program office approved, the budgets for major program activities decided and the arrangements for the program closure evaluation and summary of experience at the end of 2012 determined. The meeting required that the international organizations accelerate the appropriation of funds to ensure the completion of the program by the end of 2012. The program institutions should enhance the execution of the program, sum up achievements, formulated sustainable plans, promote the transformation of the program outcomes into policies and enlarge the coverage. On September 6, the second executive committee meeting was held in Beijing. The meeting discussed the relevant issues over the completion of the program. It was clarified that the terminal appraisal and the summary meeting should lay emphasis on summary of experience, discovery of exemplary cases, popularization of the best practice to provide practical grounds and policy suggestions for Chinese government and to improve nutrition, food safety and food security for China's most vulnerable women and children. The meeting required that all the sides accelerate the speed and the appropriation, complete the terminal appraisal and summary, and carry out publicity and popularization of the program's experience in accordance with working priorities of each department. Director of the International Cooperation Department of MOH and Chinese chair of the program Ren Minghui, WHO Representative in China and the international chair Dr. Michael O'Leary, representatives from 8 UN agencies in China, and the relevant personnel from China's program implementation departments and research institutions attended the two meetings.

(Qu Yang)

18. China/WHO Cooperation Projects of the Annual Budget Planning (2012-2013) was Launched

From February 9-10, 2012, the launching meeting of China/WHO Cooperation Projects of the Annual Budget Planning (2012-2013) was held in Beijing. The meeting summed up the experience of the 2010-2011 projects and introduced the rules for the formulation of the 2012-2013 plans, the priorities, the features of fund allocation and the requirements for the project departments in 2012-2013.The meeting also listened to the result of the external appraisal on the project implementation and the report on the general situation of 2012-2013 projects. In addition, World Health Organization Representative Office in China gave an introduction to the strategies and directions of WHO and the action plans for the health campaigns in western China. In addition, training for the program departments of 2012-2013 on program implementation and management was also organized by the office. Over 260 participants from Beijing Health Bureau, Shanghai Health Bureau, China's CDC, Chinese Academy of Medical Sciences, World Health Organization Representative Office in China, the collaborating centers of WHO in China, the implementation departments of the 2012-2013 projecs and the relevant departments and bureaus of Chinese Ministry of Health attended the meeting.

(Qu Yang)

19. The Global Fund Cooperation Program in China

The Global Fund Cooperation Program in China went basically well in 2012. Due to the sespension of fund by the Secretariat of the Global Fund in May- August in 2011, the appropriation of fund in 2012 was behind the schedule and the executive rate of the first two seasons was comparatively low. The total disbursement of the program was $ 135,000,000 in 2012. From 2003-2012, $762,000,000 was allocated for cooperative programs with China. At present, the first stage of NSA for malaria and the sixth round of malaria program would end at the middle of 2012. The provincial projects of AIDS program would end on December 31, 2012. And only the social organization's program would be continued until the end of 2013. The tuberculosis program went basically well and the extension application had been filed to the Global Fund due to lack of fund.

On February 28, 2012, the launching meeting of the 10th Round of China-the Global Fund Program on Malaria was held in Mang City, Dehong Prefecture, Yunnan. Approximately 70 participants from the International Cooperation Department of Chinese Ministry of Health, China's CDC, the Health Department of Yunnan, the People's Government of Dehong Prefecture, and the Ministry of Health of Myanmar attended the meeting. The 10th round of China program on malaria was granted by the Board of the Global Fund in December 2010. The implementation agreement was official signed in December 2012 and the program was implemented in January 2012 and would last for 2 years with a maximum fund of $ 5,080,000. The program would cover 7 counties of 3 prefectures in Yunnan, five special regions in Myanmar along the Chinese borders, mainly aiming to lower the burden of malaria in the five special regions in Myanmar, monitor the artemisinin resistance, control the imported cases and promote the eradication of malaria in China. 70% of the program fund would be used for the activities in Myanmar. China's CDC was the principal recipient(PR) and the Yunnan Health Department was the national program office, which was in charge of the specific program management and implementation. The sub-recipients were Yunnan Institute of Parasitic Diseases, Health Unlimited(HU) representative office in Yunnan and Yunnan Entry-Exit Inspection and Quarantine Bureau.

(Qu Yang)

20. China-Japan Program on Public Health Policy Planning and Management

IN 2012, according to *the Minute of Chinese Ministry of Health–Japan International Cooperation Agency(JICA) on Implementation Plans for China-Japan Technical Cooperation,* the EPI meeting was held once, ten research students for EPI were sent abroad, a Japanese expert was sent to China and two research students for tuberculosis were sent abroad.

(Qu Yang)

21. Program of China-ASEAN Public Health Cooperation Fund

China-ASEAN Public Health Cooperation Fund was an initiative of the Chinese government, aiming to support the health cooperation between China and ASEAN to fight against the regional infectious diseases with a total budget of 10,000,000 yuan. By November of 2012, with the application of Ministry of Health, 14 programs were approved by Ministry of Foreign Affairs after consulting Ministry of Finance. In 2012, 3 of the programs were implemented. 2012 China-ASEAN Symposium on Harmonious Policies and Operating Procedures of Traditional Chinese Medicine was held in Beijing from April 15-21. 17 participants from the 10 ASEAN member countries attended the symposium and exchanged experience over the harmonious policies and time operating procedures of traditional Chinese medicine. The 3rd China-ASEAN Forum on Dentistry, sponsored by MOH and the People's Government of Guangxi Zhuang Autonomous Region and organized by College of Stomatology of

Guangxi Medical University, was held in Nanning, Guangxi. The 1st Forum on Human Resources for Health in Asia-Pacific Region was held in Nanning from November 29-30, 2012. The forum aimed to implement China's national leaders' proposals at the East Asia Summit and share experience of the practical cases in human resource development and management to provide support to the administrative departments to formulate the health human resource strategies and planning.

(Qu Yang)

22. Program of China-ASEAN Cooperative Fund

East Asia was a place with a high incidence of human influenza, animal influenza and bird influenza and was the source of several influenza epidemics. In order to share the experience of influenza prevention and control in Asian countries, improve the testing ability of the laboratories in the influenza prevention and control departments in these nations and set up the regular communication and long-term cooperation mechanism, Ministry of Health applied for support from Ministry of Foreign Affair for the program "Cooperation on Flu Monitoring in Asia" and requested for a fund of 1,280,000 yuan.

(Qu Yang)

23. Program of the ASEAN Plus China, Japan and South Korea(10+3) Cooperation Fund

In order to share experience of influenza prevention and control with other countries, push forward the influenza monitoring in ASEAN countries and other Asian states, improve the testing ability of the laboratories in the influenza prevention and control departments of these nations and set up the regular communication and long-term cooperation mechanism, Ministry of Health applied for support from Ministry of Foreign Affair for the program "China-ASEAN Symposium on Response to Emerging Infectious Diseases" and requested for a fund of 599,500 yuan.

(Qu Yang)

Section 6   Collaborations with Hong Kong, Macao and Taiwan

Vice Health Minister Wang Guoqiang Attended the Meeting of Consortium of Globalization of Chinese Medicine in Macao

From August 21-23, 2012, Vice Health Minister and Commissioner of State Administration of Traditional Chinese Medicine Wang Guoqiang with the delegation headed by him visited Macao. During his stay in Macao, he attended the 11th Meeting of Consortium of Globalization of Chinese Medicine and made a speech. He indicated that after Macau returned to China, the Macau SAR government had valued greatly the development of Chinese Medicine, and the Health Bureau of Macau and Consortium of Globalization of Chinese Medicine had made tremendous efforts to create a good environment for the development of Chinese Medicine. The professionals of Chinese Medicine in Macau had united their strengths and worked very hard. He thanked them for their commitment and dedications. Chinese Medicine in Macau had gained impressive growth, especially in the standardization, regulation, and modernization of Chinese Medicine. A unique way of development had formed in advancing Chinese medicine in Macau and had gained wide recognition from the local community. University of Macau, Macau University of Science and Technology, and other higher education institutions in Macau had been long committed to nurturing talents in Chinese medicine, and had continuously improved their academic research quality. Wang Guoqiang pointed out that more scientific innovations should be made so Chinese Medicine could be part of super science era and yield more fruits. Consortium of Globalization of Chinese Medicine(hereinafter referred to as CGCM) was founded in December of 2003 and the secretariat is located in the School of Medicine, the University of Hong Kong. CGCM aims to integrate the wisdom and strength of Chinese medicine research in academia and industry worldwide and to promote the internationalization of Chinese medicine research and cooperation, so that traditional Chinese medicine could benefit all mankind. Well-known teaching and research institutions and pharmaceutical companies from more than 20 countries and regions have joined. Currently CGCM have more than 120 existing members. CGCM would hold an annual academic meeting and has received much more attentions from the international pharmaceutical industries. During the stay in Macao, the delegation headed by Wang Guoqiang, visited the Health Bureau of Macao, Macau University of Science and Technology, the State Key Laboratory of Quality Research in Chinese Medicine of Macau University of Science and Technology and other relevant organizations.

(Qu Yang)

Chapter XVII　Construction of Spiritual Civilization

Construction of Spiritual Civilization in 2012

In 2012, the following aspects of work in construction of spiritual civilization were done by centering around the central task of deepening medical reform, basing on the construction promotion of the socialist core value system, aiming at the enhancement of civilization quality for the workers and civilization degree for units, starting from the creation activities of the masse, and combining with the activities of deepening the activity of creating the first and striving for the excellence and of welcoming and celebrating the successful opening of the 18th CPC National Congress. The first one is to give full play to the leading function of the central group learning, promote sturdily the construction of the Party organization of the learning type, continuously arm the Party members with the theoretical system of socialism with Chinese characteristics, enhance study, propaganda and education of the theoretical system of socialism with Chinese characteristics and socialist core value system and intensify the self-consciousness and firmness of all Party members, cadres and workers in adhering to the socialist road with Chinese characteristics, theoretical system and institutions in accordance with the requirements of arming brains, guiding practice and pushing work. The second one is to continuously carry out the activity of creating the first and striving for the excellence and intensify the guidance of the activity of creating the first and striving for the excellence in national medical and health system, stick to the classified guidance, highlight the key service of "creating the first and striving for the excellence for people", guide the Party organizations and the Party members to strive for quality service window and outstanding medical models, and create the atmosphere of learning from the advanced, advocating the advanced and striving for the advanced. Conference on summarization and rewarding of creating the first and striving for the excellence in national health system was held to fully and systematically summarize the main achievements and experience in the activity of creating the first and striving for the excellence in national medical and health system. The advanced collectives, the excellent individuals and the guiding workers in the activity of creating the first and striving for the excellence were solemnly commended. The third one is to carry out the great discussion in national medical health system aiming at "education for thought, sublimation in spirit, and improvement in quality and work", rigorously study, discuss and condense medical health professional spirit fully reflecting socialist core values, and a preliminary expression scheme of professional spirit of medical health was formed. The fourth one is to organize national health system to deeply carry out special education and governance activities aiming at the outstanding problems in moral domain, *Implementation Scheme for Health System to Carry out Special Education and Governance Activities Aiming at the Outstanding Problems in Moral Domain* was formulated, printed and distributed, organize to find out the prominent problems of medical ethics reflected by the masses, analyze the reasons, and put forward rectification measures by means of improving service attitude optimizing service progress, upgrading service and standardizing behaviors of diagnosis and treatment.

(Ji Chenglian)

Part IV
Academic and Civil Societies

▌Chapter I   Chinese Medical Association

Work of Chinese Medical Association in 2012

I. Bringing the Advantages of Association into Full Play, and Promoting Academic Communication, Popularization of Health Knowledge and Talent Growth

(1) Academic Communication

Chinese Medical Association (hereinafter referred to as Association) held 434 academic conferences of all kinds in 2012, in which there were 58 annual academic meetings or national academic meetings, 9 international, regional or bilateral academic meetings, 20 academic meetings for the young and middle-aged, 182 symposiums and 165 learning classes, training classes and meetings for theses collection. The number of the representatives was 116,000, the number of the theses received was 83,600, 15,720 theses were exchanged and 88 books of the theses were edited and assembled.

(2) Publication and Distribution

Now, the number of all kinds of series magazines and electronic journals sponsored by Chinese Medical Association was 157 (in which the number of the kinds of paper journals of Chinese series was 87, 15 kinds of China and 24 kinds of international publication). Annually, about 1,400 issues of paper magazines are published, as well as 93 version numbers of electronic audio & video publications and 223,000 copies of disks. 13 kinds of magazines were selected as the quality journals of science & technology of China Association for Science and Technology in 2012. English Version of Chinese Medical Journal was given the second prize of Excellent International Journal of Science and Technology in 2012 by China Association for

Science and Technology with special prize money of 1,000,000 yuan (3 years in a row) support for ability improvement of Association. The audio and video publications of 2010 Version of Interpretation and Demonstration for Cardiopulmonary Resuscitation (CPR) Guidelines (base version) obtained financial support from Beijing Publishing Fund. Electronic Audio and Video Press Co., LTD was awarded as "2012 Advanced Group of Beijing News Publishing and Copyright".

(3) Popular Science Propaganda

Chinese Medical Association organized the participation into popular science propaganda activities — "National Day of Popular Science", "Popular Science Month by China Association for Science and Technology and Luliang City" and "Well-known Experts in Community — Eye Health Care", organized 22 experts from many hospitals to attend the activities of "Train Tour to Qinghai for Revitalization of the Plateau, and Service for Agriculture, Rural Areas, and Farmers" in Xining City and other counties to see patients on a volunteer basis, make consultations for common diseases and frequently-occurring diseases, and give professional training and lectures on popular science. The association continued the cooperation with Johnson & Johnson for "Academic Lectures in West Areas by Chinese Medical Association and Johnson & Johnson", organized experts to give trainings and lectures in 9 districts in the west, such as Beihai, Guangxi, Xichang, Sichuan, Yuxi, Yunnan and so on, and jointly continued "China Plan for Education of Glycosylated Hemoglobin" with the center for clinical examination of Ministry of Health. About 9,000 grassroots medical members of general practice, internal medicine, endocrinology department and laboratory medicine were trained.

(4) Continuing Education

Chinese Medical Association performed functions of national office for continuing medical education committee, organized the experts to appraise and popularized reported projects of national continuing medical education programs in 2012, collected and accepted reported projects of national continuing medical education programs in 2013, launched "Chinese Medical Association Training Project for Standardized Treatment for Tumor Ablation" and many other programs for continuing medical education.

(5) Appraisal of "Award for China Medical Science and Technology"

Donated and advocated by President of Chinese Medical Association, Chen Zhu, "Health Policy Award was added to "Award for China Medical Science and Technology" since 2012. In 2012, by means of formality examination, preliminary examination, publicity, and final judgment, 85 projects won "Award for China Medical Science and Technology", in which there were 8 items winning the first prize, 25 items of the second, 47 items of the third, 2 items of health management, 2 items of popularization of medical science and 1 item of Health Policy. Since 2011, Chinese Medical Association recommended 8 items of the first and second prizes of "China Medical Science and Technology in 2011" by merits, of which 2 items won the second prize of National Award for Science and Technology Progress.

(6) International Exchange

In 2012, Chinese Medical Association organized 54 visits of 22 batches to attend the 191st and 192nd Council Meeting of World Medical Association and the Annual European Meeting on Interventional Cardiology, other multi-lateral international meetings, the annual meetings of American Medical Association and British Medical Association and the 32nd Sino-France Day of Medicine and other bilateral meetings. 21 persons/times of 3 batches from foreign delegations on invitation were received. "The 14th Medical Exchange between Beijing and Hong Kong" and "2012 Seminar by Hong Kong Hospital Authority" and other meetings were jointly held with Hong Kong, Macao and Taiwan regions.

II. Playing a Role of Assistant and Promoting Scientific Decision-making of the Government and the Development of Medical Health Reform

Chinese Medical Association succeeded in project appraisal on 9 specialties, key experiments and private hospitals, undertook and completed more than 10 consulting assignments deployed by Ministry of Health and other superior departments, including the argumentation of multiple technologies, and the making and amendment of standardized documents, accelerated the promotion of the standardized formulation of diagnosis and treatment of 20 diseases in medical institutions at the level of county city entrusted by Ministry of Health. 151 entrusted cases of technical appraisal for the medical negligence in the whole year were given argumentation, and 27 cases were given appraisal. Appraisal conclusion of medical accidents accounted for more than 89%. *Guiding Opinions of Chinese Medical Association Encouraging Private Hospitals to Participate in the Association Activities* were formulated and implemented. Research on special topics of core values in medical profession was actively carried out and the result was reported to Ministry of Health.

III. Strengthening Self-construction and Consolidating Development Foundation of the Association

Chinese Medical Association held the conference attended by all Party members on Feb. 8, 2012, at which a new term of Party Committee and Discipline Inspection Commission were elected. 5 times of standing council meetings of various kinds were held successively by the Association. 2012 National Work Conference of Secretary General of Local Medical Association was held in Guangzhou in April, and more than 120 secretaries general and office directors from medical associations in deputy provincial cities around the whole country attended the meeting. In 2012, 4,436 new members of specialized branches were enrolled and the accumulative number of the members in specialized branches is 7,474. 30 new members of experts were enrolled and the accumulative number is 230. In March, 2012, work conference of chairman of committee and secretary general from specialized branches was held in Beijing, at which the concrete requirements for the future work of the branches were put forward. More than 200 chairmen of committee and secretaries general from specialized branches affiliated to Chinese Medical Association attended the conference. By sticking to organizational structure of "former, current and designated chairman of committee", the Association completed the changes of term office in 36 specialized branches beyond expiration of the term office, the establishment and term office changes in youth assemblies of 25 specialized branches and the establishment and term office changes in 107 professional groups of 14 specialized branches. The system check and acceptance of informatization construction was fully completed, the online information service of 68 series of magazines was realized and the system for manuscript examination and approval of 105 editorial offices was put in use.

(Ji Chenglian)

Chapter II   Chinese Association of Preventive Medicine

Work of Chinese Association of Preventive Medicine in 2012

In 2012, 91 academic conferences were held by Chinese Association of Preventive Medicine (hereinafter referred to as Association), of which 2 conferences were international ones held in Hong Kong, Macao and Taiwan regions. 17,793 scholars attended the conferences and 2,994 theses were exchanged.

I. Establishing Branches and Membership

Chinese Association of Preventive Medicine completed the changes of term office and the reelection of "Professional Committee of Rural Improvement in Drinking Water and Lavatories", "Professional Committee of Radiological Health" and "Branch of Disinfection", established "Professional Committee of Birth Defect Prevention and Control" and "Branch of Health Emergency". Approved by Ministry of Civil Affairs, "Professional Committee of Intelligence of Preventive Medicine" was renamed as "Professional Committee of Information of Preventive Medicine". Basing on pilot work launched by the branches of "Professional Committee of Health Risk Assessment and Control" and "Branch of Stroke Prevention and Control", "Branch of Medical Parasites" and "Chronic Disease Prevention and Control" re-registered the members of the specialized branches.

II. Carrying out the Popularization of Health Science and Telephone Hotline Service

During the period of the 14th Annual Conference of China Association for Science and Technology held in Shijiazhuang from September, 9 to 10, Chinese Association of Preventive Medicine hosted the 7th Popular Science Exhibition—"Science Carnivals of Disease Prevention and Scientific Living" since itinerant exhibition in 2006. More than 200 panels on disease prevention knowledge were displayed. Health care professionals of disease prevention and control, health supervision and emergency rescue were organized to offer the on-the-spot consultation service and advocate the citizens to take healthy lifestyle. The activity benefited more than 30,000 persons/times. The Association succeeded in the declaration of sub-project of Research and Application of Universal Technology for Frequently-occurring Infectious Disease Prevention covered in the project of Research of Public Health Knowledge and

Technical Screening and Evaluation in "the Twelfth-five-year" national supporting plan of science and technology, organized the experts to compile and make posters and foldings for prevention of epidemic cerebrospinal meningitis, such as, *Know More about Epidemic Cerebrospinal Meningitis Prevention, Do You Know —about Epidemic Cerebrospinal Meningitis?* More than 200,000 copies were given out freely to vaccination stations for prevention and immunization in communities around China. Special websites and consultation hotline were established for the publicity of knowledge about pneumococcal disease prevention. The number of page views in the whole year is 780,000 times. The number of the answers to hotline telephone is more than 1,200 per month, the number of advisory messages is over 4,000 per month and 1,100 parents' awareness of "hazard of pneumococcal disease was investigated around the country.

III. Paying Special Attention to the Continuing Medical Education and Launching Training for Grassroots Health Workers

In 2012, the Association completed 32 projects of continuing medical education at state level and 125 projects at association level and 71,551 persons were given training of continuing education, which increased 13.6%, compared with that of 2011. The training project of "Energetic China" was launched. 20 academic seminars were held around the country, involving more than 3,000 clinicians and general medical practitioners of cardiology department, endocrinology department, and neurology department. 95 times of continuing medical education about awareness and technology of pneumococcal disease prevention were given and 11,000 persons/ times were trained. 44 issues of training classes on poliomyelitis, DPT and infectious diseases of haemophilus influenzae B were held in 25 cities and 7,000 grassroots persons/times were trained. 7 issues of training seminars on prevention and control of respiratory infectious diseases of measles, rubella, parotiditis, chicken pox and seasonal influenza, and diseases of digestive tract of hepatitis A, rotavirus diarrhea and typhoid fever were held and more than 900 persons were trained.

IV. Formulating Guidance to Technology for Disease Prevention and Control

The Association organized more than 20 experts of disease prevention & control and pediatric clinics to formulate *Guidance to Application Technology of Vaccine in Pneumococcal Diseases (2012 version)*, and published it in *China Epidemiology* in November.

V. Writing Report for Subject Development and Carrying out Project Research

Discipline Development Reports on Public Health and Preventive Medicine 2011-2012 Volume were compiled, including 1 "general report" and 12 "special reports" of about 140,000 words. The subject research of *2049 Science & Technology and Social Outlook— Preventive Medicine and Life Quality* was launched and 5 times of expert assemblies were held to discuss the framework, structure and content.

VI. Carrying out Pilot Projects, and Academic Investigation and Research

Research on "main burdens of the chronic diseases and research of prevention and control strategies in China west rural areas" has been done for 3 years and it is near to the final conclusion. The pilot work of *Infectious Disease Management Specification and Assessment Criteria in Medical Institutions* was carried out. 300 vaccination units in relevant cities around the country launched investigation twice on vaccine of pneumococcal disease prevention and other vaccines associated with pneumonia disease prevention and made investigation and research on 31,800 samples. "Grassroots Research Project of Ability Construction of Polio Prevention and Control" was carried out in 7 cities around the country. Theoretical support was provided for governmental administrative departments to formulate and adjust scientifically and reasonably the mid-term and long-term control policies for polio.

VII. Organizing and Carrying out Award Appraisal and Result Declaration on Science and Technology of Preventive Medicine

Chinese Association of Preventive Medicine held awards ceremonies for "Science and Technology Award of Chinese Association of Preventive Medicine" and "Contribution Award for Development of Public Health and Preventive Medicine of Chinese Association of Preventive Medicine". Check and acceptance of the projects supported by scientific research funding in 2010 was carried out and new projects supported by scientific research funding were evaluated, of which 13 projects passed the check and acceptance. 47 theses were published and 4 projects were declared for achievement rewards.

VIII. AIDS Cooperation Projects

The year of 2012 is the last year for AIDS activities covered in China-Gates AIDS Program. Chinese Association of Preventive Medicine held successively annual conference on China-Gates AIDS Program, training for the management of positive cases, ability construction at provincial city level covered in China-Gates AIDS Program, appraisal of one-time communication activity entrusted by China-Gates AIDS Program and the construction of organizational ability in communities of China-Gates AIDS Program. The year of 2012 is also the final year for the implementation of Sino-German AIDS Online Education Program. Chinese Association of Preventive Medicine held completion of face-to-face training of the online education and seminar on assessment of the old students.

IX. Participating Actively in the United Nations Counseling Activities

Chinese Association of Preventive Medicine has been acting as the Office of the United Nations counseling activities of life and health (CCLH), and China Association for Science and Technology. In April, CCLH delegation of China Association for Science and Technology attended the 46th Annual Conference hosted by Executive Committee of Public Health Alliance and the Alliance. In July, CCLH delegation of China Association for Science and Technology attended the 19th National AIDS Conference held in Washington Convention Center, USA, at which 1,200 copies of brochures were given out to propagandize the work done by China government in AIDS prevention, especially the important role of the non-governmental organizations in AIDS prevention.

X. Participating Actively in Preparation Service of International Conferences

In April, Chinese Association of Preventive Medicine attended the 13th World Conference on Public Health and the 46th Annual Conference of Alliance held in Ethiopia, acted as the Secretariat of Liaison Office of World Public Health Alliance in West Pacific Region, and assisted Vietnamese Public Health Association with the preparations for the 4th Public Health Conference of World Public Health Alliance in Asia-Pacific Region. Entrusted by World Public Health Alliance, the Association gave out the questionnaires on professional abilities of all associations to the member countries.

XI. Doing a Good Job in Journal and Magazine, Strengthening Network Construction, and Starting the Transformation into Enterprise

Chinese Association of Preventive Medicine hosts 69 kinds of series magazines and 1 newspaper. In 2012, 43 kinds of magazines hosted by Chinese Association of Preventive Medicine were included in "Journals of Statistic Source" of China science and technology papers by selection and 22 kinds of magazines in "Chinese Core Periodicals". In 2012, Chinese Association of Preventive Medicine began the transformation of newspapers and periodicals into enterprises and planned to declare parts of the electronic journals. The Association established the website of "2012 China Annual Conference of Rabies —Conference Service Platform" to provide convenient and efficient service. 9 issues of *Work Communication* were compiled and distributed. And more than 50% branches established their own websites or webpage.

(Ji Chenglian)

Part V
Figures in the Health Field

▌ Chapter I   The System of Ministry of Health

Minister and Vice-ministers of Ministry of Health

Minister: Chen Zhu
Vice-minister: Zhang Mao
Huang Jiefu
Wang Guoqiang
Ma Xiaowei
Chen Xiaohong
Li Xi
Shao Mingli (dismissed in Feb. 2012)
Liu Qian
Yin Li
Xv Ke (female, in tenure since May, 2012)

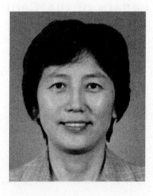

Xv Ke, Vice-minister

Xv Ke, female, Han Nationality, born in July, 1956. She entered the service in June, 1974 and joined the Party in July, 1975. She graduated from the major of medical treatment of Department of Clinical Medicine, Norman Bethune Medical University with Bachelor of Medicine and the major of Political Science & Political Administrative Department of Political Science Theory with Master of Law. From June, 1974 to December, 1976, she worked in Longjiapu Commune in Jiutai County, Jilin Province as an educated youth. From December, 1976 to April, 1977, she worked in the Party Committee Office of Jiutai County. From April, 1977 to October, 1978, she worked in the Municipal Party Committee Office of Changchun City, Jilin Province. From October, 1978 to August, 1983, she studied in Department of Clinical Medicine, Norman Bethune Medical University. From August, 1983 to September, 1990, she was the secretary in charge and deputy director general in Personnel Department of Health, Jilin Province. From September, 1990 to September, 1992, she was deputy head of Nanguan District in Changchun City, Jilin Province. From September, 1992 to June, 2001, she was deputy director general and member of the Party Group of Health Department in Jilin Province. From June, 2001 to May, 2002, she was deputy director of Disease Control Department in Ministry of Health (Office of National Patriotic Sanitation). From May, 2002 to February, 2004, she was director of Health Supervision Center of Ministry of Health. From February, 2004 to March, 2010, she was the director of Rural Health Management Division of Ministry of Health. From March, 2010, she was the director of Personnel Department of Ministry of Health. And from May, 2012, she was vice minister and a member of the Party Group of Ministry of Health.

Chapter II　System of State Food and Drug Administration

Directors General and Deputy Directors General of State Food and Drug Administration and Discipline Inspection Group Leaders of the Central Commission for Discipline Inspection

Director General and Secretary of the Party Group: Shao Mingli (dismissed in Feb. 2012)

Director General and Secretary of the Party Group: Yin Li (in tenure since May, 2012)

Deputy Director and a Member of the Party Group: Wu Zhen

Deputy Director and a Member of the Party Group: Li Jiping (dismissed in June. 2012)

Deputy Director and a Member of the Party Group: Bian Zhenjia

Team Leader of the Central Commission for Discipline Inspection in Ministry of Health and a Member of the Party Group: Yu Xiancheng

Deputy Director and a Member of the Party Group: Sun Xianze (in tenure since August, 2012)

Deputy Director: Jiao Hong (in tenure since August, 2012)

Chapter III The System of State Administration of Traditional Chinese Medical Science and Medicine

Leaders of the System of State Administration of Traditional Chinese Medical Science and Medicine

Members of the Party Group, Director General and Deputy Directors General of the System of State Administration of Traditional Chinese Medical Science and Medicine

Secretary of the Party Group and Director General: Wang Guoqiang

Member of the Party Group and Deputy Director General: Wu Gang

Deputy Director General: Yu Wenming

Member of the Party Group and Deputy Director General: Li Daning

Member of the Party Group and Deputy Director General: Ma Jianzhong

Member of the Party Group and Secretary of the Party Committee of China Academy of Traditional Chinese Medicine: Wang Zhiyong

(Ji Chenglian)

Part VI
Health Statistics

China Health Statistics Work in 2012

In 2012, China statistics work focused on health monitoring and evaluation, and health informatization construction, the construction of system and ability was strengthened and positive progress was made in all the work.

I. Completion of Monitoring Tasks of Medical Reform Progress

In 2012, 3 issues of monitoring were completed, and the 3 issues of *Monitoring Report* were made. Statistics Information Center of Ministry of Health revised monitoring program of medical reform, whose focus was on major disease protection, bidding and distribution of the basic drugs and the progress of comprehensive reforms in county-level hospitals and adjusted quantitative index to system collection of the regular statistics. According to the new monitoring program, 2,857 county districts, 340 prefectural cities and 31 provinces reported monitoring data and the quality of monitoring data was improved constantly.

II. The Important Role of Assessment on Medical Reform

Based on periodic assessment requirements for the two-year implementation of medical reform, Statistics Information Center of Ministry of Health completed the composition of the research reports on special project assessment of medical reform progress. *2003-2011 Research on Health Service and Accessible Trend of Fiscal Guarantee* was published in Scalpel. The three-year progress of deepened medical reform in Zichang County, Shaanxi Province was assessed. Good results were obtained in innovation mechanisms of employment, performance appraisal and distribution, and sustainable financial compensation, and valuable experience was accumulated, which has played a positive role in promoting county-level medical reform. In 2012, the Center and Beijing University jointly made investigation on residents' satisfactory degree. And the result shows that about 70% residents are generally satisfied with medical reform, 83.7% residents think that there is an overall improvement in medicine and health than that before medical reform and 85.5% believe that the general service provided by hospitals is better than that before medical reform.

III. New Progress in the Establishment of Health Information Standards

In 2012, Statistics Information Center of Ministry of Health organized and completed the examination and approval of 134 standards, and formally issued 64 industrial standards for implementation. By strengthening standard implementation, and supervision and administration, the Center studied and formulated management method, standard and assessment plan for conformance testing of national health information standards. 4 provinces and cities and 6 hospitals like Shanghai, Zhejiang, Sichuan and Chongqing were made the first batch of pilots for standardized maturity assessment in order to guide medical health institutions and enterprises of health information technology to exploit and utilize products meeting the national standards of information system and promote the realization of interconnection and interworking, and information sharing.

IV. Steady Promotion of Health Card for Residents

Based on previous 15 items in 6 categories of management methods and standards of residents' health cards, 8 sets of management methods and technical standards were revised and perfected, 3 technical standards of *Basic Function Specification of Residents' Health Cards Registration Management System* were added and formulated, and 5 working standards and working process, such as *Guides for Construction of Residents' Health Cards* were formulated. The construction of residents' health card product testing and certification management system was studied, the third-party detection institution of fixed points for residents' health cards was confirmed, and health card product testing and qualification for the record were initiated smoothly. The construction of secret key management system to residents' health cards and SAM Card system was completed and passed the check of the tests and security audit given by national secret bureau. Currently, 10 provinces have set up province-level secret key system and got province-level secret keys. By the end of 2012, the pilot provinces have given out 806,000 cards and more than 10,000,000 residents' information has been verified and their cards are in the production process.

V. Significant Progress in Information Platform Construction

National health information platform of comprehensive management has run 9 integrated functional modules, completed the access of direct reporting system of statistics and emergency command system of public health emergencies, and realized the online aggregation of statistical data of medical health institutions and all-level health administrative departments. The regional health information platforms of Beijing and Shanghai, as the pilot cities in the early stage, have been successfully made accessible to national platform. Thus information submission, instruction relay and information resource sharing were realized. Provincial level health information platforms of comprehensive management of varying degrees have been built in Shanghai, Jiangsu, Zhejiang, Fujian provinces and regional health information platforms of comprehensive management of varying degrees have been built in 134 prefectures and 397 county districts. By means of national health comprehensive management information platform, more than 54,690,000 pieces of infectious disease information, more than 190,000 pieces of public health emergencies, health archive data of more than 4,690,000 persons, more than 38,420,000 data of new rural cooperative medicine of 3,450,000 persons and data of diagnosis and treatment of 11,080,000 persons have been collected. Resource pool of electronic health records was established in 12 provinces, like Beijing, Shanghai and Anhui. The average filing rate of the standardized electronic health records is over 70% in east areas.

VI. Sturdy Promotion of Information Security and Confidentiality

In accordance with *Guiding Opinions on Information Security Rank Protection of Health Industry*, and basing on work of information security rank protection, reinforcement and modification, all places deployed all kinds of safety aids, formulated safety management system, and established preliminarily security technology system, security service system and safety management system required by the third level protection. According to *Management Methods of Electronic Certification Service of Health System*, the construction of electronic certification service system has been improved. 22 CA institutions, passed re-check and test in 4 batches, which were listed in the institutions of electronic certification service of health system and made accessible to digital certificate supervision service platform of Ministry of Health. 144,983 digital certificates (personal certificate, certificate of unit and digital ID of server) were signed and issued to health system by all CA institutions around the country, and 35,846 certificates were updated. The total number of certificates is 180,829.

VII. Full Implementation of Informatization Construction in Grassroots Medical Health Institutions

In 2011, National Development and Reform Commission and Ministry of Health selected 10 provinces to launch pilot construction of grassroots medical and health management system, perfect informatization infrastructures, promote grassroots medical and health management system basing on electronic health archive and integration of urban and rural planning as a whole. After that in 2012, National Development and Reform Commission continued the input of more than 3,000,000,000 yuan for the full project implementation of grassroots medical health management system construction across the country. At present, 29 provinces and cities have obtained subsidies of special funds to launch informatization construction in grassroots medical health institutions in province unit, covering functions of residents' health management, standardization of diagnosis and treatment, and performance assessment, realized the effective connection to related systems of health, medical insurance, and drug supervision, and upgraded service quality and standardization in grassroots medical health institutions.

VIII. Issue and Implementation of Statistical Investigation System of New Edition, and Completion of Preparations for National Health Service Survey

In 2012, 5 sets of survey systems for national health resources, medical service, disease control, health supervision, women and children's health and new rural cooperative medicine were organized for the amendment. The database for birth information of medicine and rural doctor information was created and included in statutory statement. Authorized by State Statistics Bureau, Ministry of Health printed and distributed them for the implementation by step. The survey systems of health resources and health service are taking the lead in execution around the country. Nearly 900,000 medical health institutions have submitted annual reports and monthly repots through direct statistical reporting system, and the dynamic information base of medical health institutions, and health manpower was established. The preparations for the survey plan design of the 5th national health service were finished smoothly. In June, 2013, field survey will be launched, which reviews and summarizes health work in the previous 5 years, predicts residents' needs and demand for health service, and long-term health problems and provides the base for the assessment of medical reform and the formulation of the "Thirteenth Five-year" health planning.

IX. Strengthened Utilization of Data Analysis

The Center of Statistics Information of Ministry of Health released 11 issues of monthly statistical materials, health statistical abstracts, health statistical yearbooks, briefs of China health development in 2012, and 2 issues of statistical materials of Chinese traditional medicine. The website of Ministry of Health published statistical bulletins, and monthly and seasonal information of medical service, which provide the significant data support for decision-making by the government. 11 issues of *Report of Health Statistics* were compiled and printed, and the contents cover the utilization of medical service, patients' medical expenditure, the development of non-public medical institutions and life expectancy analysis.

(Ji Chenglian)

图书在版编目（CIP）数据

中国卫生年鉴.2013：英文/陈竺主编；王琁译.
—北京：人民卫生出版社，2015
ISBN 978-7-117-20062-2

Ⅰ.①中…　Ⅱ.①陈…②王…　Ⅲ.①卫生工作–中
国–2013–年鉴–英文　Ⅳ.①R199.2-54

中国版本图书馆CIP数据核字（2014）第278703号

人卫社官网　**www.pmph.com**	出版物查询，在线购书	
人卫医学网　**www.ipmph.com**	医学考试辅导，医学数据库服务，医学教育资源，大众健康资讯	

2013 中国卫生年鉴（英文）

主　　编：陈　竺
出版发行：人民卫生出版社（中继线 010-59780011）
地　　址：中国北京市朝阳区潘家园南里 19 号
邮　　编：100021
网　　址：http://www.pmph.com
E – mail：pmph @ pmph.com
购书热线：010-59787592　010-59787584　010-65264830
开　　本：787×1092　1/16
版　　次：2015 年 2 月第 1 版　2015 年 2 月第 1 版第 1 次印刷
标准书号：ISBN 978-7-117-20062-2/R·20063
打击盗版举报电话：**010-59787491　E-mail：WQ @ pmph.com**
（凡属印装质量问题请与本社市场营销中心联系退换）